Basic Techniques of Ophthalmic Surgery

Executive Editors
James P. Dunn, MD
Paul D. Langer, MD, FACS

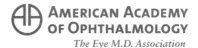

AMERICAN ACADEMY
OF OPHTHALMOLOGY
The Eye M.D. Association

Supported by an
educational grant from

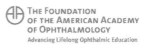

THE FOUNDATION
OF THE AMERICAN ACADEMY
OF OPHTHALMOLOGY
Advancing Lifelong Ophthalmic Education

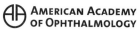
**AMERICAN ACADEMY
OF OPHTHALMOLOGY**
The Eye M.D. Association

P.O. Box 7424
San Francisco, CA 94120-7424

Clinical Education Secretaries
Gregory L. Skuta, MD, *Senior Secretary
for Clinical Education*
Louis B. Cantor, MD, *Secretary
for Ophthalmic Knowledge*

Academy Staff
Richard A. Zorab, *Vice President,
Ophthalmic Knowledge,
Clinical Education Division*
Hal Straus, *Director of Print
Publications*
Kimberly Torgerson, *Publications
Editor*
D. Jean Ray, *Production Manager*
Denise Evenson, *Design*

Acquisitions
Tina-Marie Gauthier

Illustration
Mark M. Miller

Printed in Colombia.

Library of Congress Cataloging-in-Publication Data

Basic techniques of ophthalmic surgery / executive editors, James P. Dunn, Paul D. Langer.
   p. ; cm.
  Includes index.
  ISBN 978-1-56055-983-2
  1. Eye--Surgery--Handbooks, manuals, etc. 2. Eye--Surgery--Atlases. I. Dunn, James P., 1957- II. Langer, Paul D., 1963- III. American Academy of Ophthalmology.
  [DNLM: 1. Eye Diseases--surgery--Atlases. 2. Eye Diseases--surgery--Handbooks. 3. Ophthalmologic Surgical Procedures--methods--Atlases. 4. Ophthalmologic Surgical Procedures--methods--Handbooks. WW 39 B311 2009]

  RE80.B373 2009
  617.7'1--dc22
      2009005409

Financial Disclosures

The following authors and reviewers have disclosed financial relationships:

Ashley Behrens, MD: (C) Inspire Pharmaceuticals; (C, L) Aton Pharmaceuticals, Dupont Healthcare; (O, P) LumenOra LLC

Lawrence P. Chong, MD: (C) Allergan, Bausch & Lomb

Roy S. Chuck, MD, PhD: (C) IOP, WMR Biomedical; (C, L) Alcon Laboratories

Elizabeth Davis, MD: (C) Advanced Medical Optics, Bausch & Lomb, STAAR Surgical Company, Ista Pharmaceuticals; (S) Allergan, Inspire Pharmaceuticals

Steven C. Dresner, MD: (P) Porex Surgical

James P. Dunn Jr, MD: (C) Allergan

Steven J. Gedde, MD: (C) Alcon Laboratories; (L) Merck

John B. Holds, MD: (C) QLT Phototherapeutics

Daniel A. Johnson, MD: (C, L) Alcon Laboratories; (L) Bio-Tissue

Paul D. Langer, MD, FACS: (C) Allergan

W. Barry Lee, MD, FACS: (C, L) Allergan

Jennifer I. Lim, MD: (C) Allergan, Bausch & Lomb Surgical, Novartis Pharmaceuticals, Quark; (L) Heidelberg Engineering, Optovue; (S) Icon Bioscience, Pfizer Ophthalmics, QLT Phototherapeutic; (C, L, S) Genentech

Scott M. MacRae, MD: (C) AcuFocus; (C, L) Bausch & Lomb

Joseph A. Mauriello Jr, MD: (P) Lippincott Williams & Wilkins

John D. McCann, MD, PhD: (E, O) McCann Medical Matrix

Shahzad I. Mian, MD: (C) Allergan

Kevin M. Miller, MD: (S) Hoya; (L, S) Alcon Laboratories

Yasaman Mohadjer, MD: (L) Allergan

Roberto Pineda II, MD: (L) Alcon Laboratories

Christopher J. Rapuano, MD: (L) Alcon Laboratories, Inspire, Vistakon Johnson & Johnson Visioncare; (O) Rapid Pathogen Screening; (C, L) Allergan

Ivan R. Schwab, MD, FACS: (C) Inspire

Gail Schwartz, MD: (C, L, S) Pfizer Ophthalmics: (S) Alcon Laboratories, Allergan

Scott D. Smith, MD, MPH: (L) Allergan, Pfizer Ophthalmics; (C, L) Alcon Laboratories

Agnieszka Trzcinka, MD: (S) Student Biomedical Research Program

Rudolph S. Wagner, MD: (C, L) Alcon Laboratories

Sonia H. Yoo, MD: (S) Carl Zeiss Meditec; (C, L) Alcon Laboratories; (C, S) Advanced Cell Technology, Foundation Fighting Blindness; (L, S) Advanced Medical Optics

Marco A. Zarbin, MD, PhD, FACS: (C) Novartis Pharmaceuticals, Wyeth-Ayerst Pharmaceuticals; (P) University of Medicine & Dentistry of New Jersey.

C	Consultant fee, paid advisory boards, or fees for attending a meeting (for the past 1 year)
E	Employed by a commercial entity
L	Lecture fees (honoraria), travel fees, or reimbursements when speaking at the invitation of a commercial entity (for the past 1 year)
O	Equity ownership/stock options of publicly or privately traded firms (excluding mutual funds) with manufacturers of commercial ophthalmic products or commercial ophthalmic services
P	Patents and/or royalties that might be viewed as creating a potential conflict of interest
S	Grant support for the past 1 year (all sources) and all sources used for this project if this form is an update for a specific talk or manuscript with no time limitation

The other authors and reviewers do not state significant financial interest or other relationship with the manufacturer of any commercial product discussed in the chapters that they contributed to this publication or with the manufacturer of any competing commercial product: Esen K. Akpek, MD; Robert S. Bailey Jr, MD; Rhonda V. Barrett, MD; Neelakshi Bhagat, MD, MPH, FACS; James C. Bobrow, MD; Kathryn E. Bollinger, MD, PhD; Geoffrey Broocker, MD, FACS; Irina Bykhovskaya Ganelis, MD; Walter Camacho, MD; Susan R. Carter, MD;

Contributors

Executive Editors
James P. Dunn, MD
Paul D. Langer, MD, FACS

Section Editors
Neelakshi Bhagat, MD, MPH, FACS, vitreoretinal surgery (co-editor)

James P. Dunn, MD, anterior segment, refractive, and glaucoma surgeries

Suqin Guo, MD, strabismus surgery (co-editor)

Paul D. Langer, MD, FACS, ophthalmic plastic surgery, trauma surgery

Rudolph S. Wagner, MD, strabismus surgery (co-editor)

Marco A. Zarbin, MD, PhD, FACS, vitreoretinal surgery (co-editor)

Authors
Esen K. Akpek, MD, Baltimore, Maryland

Robert S. Bailey, MD, Wyndmoor, Pennsylvania

Rhonda V. Barrett, MD, Slingerlands, New York

Ashley Behrens, MD, Baltimore, Maryland

Neelakshi Bhagat, MD, MPH, FACS, Newark, New Jersey

Kathryn E. Bollinger, MD, PhD, Cleveland, Ohio

Geoffrey Broocker, MD, FACS, Atlanta, Georgia

Irina Bykhovskaya Ganelis, MD, Los Angeles, California

Walter Camacho, MD, Baltimore, Maryland

Susan R. Carter, MD, Warren, New Jersey

Lawrence P. Chong, MD, Los Angeles, California

Roy S. Chuck, MD, PhD, Baltimore, Maryland

Elizabeth Davis, MD, Bloomington, Minnesota

Steven C. Dresner, MD, Santa Monica, California

James P. Dunn, MD, Baltimore, Maryland

Justis P. Ehlers, MD, Philadelphia, Pennsylvania

Christina Flaxel, MD, Portland, Oregon

Anat Galor, MD, Miami, Florida

Roberta E. Gausas, MD, Philadelphia, Pennsylvania

Steve J. Gedde, MD, Miami, Florida

Emily Graubart, MD, Atlanta, Georgia

Suqin Guo, MD, Newark, New Jersey

Pankaj C. Gupta, MD, Augusta, Georgia

Kristin M. Hammersmith, MD, Philadelphia, Pennsylvania

Peter S. Hersh, MD, Teaneck, New Jersey

Holly B. Hindman, MD, Rochester, New York

John B. Holds, MD, St. Louis, Missouri

Camille Hylton, MD, Phoenix, Arizona

Daniel A. Johnson, MD, San Antonio, Texas

David R. Jordan, MD, Ottawa, Ontario, Canada

Albert Jun, MD, PhD, Baltimore, Maryland

Robert Kersten, MD, Denver, Colorado

John J. Kim, MD, Bronx, New York

Krista Kinard, MD, Salt Lake City, Utah

Paul D. Langer, MD, FACS Newark, New Jersey

W. Barry Lee, MD, FACS, Atlanta, Georgia

Jennifer I. Lim, MD, Chicago, Illinois

Scott M. MacRae, MD, Rochester, New York

Joseph A. Mauriello Jr, MD, Summit, New Jersey

Louise Mawn, MD, Nashville, Tennessee

John D. McCann, MD, PhD, Salt Lake City, Utah

Alan W. McInnes, MD, Santa Monica, California

Dale R. Meyer, MD, FACS, Slingerlands, New York

Shahzad I. Mian, MD, Ann Arbor, Michigan

Mark D. Mifflin, MD, Salt Lake City, Utah

Kevin M. Miller, MD, Los Angeles, California

Yasaman Mohadjer, MD,
Largo, Florida

Parveen K. Nagra, MD,
Ashland, Kentucky

Parag Parekh, MD, MPA,
Boston, Massachusetts

Roberto Pineda II, Boston,
Massachusetts

Jed T. Poll, MD, Houston,
Texas

N. Venkatesh Prajna, MD,
Maduraii, Tamilnadu, India

Pradeep Y. Ramulu, MD,
PhD, Baltimore, Maryland

Ivan, R. Schwab, MD,
Sacramento, California

Gail Schwartz, MD,
Baltimore, Maryland

Scott D. Smith, MD, MPH,
New York, New York

Walter J. Stark, MD,
Baltimore, Maryland

Leejee H. Suh, MD, Miami,
Florida

Bradford L. Tannen, MD,
Madison, New Jersey

Christopher K. Thiagarajah,
MD, Denver, Colorado

Jennifer E. Thorne, MD, PhD,
Baltimore, Maryland

Agnieszka Trzcinka, MD,
Ann Arbor, Michigan

Roger E. Turbin, MD, FACS,
Newark, New Jersey

M. Reza Vagefi, MD,
Philadelphia, Pennsylvania

Deborah K. VanderVeen, MD,
Boston, Massachusetts

Rengaraj Venkatesh, MD,
Thavalakuppam,
Pondicherry, India

Rudolph S. Wagner, MD,
Newark, New Jersey

Scott M. Warden, MD, New
York, New York

Robert S. Weinberg, MD,
Baltimore, Maryland

Edward J. Wladis, MD,
Slingerlands, New York

Michael T. Yen, MD,
Houston, Texas

Sonia H. Yoo, MD, Miami,
Florida

Marco A. Zarbin, MD, PhD,
FACS, Newark, New
Jersey

Contents

Foreword

For the past several years, a group of talented and dedicated ophthalmologists, under the direction of James P. Dunn, MD, and Paul D. Langer, MD, FACS, have undertaken a huge effort to explain and illustrate more than 75 of the most common surgical procedures performed by ophthalmologists and to describe the skills needed for surgical proficiency. Their collaboration has resulted in *Basic Techniques of Ophthalmic Surgery*, the book you have before you today. This is the second volume of a pair of books intended to improve surgical training in ophthalmology residency programs. The first book, *Basic Principles of Ophthalmic Surgery*, was published in 2006. Together, the two volumes provide a solid overview of the wide range of principles and procedures that will be covered throughout the residency training program.

The Accreditation Council for Graduate Medical Education (ACGME) noted in its 2008 program requirements: "The education of surgeons in the practice of general surgery encompasses both didactic instruction in the basic and clinical sciences of surgical diseases and conditions, as well as education in procedural skills and operative techniques. The education process must lead to the acquisition of an appropriate fund of knowledge and technical skills, the ability to integrate the acquired knowledge into the clinical situation, and the development of surgical judgment."

For ophthalmology, surgery is a core and complex competency, and surgical training remains a process equally daunting for teacher and student alike. From the start the authors' objective has not been to supplant the role of individual mentor-to student surgical instruction, but to compile many of the key elements of the surgical process and environment into a valuable complement to the overall learning program. We believe they have succeeded, crafting a volume that should be on the desk of every resident.

As part of the American Academy of Ophthalmology's ongoing commitment to resident education, we are underwriting most of the cost of this book, so that it can be provided at a low price to ophthalmology residents and practicing ophthalmologists.

As surgeons, we have a profound obligation to our patients. They honor us by entrusting us with their sight and sometimes their lives. This text acknowledges the complexity and scope of that obligation.

DAVID W. PARKE II, MD
Executive Vice President and CEO
American Academy of Ophthalmology

H. DUNBAR HOSKINS JR, MD
Executive Vice President Emeritus
American Academy of Ophthalmology

Preface

Basic Techniques of Ophthalmic Surgery is a companion to *Basic Principles of Ophthalmic Surgery*, a book edited by Anthony Arnold, MD, and published in 2006 by the American Academy of Ophthalmology. *Basic Techniques* is intended to be a quick reference source for residents who will be assisting in a particular type of surgery and a review for more senior residents and beginning surgeons who will be performing surgery themselves.

This book is composed of step-by-step procedures of the most commonly performed surgeries performed by ophthalmologists. We have confidence that not only residents, but also ophthalmologists who are honing their surgical or teaching skills, will find the summaries of these procedures helpful in their preparation. The chapters are not meant to be exhaustive. The reader should recognize that even the simplest surgery has as many variations, large or small, as there are surgeons who perform it. With cataract surgery, for example, numerous machine settings may be used in phacoemulsification. Even such apparently basic steps as preoperative dilation, prepping and draping (including the use of povidone-iodine on the skin and eye), or postoperative care may vary widely among surgeons. To try to list them all would not only be impractical, it would distract the reader from the fundamental purpose of the book.

Similarly, certain "steps" in a procedure are so basic as to merit exclusion from each chapter. It goes without saying that appropriate informed consent should be obtained prior to any surgery, and that the correct eye or specific tissue be correctly identified in accordance with the guidelines of the hospital, clinic, or surgery center in which it is performed. These critical aspects of surgery are therefore not listed in each chapter, although some informed consent procedures merit additional discussion and thus are included in the text. For purposes of space, we have also avoided listing "obvious" steps, such as removing a lid speculum at the end of a procedure.

We would consider our job well done if, at the completion of training, a resident or fellow has deleted certain sections of various chapters and added extensive handwritten margin notes to others. To do so would mean that the resident has thought critically about each step and developed, through observation and personal experience, his or her own approach to a certain technique.

Any surgical text is to some extent outdated by the time it is published. In the time it took for this book to be conceived, written, edited, and published, certain procedures that were initially performed only by a select few specialists, such as Descemet's stripping and endothelial keratoplasty, have become almost routine. Given the rapid evolution within many ophthalmic subspecialties, no doubt we have failed to include chapters about procedures that will largely supplant those that are in vogue today. The reader who does not simply memorize the steps of a given procedure but constantly considers why each particular step is listed (and what complications can occur) is much more likely to be able to adapt to more advanced or entirely new techniques and technologies.

Finally, we have consistently used generic names of drugs and equipment, such as sutures. In some cases, however, the brand name is so pervasive (eg, Vicryl) that many readers will not immediately recognize the generic (polyglactin). In such instances, we have listed the generic name first and the brand name in parentheses afterwards the first time it is mentioned in a given chapter, and the generic name thereafter. We chose this approach as a nod to practicality rather than any commercial bias.

We hope this book becomes a valuable addition to the residency program educational process and eventually finds a permanent place in the libraries of practicing ophthalmologists.

Acknowledgements

This book represents the cumulative efforts of a great number of people, including most obviously the authors. We are especially indebted as well to Kim Torgerson and Tina Gauthier for their exceptional patience and editing skills, Richard Zorab and Hal Straus of the Academy for their guidance and support, and Mark M. Miller for his superb art work. His illustrations appear in chapters 1–8, 10–15, 19–20, 22–25, 28, 29, 32–50, 52–57, 62–74, 75 (1), and 76. The following Chairs of the Academy's *Basic and Clinical Science Course* provided valuable suggestions and proofreading: James C. Bobrow, MD; John B. Holds, MD; Ramana S. Moorthy, MD; Edward L. Raab, MD; Christopher J. Rapuano, MD; and Hermann D. Schubert, MD. To all of them, thank you for your time, generosity, and commitment.

JAMES P. DUNN, MD
Associate Professor of Ophthalmology
Director of the Division of Ocular Immunology
SOCA Clinical Director and Residency Education Director
The Wilmer Eye Institute–Johns Hopkins
Baltimore, Maryland

PAUL D. LANGER, MD, FACS
Associate Professor
Director, Residency Training Program
Chief, Division of Ophthalmic Plastic and Reconstructive Surgery
New Jersey Medical School
Newark, New Jersey

Part I

Anterior Segment

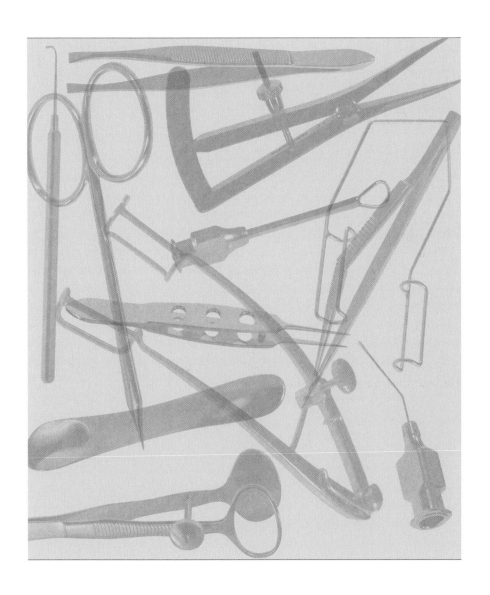

Chapter 1

Divide-and-Conquer Phacoemulsification and Nd:YAG Laser Capsulotomy

Kevin M. Miller, MD
James P. Dunn, MD

Cataract surgery is indicated when visual function no longer meets a patient's needs and surgery provides a reasonable likelihood of improvement. It is also indicated when the lens opacity inhibits optimal management of posterior segment disease or the lens causes inflammation, angle closure, or medically unmanageable open-angle glaucoma. Surgery should not be performed if glasses or visual aids are able to provide vision that meets the patient's needs. "Divide and conquer" is the basic phacoemulsification technique that should be mastered before attempting variations that are more sophisticated. Regardless, it remains the preferred technique, even for experienced surgeons. "Phaco chop," a more advanced phacoemulsification technique, is described in Chapter 2.

This chapter also describes Nd:YAG laser capsulotomy, a procedure indicated when visual function following cataract surgery deteriorates due to opacification of the posterior capsule or contraction of the anterior capsule.

DIVIDE-AND-CONQUER PHACOEMULSIFICATION

Preoperative Steps

1. Determine the patient's desired postoperative refraction.
2. Determine the method of anesthesia (topical, intracameral, orbital injection, or general).
3. Calculate IOL power.

4. Ensure that primary and back-up IOLs are available.
5. Obtain a corneal topography map if planning refractive cataract surgery (eg, peripheral corneal relaxing incisions).

Instrumentation and Supplies

- Povidone-iodine 2.5% or 5% solution
- Topical anesthetic (lidocaine gel, bupivacaine 0.75%, tetracaine 0.5%, proparacaine 0.5%)
- Preservative-free lidocaine 1%
- Xylocaine or bupivacaine for injection
- Wire lid speculum (eg, Barraquer-Kratz or Lieberman speculum)
- Metal or diamond keratome
- Crescent blade
- 15° sharp blade
- Viscoelastic agent (viscosurgical device) of choice
- Cystotome or pre-bent 25-, 27-, or 30-gauge needle
- Capsulorrhexis forceps
- Hydrodissection cannula (27 gauge, 30 gauge, or flat tip)
- Cyclodialysis spatula or nucleus rotator
- Phacoemulsification unit
- Capsule polisher
- IOL injector
- Kuglen (iris push–pull) or similar hook
- 10-0 nylon or polyglactin (Vicryl) suture

Surgical Procedure

1. Dilate the pupil using cycloplegic drops of choice.
2. Prime and tune the phacoemulsification unit (usually done by operating room staff).
3. If using topical anesthesia, place anesthetic drops or gel just before the povidone-iodine prep to minimize patient discomfort. Sub-Tenon's, retrobulbar, or general endotracheal anesthesia may also be used, depending on patient and surgeon preference.
4. Apply pressure over the closed eye for a few minutes if using retrobulbar anesthesia to reduce positive pressure intraoperatively.
5. Prepare and drape the lids. Cover the lid margin and lashes with the drape.
6. Place the lid speculum. Do not overly separate the lids; otherwise, a blepharoptosis may develop postoperatively.

7. If using topical anesthesia, instruct the patient to fixate on a light in the operating microscope.

8. Make a 2.2- to 3.5-mm groove about 300 μm deep with the crescent blade in the peripheral clear cornea or limbus on the steep axis as determined by corneal topography if performing refractive cataract surgery, or according to surgeon's preference otherwise. The groove may also be made using a metal or diamond knife with a 300- to 450-μm footplate. Some surgeons perform this step after Step 9.

9. Create a paracentesis using a 15° blade or diamond knife 2 to 3 clock hours away, large enough to accommodate a second instrument in the nondominant hand.

10. Supplement topical anesthesia by slowly injecting up to 0.5 cc of preservative-free 1% lidocaine through the paracentesis.

11. Inject viscoelastic agent through the paracentesis to fill the anterior chamber.

12. Create a corneal tunnel incision, starting deep in the corneal groove, using a metal or diamond keratome. The incision should be 1.5 to 2 mm long and wide enough to accommodate a phacoemulsification tip.

13. Puncture the anterior capsule with the cystotome and begin tearing the capsule by raising a flap and extending it circumferentially (some surgeons prefer to tear clockwise, others counterclockwise).

14. Complete the capsulorrhexis with capsulorrhexis forceps. Always tear the flap tangentially (shearing tear) to maintain control; inward radial forces (ripping tear) may cause the capsulorrhexis to tear out peripherally.

15. Perform hydrodissection. Place the hydrodissection cannula beneath the capsulorrhexis, advance it 1 to 2 mm without wiggling, lift gently, and inject balanced salt solution (BSS) slowly to obtain a posterior fluid wave. Once the nucleus begins to rise, push it down to release the fluid pocket that is trapped behind the nucleus. Repeat as necessary in different meridians until the nucleus rotates freely.

16. Make sure the holes in the irrigating sleeve that covers the phaco needle are at right angles to the bevel on the phaco needle. Introduce the phaco needle in reflux mode.

17. Sculpt a deep vertical groove through the nucleus using low-flow and vacuum settings (Figure 1.1A). Try to get at least two-thirds to three-fourths of the way through the nucleus before attempting to crack (Figure 1.1B).

18. With the phaco probe in foot position 1 (irrigation or pressurization), introduce a second instrument (cyclodialysis spatula or nucleus rotator) through the paracentesis (Figure 1.2A). Using a cross-action

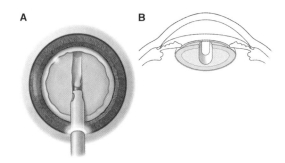

Figure 1.1. Sculpting the initial groove. (A) The phaco probe is used to sculpt a long deep trough through the center of the nucleus (surgeon's view). (B) Side view of the initial groove.

technique, anchor the 2 instruments against the walls of the groove deep in the trough. Lift and separate (Figure 1.2B), keeping the center of mass of the nucleus in the center of the pupil. Be sure to crack through the posterior plate. This may be difficult if the nucleus is dense. Propagate the crack in both directions and break all equatorial connections between the 2 halves.

19. Spin the nucleus 90° using the second instrument (Figure 1.3). Engage the nucleus as far peripherally as possible when spinning to maximize torque and minimize zonular stress.

20. Make a second trough at right angles to the first (Figure 1.4). Crack the heminucleus into 2 quadrants, then rotate and repeat for the second heminucleus.

21. Remove the quadrants one by one by phaco-assisted aspiration using high flow and high vacuum settings. Bury the tip to gain occlusion, build vacuum, and use pulse control or horizontal oscillation mode to break up and aspirate the fragments through the phaco tip. Use the

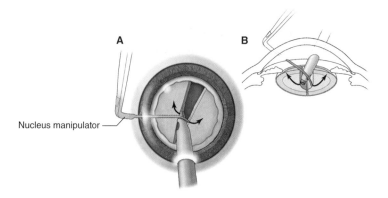

Nucleus manipulator

Figure 1.2. Cracking the initial groove. (A) The phaco probe and second instrument are lifted and separated (surgeon's view). (B) Side view showing instrument movement.

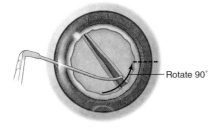

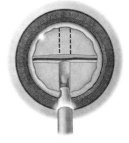

Figure 1.3. Rotation of the nucleus through the side port incision.

Figure 1.4. Sculpting a second deep groove perpendicular to the first groove.

second instrument to guide fragments to the phaco tip and keep them from chattering against the cornea (Figure 1.5). If the capsule is floppy or little cortex is present, reduce the vacuum level before the final quadrant is removed to reduce the risk of post-occlusion-break surge and capsule rupture.

22. Remove the epinuclear shell, if present, using moderate flow and vacuum settings.

23. Remove cortex using an irrigation/aspiration (I/A) probe. Always strip cortex from anterior capsule to posterior capsule rather than the other way around. Since subincisional cortex is the hardest to reach, go after it first.

24. Polish the posterior capsule, if necessary, to remove residual debris or plaque. This can be done using the I/A probe in capsule vacuum mode or using a variety of capsule polishers.

25. Inject additional viscoelastic material to reform the anterior chamber and capsular bag.

26. Inspect the IOL and make certain it is free of manufacturing defects. Load it into an injector device. Inject the IOL into the eye. Manipulate it into the capsular bag using a Kuglen hook or lens manipulator.

Figure 1.5. Use of the phaco tip to engage the first nuclear quadrant.

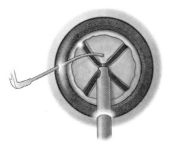

27. If the IOL is placed in the ciliary sulcus, it should be properly sized and the power reduced appropriately for the more anterior location.

28. Remove the viscoelastic material using the I/A probe. Inject a miotic agent after viscoelastic removal to prevent optic capture. Miotic agents are usually not necessary if the IOL is placed inside the capsular bag and the periphery of the IOL optic is completely covered with anterior capsule.

29. Close the phaco and paracentesis incisions by stromal hydration (injecting BSS into the walls of the incisions). Push down on the roof of the phaco incision to facilitate closure. Inject BSS into the paracentesis to raise intraocular pressure (IOP) to normal or just above normal.

30. Test the incisions and make sure they are watertight. If there is any concern about wound closure, place a single interrupted 10-0 nylon or polyglactin suture.

31. Patch and shield the eye if injection or general anesthesia was administered. Protect the eye with glasses or a shield if topical anesthesia was administered.

Postoperative Care

1. Arrange for postoperative examination the next day.

2. If no patch is applied, the patient may begin use of antibiotic and corticosteroid drops that day.

3. Postoperative regimens vary widely; common sequences are to see the patient 1 day, 1 week, and 1 month after surgery or 1 day and 2 weeks after surgery.

4. Antibiotics are usually discontinued 1 week after surgery.

5. If a nylon suture is used, it is usually removed at 1 week.

6. Corticosteroid drops are tapered and discontinued over 2 to 4 weeks.

7. A final refraction is usually performed 2 weeks to 1 month after surgery.

Complications

- Intraoperative: pain, iris atrophy or prolapse, thermal corneal injury (phaco burn), incomplete or torn capsulorrhexis, posterior capsule rupture, vitreous loss, dropped nucleus or lens fragments, suprachoroidal hemorrhage

- Early postoperative period (1 day to 1 week after surgery): blepharoptosis, extraocular muscle paresis (diplopia), wound leak, corneal edema, anterior chamber inflammation, iris trauma, paralysis, or

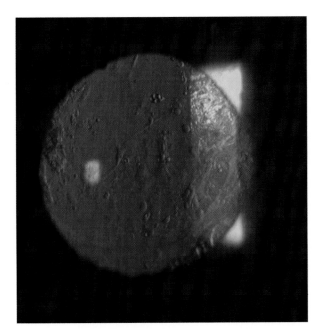

Figure 1.6. Capsular opacification as seen in retroillumination.

atrophy (polycoria), retained lens material, IOP spike, lens power calculation error, endophthalmitis, macular edema, retinal tear, macular hole, retinal vascular occlusion, retinal detachment

- Late postoperative period (greater than 1 week after surgery): binocular imbalance, corneal decompensation (pseudophakic bullous keratopathy), chronic iritis, glaucoma, lens decentration or dislocation, posterior capsule opacification (Figure 1.6), worsening of pre-existing conditions (diabetic retinopathy, macular degeneration, glaucoma, epiretinal membranes, floaters), failure to achieve or restore visual acuity to 20/20 or better; glare, halos, streaks, starbursts, light sensitivity, temporal scotomata or other problems listed as early postoperative complications

ND:YAG LASER CAPSULOTOMY

Much as with cataract surgery itself, the indication for capsulotomy is usually based not on the degree of capsular opacification or Snellen acuity, but on subjective complaints such as blurred vision, glare, and monocular diplopia.

While generally a very safe procedure, Nd:YAG laser capsulotomy poses a small risk of corneal abrasion, retinal detachment, bleeding, glare (from pitting of the IOL), and IOL dislocation (primarily with plate-haptic silicone lenses). Capsulotomy is most commonly performed for posterior capsular opacification, but may also be of benefit in cases of pupillary membrane formation or dense giant cell formation on the intraocular surface (hence, not a true "capsulotomy") or anterior capsular contraction causing IOL decentration or functional miosis. Nd:YAG laser capsulotomy is usually a "one and done" procedure, as the capsule does not regenerate, but may need to be repeated if the original capsulotomy proves too small or if there is recurrent pupillary membrane formation.

Preoperative Steps

1. Assess best-corrected visual acuity.
2. Rule out other causes of decreased vision (eg, pseudophakic cystoid macular edema).
3. Review potential risks of the procedure.
4. Be sure that patient is able to cooperate with the procedure.

Instrumentation and Supplies

- Capsulotomy lens (optional; highly recommended in patients who are light sensitive, have trouble fixating, or have ocular surface disease that diminishes focusing of the aiming beam)
- Hydroxypropyl methylcellulose (HPMC), if capsulotomy lens is used
- Topical anesthetic (eg, proparacaine 0.5%)
- Cycloplegic drops of choice (cyclopentolate 1%, tropicamide 1%)
- Iopidine 0.5% to 1%
- Balanced salt solution (if capsulotomy lens used)
- Topical corticosteroid (eg, prednisolone acetate 1%)
- Nd:YAG laser

Surgical Procedure

1. Dilate the pupil using the cycloplegic drop of choice.
2. Many clinicians instill 1 drop of Iopidine 0.5% to 1% to reduce risk of post-laser IOP spike.
3. Determine if a contact lens is to be used. Avoid topical anesthetic if a contact lens is not used, as it tends to cause epithelial drying and difficulty focusing.
4. Adjust the patient's chin and headrest to allow adequate range of vertical adjustment of focusing beam.

5. Adjust the laser settings to the desired power (usually between 0.8 to 3.0 mJ), depending on the density of the opacification, with 1 shot/burst.
6. Set the "offset" at "minimum."
7. If a contact lens is to be used, place it on the eye.
8. Adjust the width, height, and intensity of the slit beam to allow good visualization without patient discomfort.
9. Adjust the red (helium-neon) light, aiming the beam so that the 2 lights are focused sharply on the capsule or membrane to be lasered.
10. Turn the power on; always return power to "standby" when making any significant adjustments to the contact lens or patient positioning, and after the procedure is complete.
11. Adjust the joystick with one hand, with the index finger of the dominant hand on the "fire" button on top of the joystick. Never "jab" the finger to fire the laser; always use a smooth, controlled downward movement to maintain laser focus.
12. For posterior capsulotomy: focus the helium-neon beam precisely on the posterior capsule, then push the joystick very slightly forward (toward the retina) so that the 2 red dots slightly diverge before firing. This step will reduce the chances of "pitting" the IOL. An alternate approach is to set the offset at 100 μm and focus the helium-neon beam directly on the capsule before firing.
    - Circular capsulotomy technique: beginning peripherally, create a hole in the posterior capsule. Work around for 360° to create a posterior capsulotomy of about 4 to 5 mm (Figure 1.7). Be certain

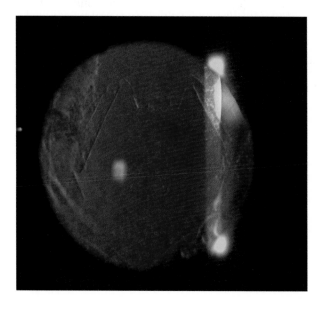

Figure 1.7. Open posterior capsule following Nd:YAG capsulotomy.

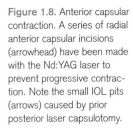

Figure 1.8. Anterior capsular contraction. A series of radial anterior capsular incisions (arrowhead) have been made with the Nd:YAG laser to prevent progressive contraction. Note the small IOL pits (arrows) caused by prior posterior laser capsulotomy.

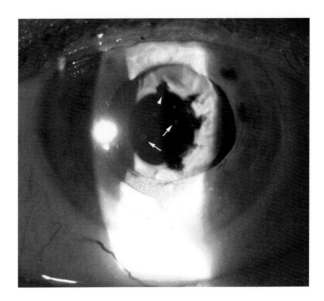

to sever all vitreous attachments. Ask the patient to look up, down, left, and right; this will allow you to see if the posterior capsule is completely separated.

- Cruciate capsulotomy technique: beginning peripherally in the vertical or horizontal midline, create a posterior capsular opening, then continue along that meridian to the opposite side (about 4 mm total length). Repeat this step in the meridian 90° to the first.

13. For pupillary membranotomy: focus the helium-neon beam precisely on the membrane. Start with a low power setting to gauge the necessary energy. Work around the membrane for 360°. Avoid the pupillary margin; fine blood vessels are often present in this area and will bleed if lased. It is acceptable to allow the lased membrane to fall into the inferior angle. For removal of large giant cell deposits on the anterior IOL surface, use very low energy (around 0.8 mJ). Focus the helium-neon beam precisely on a deposit and fire. The deposit will pop off in a "tiddlywink" fashion. Each individual deposit can be removed in this fashion, so that the anterior IOL surface is "dusted off."

14. For anterior capsulotomy: focus the helium-neon beam precisely on the membrane. The contracted anterior capsular ring is often thickest centrally and may take high energy settings (up to 5 mJ or more in some cases) to cut through. Moving peripherally along the same meridian, make 3 to 4 contiguous cuts to create a radial opening 1 to 1.5 mm long; the energy can usually be reduced as the cuts move

peripherally. Make similar radial incisions in 3 to 4 additional meridians to allow the anterior capsule to open up like a flower and prevent
further contraction (Figure 1.8).

15. Remove the capsulotomy lens if used and gently irrigate the cornea
with balanced salt solution.

16. Document the final parameters of the procedure (number of shots,
total energy) in the patient's chart.

17. Turn off the laser machine.

Postoperative Care

1. No patching or restrictions on activity are necessary.

2. Corticosteroid drops are used by some clinicians (eg, 4 times daily for
1 week), but are not needed for routine posterior capsulotomy procedures. In procedures involving a pupillary membrane or IOL deposits
(indicative of chronic, low-grade uveitis), use a topical corticosteroid
every 2 hours while awake until follow up, then taper according to
need.

3. A final refraction is usually performed 2 weeks to 1 month after the
procedure. A dilated examination should be performed to assess the
peripheral retina and macula at this time.

COMPLICATIONS

- Intraoperative: pain and blurred vision
- Early postoperative period (1 day to 1 week after surgery): floaters,
photopsias, glare, elevated IOP, blurred vision and sticky sensation
from HPMC, pitting of the IOL
- Late postoperative period (greater than 1 week after surgery): retinal
detachment, IOL decentration, cystoid macular edema

Chapter 2

Phaco Chop

Kevin M. Miller, MD

Indications for cataract surgery are discussed in Chapter 1. "Phaco chop" is a more advanced phacoemulsification technique. The surgeon should attempt it only after mastering the divide-and-conquer technique. The primary advantage of phaco chop is less phacoemulsification time and, therefore, potentially less risk of corneal endothelial compromise.

PREOPERATIVE STEPS

1. Determine the patient's desired postoperative refraction.
2. Determine the method of anesthesia (topical, intracameral, orbital injection, general).
3. Calculate IOL power.
4. Ensure that primary and back-up IOLs are available.
5. Obtain a corneal topography map if planning refractive cataract surgery (eg, peripheral corneal relaxing incisions).

INSTRUMENTATION AND SUPPLIES

- Povidone-iodine 2.5% or 5% solution
- Topical anesthetic (lidocaine gel, bupivacaine 0.75%, tetracaine 0.5%, or proparacaine 0.5%)
- Preservative-free lidocaine 1%
- Balanced salt solution

14

- Wire lid speculum (eg, Kratz-Barraquer or Lieberman speculum)
- Metal or diamond keratome
- Crescent blade
- 15° sharp blade
- Viscoelastic agent (viscosurgical device)
- Cystotome or pre-bent 25-, 27-, or 30-gauge needle
- Capsulorrhexis forceps
- Hydrodissection cannula
- Cyclodialysis spatula or nucleus rotator
- Vertical or horizontal chopper (many types available)
- Phacoemulsification unit
- Capsule polisher
- IOL injector
- Iris push–pull hook (eg, Kuglen)

SURGICAL PROCEDURE

1. Repeat Steps 1 to 16 from Chapter 1.
2. Remove the soft cortical and epinuclear material overlying the central nucleus using low flow and vacuum settings (Figure 2.1).

Horizontal Chop

1. Impale the phaco probe into the center of the nucleus. Use high vacuum to maintain adequate grip. Rock the nucleus slightly from side to side to confirm a good hold. Pull the nucleus slightly toward the incision to create space for the horizontal chopper to pass around the distal equator. Slide the horizontal chopper under the capsulorrhexis and rotate it around the equator of the lens. Be careful not to dislodge the nucleus

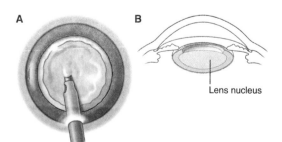

A   B

Lens nucleus

Figure 2.1. Preparation for chopping technique. (A) Removal of anterior cortex and soft epinucleus (surgeon's view). (B) Side view of the lens with the anterior cortex and the epinucleus removed.

from the phaco needle in the process. Pull the chopper toward the phaco needle, creating a full-thickness slice through the nucleus. When the 2 instruments are close to each other, separate them to propagate the crack further. It is important to propagate the separation through the posterior plate (Figure 2.2).

2. Spin the nucleus 30° to 45° to the side of the hand holding the phaco probe. Reocclude the phaco needle in the central nucleus. Pull the nucleus slightly toward the incision. Maneuver the horizontal chopper out around the distal lens equator and perform the chopping maneuver again, creating a wedge-shaped fragment of nucleus (Figure 2.3).

3. Repeat the chopping maneuver until the nucleus is segmented into 6 or more fully separate pieces. Proceed to Step 9 below (Figure 2.4).

Vertical Chop

1. Impale the phaco probe deep into the center of the nucleus. It helps to retract the silicone sleeve and expose more of the needle to facilitate

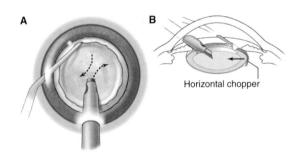

Figure 2.2. Horizontal chopping. (A) Movement of the phaco tip and the horizontal chopper to effect cracking (surgeon's view). (B) Side view of the lens with horizontal chopping instruments.

Horizontal chopper

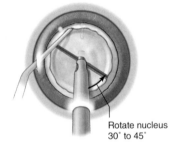

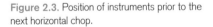

Rotate nucleus 30° to 45°

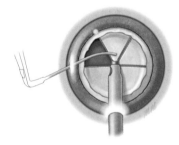

Figure 2.3. Position of instruments prior to the next horizontal chop.

Figure 2.4. Use of the phaco tip and the nucleus manipulator to engage and remove individual nuclear fragments.

a deep purchase. Use high vacuum to maintain a good grip. Rock the nucleus slightly from side to side to confirm adequate hold. Impale the vertical chopper firmly and deeply into the nucleus just in front of, or to the side of, the phaco needle. The phaco needle should provide countertraction and a slight amount of upward rotation. As a cleavage plane is established, spread the instruments sideways away from each other to propagate the crack toward the equator. It is also important to verify that the crack extends vertically through the posterior plate (Figure 2.5).

2. Spin the nucleus 30° to 45° to the side of the hand holding the phaco probe. Reocclude the phaco needle deep in the central nucleus. Pull the nucleus slightly toward the incision. Repeat the vertical chop maneuver and create a wedge-shaped fragment of nucleus (Figure 2.6).

3. Continue chopping until the nucleus is segmented into 6 or more fully separate pieces (Figure 2.7).

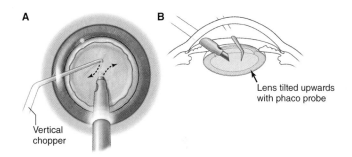

Figure 2.5. Preparation for vertical chopping. (A) Movement of the phaco tip and the vertical chopper to effect cracking (surgeon's view). (B) Side view of the lens with vertical chopping instruments.

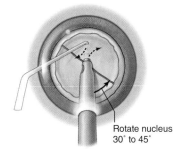

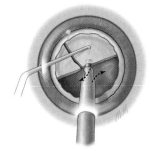

Figure 2.6. Position of the phaco tip and the vertical chopper after nucleus rotation prior to chopping of the first heminucleus.

Figure 2.7. Position of the phaco tip and the vertical chopper prior to final chopping of the remaining heminucleus.

4. Remove the quadrants one by one by phaco-assisted aspiration using high flow and high vacuum settings. Bury the tip to gain occlusion, build vacuum and pulse the ultrasound power to feed the fragments into the line. Use the second instrument to guide fragments to the phaco tip and keep them from chattering against the cornea. If the capsule is floppy or little cortex is present, reduce the vacuum level before the final nuclear segment is removed to reduce the risk of post-occlusion-break surge and capsule rupture.

5. Remove the epinuclear shell, if present, using moderate flow and vacuum settings.

6. Remove cortex using an irrigation/aspiration (I/A) probe. Always strip cortex from anterior capsule to posterior capsule rather than the other way around. Since subincisional cortex is the hardest to reach, go after it first.

7. Polish the posterior capsule, if necessary, to remove residual debris or plaque. This can be done using the IA probe in capsule vacuum mode or using a variety of capsule polishers.

8. Inject additional viscoelastic material to reform the anterior chamber and capsular bag.

9. Inspect the IOL and make certain it is free of manufacturing defects. Load it into an injector device. Inject the IOL into the eye. Manipulate it into the capsular bag using a Kuglen hook or lens manipulator.

10. Miotic agents are not necessary if the IOL is placed inside the capsular bag and the periphery of the IOL optic is completely covered with anterior capsule. If the IOL is placed in the ciliary sulcus, it should be properly sized and powered for that location. Inject a miotic agent after viscoelastic removal to prevent optic capture.

11. Remove the viscoelastic material using the I/A probe.

12. Close the phaco and paracentesis incisions by stromal hydration (injecting balanced salt solution [BSS] into the walls of the incisions). Push down on the roof of the phaco incision with a surgical sponge to facilitate closure. Inject BSS into the paracentesis to raise IOP to normal or just above normal.

13. Test the incisions and make sure they are watertight. If there is any concern about wound closure, place a single interrupted 10-0 nylon or polyglactin suture.

14. Patch and shield the eye if injection or general anesthesia was administered. Protect the eye with glasses or a shield if topical anesthesia was administered.

POSTOPERATIVE CARE

1. Postoperative care is the same as for divide-and-conquer phacoemulsi-fication (Chapter 1).

COMPLICATIONS

Intraoperative

- Pain
- Iris atrophy or prolapse
- Thermal corneal injury (phaco burn)
- Incomplete or torn capsulorrhexis
- Posterior capsule rupture
- Vitreous loss
- Dropped nucleus or lens fragments
- Suprachoroidal hemorrhage

Early Postoperative Period (1 Day to 1 Week After Surgery)

- Blepharoptosis
- Extraocular muscle paresis (diplopia)
- Wound leak
- Corneal edema
- Anterior chamber inflammation
- Iris trauma, paralysis, or atrophy (polycoria)
- Retained lens material
- Intraocular pressure spike
- Lens power calculation error
- Endophthalmitis
- Macular edema
- Retinal tear
- Macular hole
- Retinal vascular occlusion
- Retinal detachment

Late Postoperative Period (Greater Than 1 Week After Surgery)

- Binocular imbalance
- Corneal decompensation (pseudophakic bullous keratopathy)
- Chronic iritis
- Glaucoma
- Lens decentration or dislocation
- Posterior capsule opacification
- Glare, halos, streaks, starbursts, light sensitivity, temporal scotomas
- Worsening of pre-existing conditions (eg, diabetic retinopathy, macular degeneration, glaucoma, epiretinal membranes, or floaters)
- Failure to achieve or restore visual acuity to 20/20 or better
- Other problems listed as early postoperative complications

Chapter 3

Pediatric Cataract Surgery

Scott M. Warden, MD
Deborah K. VanderVeen, MD

Appropriate timing of cataract surgery in children is especially critical in order to prevent irreversible amblyopia. Visually significant congenital cataracts should be removed in the first few weeks of life when unilateral, and generally by 4 to 6 weeks of life when bilateral. Less severe cataracts may be observed and managed medically, with good outcomes if surgery is performed later. Older children (age ≥6 years) who develop cataracts are at less risk of severe amblyopia and should have surgery when the cataract(s) adversely affects the child's daily activities.

PREOPERATIVE STEPS

1. Conduct an age-appropriate evaluation to fully assess the visual significance of the cataract and to plan the surgical procedure.
   - Neonates less than 2 months of age: careful analysis of the morphology of the cataract is the primary method of assessment. Concerning signs include a cataract in the central visual axis larger than 3 mm, a posterior opacity, or a cataract that is confluent without clear zones. For smaller opacities, if there is a clear view to the macula using direct ophthalmoscopy, observation should be considered.
   - Infants and preverbal children (3 months to 2 years): in addition to the morphology of the cataract, evaluation of fixation patterns is useful. Poor or eccentric fixation, irritability when covering the

21

"better" eye, or the presence of nystagmus or strabismus indicates the presence of amblyopia and a visually significant cataract. A documented myopic shift may also signify the presence of amblyopia.

- Verbal children: in addition to the above, recognition visual acuity measures may be obtained. Visual acuity of 20/70 or worse is generally an indication for surgery. For children, the loss of accommodation from surgery is often more detrimental than the benefit of improved visual acuity when already better than 20/70.

2. Consider IOL implantation.
   - A posterior chamber IOL is usually placed at the time of cataract aspiration for children ≥2 years.
   - It is not uncommon for surgeons experienced in pediatric cataract surgery to perform IOL implantation for children age 6 months to 2 years, but implantation for infants, especially those <6 months of age, is particularly controversial because of the marked changes in the axial length of the growing eye and increased post-surgical inflammation and associated complications.
   - A target postoperative refraction is usually mild to moderate hyperopia for children ≤5 years and near emmetropia for children ≥6 years.
   - Keratometry and A-scan measurements with IOL calculations often must be performed under anesthesia in order to obtain accurate measurements.

INSTRUMENTATION AND SUPPLIES

- Cataract aspiration without IOL:
  - Colibri (.12) forceps
  - Microvitreoretinal (MVR) or 15° sharp blade
  - Ocutome/anterior vitrectomy handpiece, with or without separate anterior chamber cannula/handpiece
  - Absorbable 10-0 or 9-0 suture
- Cataract aspiration with IOL and primary capsulotomy/anterior vitrectomy:
  - Crescent knife
  - Keratome
  - Cystotome
  - Capsulorrhexis forceps
  - IOL folder/inserter
  - 4-0 silk and 8-0 polyglactin sutures

SURGICAL PROCEDURE

The soft, elastic nature of a child's eye and lens requires some adjustment from adult techniques. The main variations from adult cataract surgery are described here.

1. General endotracheal anesthesia is used. No supplemental injections are necessary.
2. Biometry and IOL calculations must be performed under anesthesia; immersion biometry is recommended, using Holladay or Hoffer Q formulas for IOL calculations for short eyes.
3. Prep and drape.
4. Place an appropriately sized lid speculum.

For Infants With No IOL Placement

1. Make side port incisions at 10 and 2 o'clock, and inject viscoelastic.
2. Introduce the irrigating cannula or handpiece into 1 side port and the Ocutome into the other (Figure 3.1A). Alternatively, create a single 2.5-mm superior incision large enough to accommodate the combined irrigation/aspiration handpiece (Figure 3.1B).
3. The anterior capsule is opened by turning the cutting port posteriorly. Place the tip of the Ocutome through the capsular opening and rotate anteriorly, to cut a circular opening in the anterior capsule (Figure 3.2).
4. Aspirate the cataractous lens. All cortical material must be removed to reduce inflammation and prevent lens reproliferation and opacification of the visual axis.

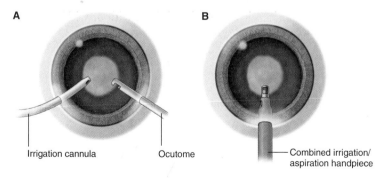

Figure 3.1. Instrument placement shown through (A) 2 side port incisions or (B) a single incision.

Figure 3.2. Opening the anterior capsule using the Ocutome ("vitrectorrhexis").

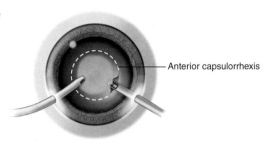

Anterior capsulorrhexis

Figure 3.3. Performing anterior vitrectomy.

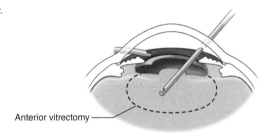

Anterior vitrectomy

5. Use the Ocutome to cut a circular opening in the posterior capsule, leaving a rounded border without radial tears.
6. Perform anterior vitrectomy, using a high cut rate and low aspiration (Figure 3.3).
7. Inject acetylcholine to confirm a round pupil with no vitreous in the anterior chamber.
8. Close the wound(s) with absorbable suture.

For Children With IOL Placement and Requiring Anterior Vitrectomy (Pars Plana Approach)

1. Repeat Steps 1 to 4 above.
2. Place 4-0 silk suture at the superior rectus.
3. Perform a conjunctival peritomy to allow creation of scleral tunnel wound and sclerotomy (Figure 3.4).
4. Cauterize sclera for hemostasis.
5. Create a scleral tunnel large enough to accommodate a foldable IOL, and enter the anterior chamber with a keratome.
6. Create 1 or 2 side port incisions, and inject a highly cohesive viscoelastic to allow better flattening of the elastic anterior capsule of young patients.

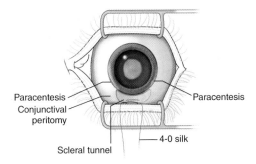

Figure 3.4. Performing conjunctival peritomy and creating a scleral tunnel incision.

Paracentesis
Conjunctival
peritomy
Paracentesis
4-0 silk
Scleral tunnel

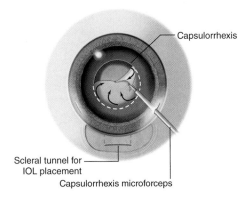

Figure 3.5. Creating a continuous curvilinear capsulorrhexis.

Capsulorrhexis

Scleral tunnel for
IOL placement
Capsulorrhexis microforceps

7. Create a continuous curvilinear capsulorrhexis with the cystotome and capsulorrhexis forceps. While guiding the leading edge of the capsular flap around, pull toward the center of the pupil to help prevent the elastic capsule from running outward (Figure 3.5). Avoid loss of viscoelastic by minimal manipulation of the wound and frequent regrasping of the capsular flap; add viscoelastic as necessary to keep the anterior capsule flattened. In young children, aiming for a smaller opening when starting the capsulotomy will still generally result in a 5- to 6-mm opening. If the flap runs outward, use the Ocutome to complete a circular opening.

8. Aspirate the cataract with the Ocutome handpiece.

9. Reform the capsular bag, enlarge the scleral wound slightly, and insert the IOL. Most pediatric ophthalmologists prefer acrylic foldable lenses.

10. Partially close the scleral tunnel with absorbable suture (9-0 or 10-0), remove the viscoelastic from the anterior chamber, and close 1 side port incision.

11. Create a pars plana sclerotomy site with the MVR blade (usually ≤3 mm from the limbus, depending on eye size), and pre-place an 8-0 polyglactin suture in a figure-eight shape.

12. Insert the Ocutome into the anterior vitreous cavity, with irrigation via the side port incision, and cut a round posterior capsulotomy and perform partial vitrectomy (Figures 3.6A, 3.6B).

13. Close the scleral wound with the pre-placed suture and check for leaks.

14. Remove the irrigating cannula and close the side port incision with a 9-0 or 10-0 absorbable suture.

15. Confirm the appropriate IOL position, and inject acetylcholine to constrict the pupil if desired.

16. Close the conjunctiva.

17. Subconjunctival injections of corticosteroid with or without antibiotic are given.

POSTOPERATIVE CARE

1. Minimize inflammation with the use of topical corticosteroids (and a cycloplegic, such as atropine for aphakic patients).

2. Manage aphakia with contact lens placement as early as 1 week after surgery. Spectacle correction with a bifocal for IOL patients should

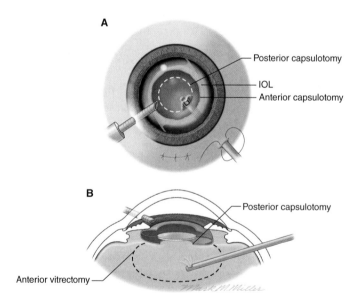

Figure 3.6. Performing pars plana posterior capsulotomy and anterior vitrectomy. (A) Surgeon's view. (B) Side view of instruments.

be done once the refractive error has stabilized, about 1 month after surgery, after sutures have absorbed.

3. Amblyopia therapy should be instituted as necessary after the operated eye has full contact lens or spectacle correction.

COMPLICATIONS

- Incomplete vitreous removal or prolapse into the anterior chamber
- Wound leak or dehiscence
- Glaucoma
- IOL prolapse or dislocation, including that caused by prolapsed vitreous or later dislocation from iris/capsule adhesions
- Posterior capsule opacity, or reproliferation of lens material
- Endophthalmitis
- Retinal detachment

All wounds should be sutured, and careful passage of the needle will prevent leaks from the suture track or from "cheese-wiring" of the tissues with the suture.

Early glaucoma may be due to severe inflammation or pupillary block. Corticosteroid response glaucoma is not uncommon in children. Aphakic glaucoma may occur in up to 30% of infants undergoing early surgery and often manifests early but may occur years after cataract surgery.

Posterior capsule opacification is common when the posterior capsule is left intact at the time of cataract aspiration, requiring future YAG capsulotomy or surgery.

Chapter 4

Gundersen Flap

Daniel A. Johnson, MD

A Gundersen flap provides a durable, vascularized epithelial covering for a diseased or damaged cornea. Historical indications for the procedure include medically resistant microbial keratitis, painful bullous keratopathy in an eye with limited or no vision, neurotrophic keratopathy, and even recurrent corneal erosions. Its use over the past several years has declined due to advances in the therapy of such disorders, including the development of newer antimicrobial agents, hypertonic solutions, bandage contact lenses, the availability of donor corneal tissue, and limbal and amniotic membrane grafts. Nonetheless, the Gundersen flap continues to be a useful technique.

PREOPERATIVE STEPS

1. Examine the conjunctiva carefully at the slit lamp for evidence of prior conjunctival surgery or scarring that may hinder conjunctival dissection.
2. In instances where the superior bulbar conjunctiva has limited mobility, it may be necessary to harvest tarsal conjunctiva in addition to bulbar conjunctiva.
3. It is essential to obtain a proper informed consent, including a thorough discussion of other treatment options.

INSTRUMENTATION AND SUPPLIES

- Povidone-iodine 5% solution
- Marking pen or gentian violet
- Lid speculum
- Muscle hook
- Nontoothed forceps (conjunctival, Bishop-Harmon, others)
- Blunt Westcott scissors
- Syringe with balanced salt solution or lidocaine (1% to 2%) with epinephrine
- 8-0 polyglactin suture on a spatulated needle
- Crescent blade
- Cellulose sponges
- Absolute alcohol (optional)
- Desmarres retractor (for supratarsal conjunctival dissection)

SURGICAL PROCEDURE

1. Anesthesia: although retrobulbar anesthesia may suffice, general anesthesia may be preferable since there will be less resistance to globe rotation.
2. Prep the conjunctival fornix, lashes, and periorbital skin with povidone-iodine solution.
3. Drape the lashes out of the surgical field (unless tarsal conjunctiva will need to be harvested).
4. Rotate the globe inferiorly with the use of either a bridle suture at the superior limbus or a muscle hook placed in the inferior fornix.
5. Mark a line 14 to 16 mm superior to the upper edge of the corneal limbus, approximately 3 cm long (Figure 4.1).
6. Incise the marked line (Figure 4.2).

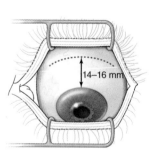

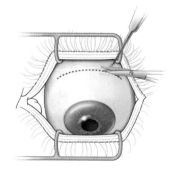

Figure 4.1. Marking the conjunctiva prior to the incision.

Figure 4.2. Incising the conjunctiva.

7. Perform a 360° limbal peritomy with Westcott scissors.
8. Denude the corneal and limbal epithelium with the crescent blade (Figure 4.3) or absolute alcohol to allow adherence of the graft. Leaving the limbal epithelium untouched may allow subsequent, albeit difficult, reversal for future corneal surgery; however, the risk of inclusion cysts may be increased.
9. Balloon the conjunctiva and Tenon's by injecting balanced salt solution or lidocaine with epinephrine beneath the epithelium, using caution not to allow the needle to pierce the desired graft (Figure 4.4).
10. Using a nontoothed forceps and Westcott scissors, dissect the conjunctival flap anteriorly and complete the incision circumferentially along the superior limbus (Figure 4.5). The goal is to create a thin flap without buttonholes that is large enough to cover the cornea without significant traction. Buttonholes can subsequently enlarge and contribute to graft retraction.
11. Pull the conjunctival flap over the cornea and suture with interrupted 8-0 polyglactin sutures. The superior edge of the flap should be sutured to the superior limbus and the inferior edge to both the inferior limbus and inferior edge of the peritomy (Figure 4.6).

Figure 4.3. Creation of a 360° limbal peritomy and removal of corneal epithelium.

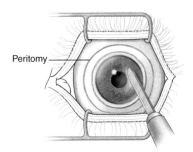

Peritomy

Figure 4.4. Ballooning the conjunctiva prior to dissection.

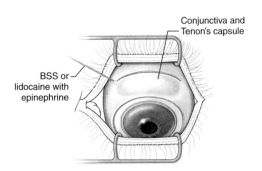

Conjunctiva and Tenon's capsule

BSS or lidocaine with epinephrine

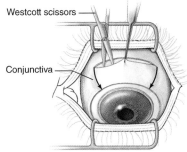
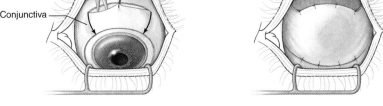

Figure 4.5. Dissection of a thin conjunctival flap.

Figure 4.6. Movement of the conjunctival flap over the cornea and suture placement.

12. Buttonholes should be sutured closed with 10-0 nylon to deeper tissue (corneal stroma or episclera) and positioned off the cornea if possible.
13. Apply an antibiotic-corticosteroid ointment, a cycloplegic drop, a pressure patch, and a shield.

MODIFICATIONS

Inadequate Bulbar Conjunctiva

1. If it is suspected preoperatively that there will be inadequate superior bulbar conjunctiva to cover the cornea, prior to placing the lid speculum, use a Desmarres retractor to evert the upper lid.
2. The supratarsal conjunctiva is ballooned using lidocaine with epinephrine (Figure 4.7).
3. Incise the conjunctiva along the superior border of the tarsal plate and dissect toward the fornix (Figure 4.8).
4. Once at the fornix, place the lid speculum and carry the dissection to completion at the limbus.

Dissection Alternative

1. Create 10 to 15 radial rows of dots on the superficial conjunctiva between the limbal and forniceal borders of the future flap, using a sterile marking pen or gentian violet (Figure 4.9).
2. Holding the limbal edge of the flap taut with a nontoothed forceps, create a series of radial dissection tunnels beneath each row of dots by

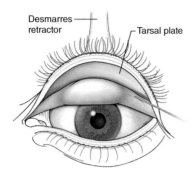

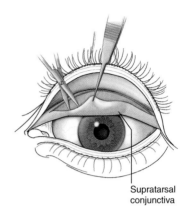

Figure 4.7. Preparation of the supratarsal conjunctiva and ballooning the superior tarsal conjunctiva with lidocaine.

Figure 4.8. Dissection of the tarsal conjunctiva toward the fornix.

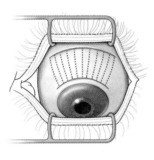

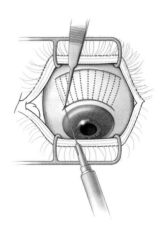

Figure 4.9. Conjunctival marks from the sterile marking pen.

Figure 4.10. Creation of radial tunnels with a 25-gauge needle.

infusing lidocaine with epinephrine from a syringe with a 25-gauge needle (Figure 4.10). Advance the needle beneath the conjunctiva from the limbal side to the forniceal side.

3. Once the needle is withdrawn, widen the path with scissors. Adjacent paths so created are then connected by cutting the Tenon's fibers that separate the 2 adjacent tunnels.

4. Continue the process until all of the tunnels have been created, connected, and the flap is free from the underlying Tenon's tissue (see Figure 4.7).

Flap Alternative

1. If superior or inferior scarring prevents those portions of the conjunctiva from being used, or if it would be helpful to avoid the action of the lid causing the flap to dehisce, a flap may be taken from the temporal conjunctiva and pulled nasally across the cornea.
2. The technique of suturing to the temporal limbus and to the peritomy and sclera nasally is the same, but the result is a flap that will not be susceptible to vertical displacement by the lid.

POSTOPERATIVE CARE

1. A reasonable postoperative regimen includes a topical antibiotic (eg, moxifloxacin 0.5%, gatifloxacin 0.3%) and topical corticosteroid (eg, prednisolone acetate 1%) 4 times daily.
2. The antibiotic can be discontinued when the ocular surface has re-epithelialized. The topical corticosteroid can be tapered by 1 drop per day each week over the ensuing month.

COMPLICATIONS

- Conjunctival buttonholes
- Graft retraction
- Hemorrhage beneath the flap
- Conjunctival inclusion cysts
- Bleeding
- Infection
- Pain
- Ptosis

Chapter 5

Corneal Gluing

Leejee H. Suh, MD
Esen K. Akpek, MD

Tissue adhesives (cyanoacrylate glues) have been widely used as topical skin adhesives and are readily available in the United States. Although not approved by the United States Food and Drug Administration for ophthalmic use, cyanoacrylate glues have been successfully used for closure of impending or frank small corneal perforations measuring 1 to 2 mm, descemetoceles, leaking filtering blebs, and wound leaks. The various preparations available for clinical use are butyl-2-cyanoacrylate (Indermil, Sherwood, Davis, and Geck, St Louis, Missouri), N-butyl-2-cyanoacrylate (Histoacryl Blue, B. Braun AG, Melsungen, Germany), N-butyl-cyanoacrylate (Nexacryl, Closure Medical, Raleigh, North Carolina), and 2-octyl-cyanoacrylate (Dermabond, Closure Medical, Raleigh, North Carolina).

Early application of cyanoacrylate glue can effectively manage small corneal perforations, improve visual outcome, and possibly avoid the need for tectonic penetrating keratoplasty. Application of the tissue adhesive can be performed either at the slip lamp or under an operating microscope. Cyanoacrylate glues have been shown to prevent re-epithelialization into the area of damaged stroma, thereby halting entrance of collagenase proteins and further corneal melting. The glues have bacteriostatic activity against gram-positive organisms. Corneal gluing, however, only temporarily addresses the problem; repeat applications of glue or surgery are often necessary.

PREOPERATIVE STEPS

1. Once a perforation is diagnosed, the wound should be glued as soon as possible to prevent further collapse of the anterior chamber.
2. Obtain informed consent. The patient should provide consent for corneal gluing and also for possible future procedures. The patient should also understand that, although corneal gluing may be recommended, it is not an FDA-approved use of the adhesive.

INSTRUMENTS AND SUPPLIES

- Topical proparacaine 0.5%
- Topical broad-spectrum antibiotic (eg, moxifloxacin 0.5% or gatifloxacin 0.3%) or specific anti-infective based on culture results (eg, cefazolin, 50 mg/mL)
- Povidone-iodine 5% solution (stock 10% solution diluted 1:1 with balanced salt solution)
- Lid speculum
- Cellulose sponges
- Filter for syringe
- Cyanoacrylate glue
- 15° sharp blade
- Crescent blade
- 27-gauge needle
- 30-gauge needle (2)
- Tuberculin syringe (2)
- Bandage soft contact lens

SURGICAL PROCEDURE

1. Apply 1 drop of topical anesthetic and 1 drop of antibiotic. Place 1 drop of 50:50 mixture of povidone-iodine solution into the conjunctival fornix and clean lashes and periocular skin.
2. Prepare the aseptic working field.
3. Gently place the lid speculum.
4. Dry the ocular surface with sponges and examine the eye (Figure 5.1).
5. If the anterior chamber is flat, make peripheral paracentesis with a 15° blade. Use a 30-gauge needle attached to empty tuberculin syringe to

inject a small amount of filtered air into the anterior chamber (Figure 5.2). Take care not to inject too much air, as it may cause discomfort.

6. Remove epithelium 2 mm on either side of perforation with a crescent blade (Figure 5.3).

7. Dry the corneal surface thoroughly with cellulose sponges (Figure 5.4). The glue will not attach to the surface if it is not dry.

8. Draw cyanoacrylate glue with the 27-gauge needle attached to the tuberculin syringe.

9. Switch to the 30-gauge needle and bring up a small amount of glue to bevel (Figure 5.5).

10. Apply 1 drop onto the area of perforation (Figure 5.6) and quickly withdraw the needle. The goal is to leave the glued surface as flat and smooth as possible.

11. Allow glue to completely dry on the corneal surface.

12. Place the bandage contact lens.

13. Start or resume a topical antibiotic.

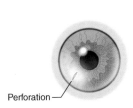

Perforation

Figure 5.1. Corneal perforation.

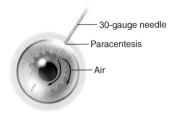

30-gauge needle

Paracentesis

Air

Figure 5.2. Injection of air through the side port incision into the anterior chamber.

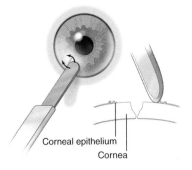

Corneal epithelium
Cornea

Figure 5.3. Removal of epithelium surrounding the perforated area.

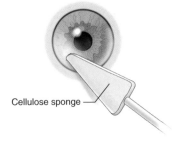

Cellulose sponge

Figure 5.4. Drying of the corneal surface with cellulose sponge.

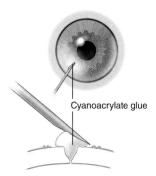

Cyanoacrylate glue

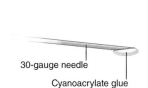

30-gauge needle

Cyanoacrylate glue

Figure 5.5. Exposure of a small amount of glue at the tip of the needle bevel.

Figure 5.6. Application of glue onto the perforated area.

POSTOPERATIVE CARE

1. Follow up in 1 day and then as needed, depending on the clinical status.
2. With each visit, check for wound leak (Seidel test) and anterior chamber depth.

COMPLICATIONS

- Reperforation due to separation or loss of glue from the perforation site
- Elevated IOP
- Hypotony
- Keratitis
- Endophthalmitis
- Tissue toxicity due to direct contact with corneal endothelium or lens
- Dislodging of the contact lens with irritation of palpebral conjunctiva from glue

Chapter 6

Conjunctival Biopsy

Jennifer E. Thorne, MD, PhD

A conjunctival biopsy may be utilized in the management of conjunctival disease to establish a diagnosis and institute appropriate therapy. Conjunctival biopsies may be useful in establishing a cause of conjunctival nodules, dysplasia, or chronic inflammation with or without scarring.

PREOPERATIVE STEPS

1. Consult with the pathologist about tests to be performed on the specimen.
2. Obtain necessary transport media.
3. Obtain informed consent.

INSTRUMENTATION AND SUPPLIES

- Topical proparacaine 0.5%
- 1% lidocaine with epinephrine 1:100,000 in a tuberculin syringe and 30-gauge needle
- Sterile 0.12 forceps
- Sharp Wescott scissors
- Transport media
- Antibiotic ointment

SURGICAL PROCEDURE

1. Anesthetize the inferior cul-de-sac in the area planned for biopsy, using a cotton-tipped applicator soaked with topical proparacaine (Figure 6.1).

2. After ensuring proper anesthesia, perform a subconjunctival injection of 0.1 to 0.2 mL of 1% lidocaine with epinephrine to form a small wheal in the inferior cul-de-sac (Figure 6.2).

3. Grasp the elevated conjunctiva with the 0.12 forceps and excise approximately 2 mm of conjunctiva from the inferior cul-de-sac with sharp Wescott scissors (Figure 6.3).

4. Transfer tissue into the transport media.

5. Provide hemostasis with direct pressure, using a cotton-tipped applicator.

6. Apply antibiotic ointment to the biopsy site and place the pressure patch on the eye.

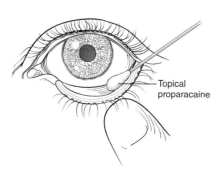

Figure 6.1. Anesthetizing the biopsy site with topical proparacaine.

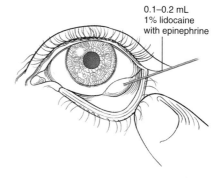

Figure 6.2. Subconjunctival anesthesia.

Figure 6.3. Obtaining the biopsy.

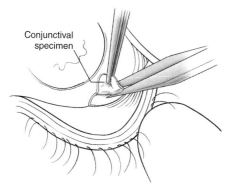

POSTOPERATIVE CARE

1. Send the specimen promptly to the pathologist and include the relevant clinical history.
2. The pressure patch may be removed after 3 to 4 hours.
3. The antibiotic ointment should be applied to the biopsied eye twice daily for 3 days.

COMPLICATIONS

- Bleeding
- Infection
- Worsening of scarring if the patient has a cicatrizing conjunctivitis (eg, mucous membrane pemphigoid)
- Loss of vision

Chapter 7

EDTA Chelation

Parveen K. Nagra, MD
Kristin M. Hammersmith, MD

Band keratopathy, or calcium deposition at the level of Bowman's membrane, may lead to pain from corneal erosions or lid irritation. In addition, decreased vision may result when the visual axis is involved. Patients may be considered for disodium EDTA chelation when the band keratopathy is visually significant; pain or irritation is not relieved by more-conservative measures, such as lubrication; or for cosmetic purposes. EDTA chelation can also be considered for asymptomatic patients when diagnostic and therapeutic procedures for the interior of the eye are compromised.

PREOPERATIVE STEPS

1. Address the underlying pathology to the extent possible. This could include control of uveitis, discontinuation of topical medications containing phosphates or mercury, or treatment of systemic diseases associated with hypercalcemia, such as sarcoidosis, hyperparathyroidism, or renal failure. Band keratopathy may also be secondary to ocular surgery, especially with silicone oil. Patients with band keratopathy and no known etiology warrant additional work-up.
2. The procedure can be performed at the slit lamp or under the operating microscope.

INSTRUMENTATION AND SUPPLIES

- Wire lid speculum
- Disodium ethylenediamine tetraacetic acid (EDTA) 2% to 3%
- Topical anesthetic (proparacaine 0.5%)
- 0.9% normal saline
- 1.0-mL tuberculin syringe
- Topical anesthetic
- Sterile scalpel or sterile cotton-tipped applicators
- Cellulose sponges
- Bandage contact lens
- Antibiotic solution (moxifloxacin 0.5%, gatifloxacin 0.3%) or ointment (erythromycin, bacitracin)
- Cycloplegic drops (atropine 1%, cyclopentolate 1% or 2%)
- Pressure patch and tape

SURGICAL PROCEDURE

1. Disodium EDTA is no longer commercially available and must be compounded. While recommended concentrations vary, in general 1 to 2 ml of a 2% to 3% solution is adequate.
2. Anesthetize the eye with topical anesthetic; if using the operating microscope and the calcium deposition is dense, consider a sub-Tenon's or retrobulbar block.
3. Place the lid speculum.
4. Debride corneal epithelium (using a sterile scalpel or sterile cotton-tipped applicator) over the area of calcium to be removed (Figure 7.1); avoid overly extensive epithelial debridement.
5. Draw up the disodium EDTA in the tuberculin syringe and saturate a cellulose sponge or cotton swab with 3% disodium EDTA, then wipe repeatedly over band keratopathy until calcium clears (Figure 7.2). This may take 10 to 45 minutes. Additional applications of topical anesthetic may be necessary during the procedure.
6. For dense calcium deposits, after initial application of EDTA, superficial debridement may be attempted with the scalpel, followed by further EDTA. Avoid scraping Bowman's layer if possible, as this contributes to corneal scarring and higher-order aberrations.
7. Irrigate the eye with normal saline to remove EDTA.

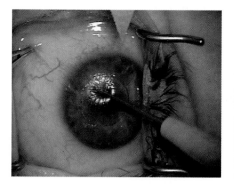

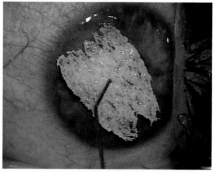

Figure 7.1. Epithelial debridement overlying band keratopathy using the edge of the crescent blade.

Figure 7.2. Use of disodium EDTA-saturated cellulose sponge to remove final remnants of band keratopathy.

POSTOPERATIVE CARE

1. Place an antibiotic ointment and a cycloplegic drop, and pressure patch eye for 24 hours. Alternatively, an antibiotic drop (eg, a fluoroquinolone) and a cycloplegic drop may be placed, followed by a bandage contact lens.
2. Pain may be a significant issue for some patients in the immediate postoperative period. Switching to a bandage contact lens if not utilized initially or repeating pressure patching, as well as use of oral analgesics (eg, acetaminophen with codeine) may help alleviate patient discomfort.
3. Patients should be followed closely until epithelialization is complete.
4. Topical corticosteroids may reduce residual anterior stromal haze but also increase the risk of infectious keratitis and should be used judiciously.

COMPLICATIONS

- Nonhealing corneal epithelial defects (debridement of a large area of corneal epithelium prior to chelation may result in absence of limbal stem cells with subsequent poor healing)
- Infectious keratitis
- Recurrent band keratopathy
- Residual anterior stromal haze

Chapter 8

Iris Suture Fixation of an Intraocular Lens

John J. Kim, MD
Walter J. Stark, MD

In the absence of capsule or zonular support, an intraocular lens (IOL) can be inserted via a small clear corneal or limbal incision and sutured to the peripheral iris using modified McCannel sutures. This technique is useful in the instances of aphakia, surgical complications such as loss of capsular support, and poor zonular support (eg, lens subluxation from conditions such as pseudoexfoliation and Marfan syndrome).

PREOPERATIVE STEPS

1. Calculate the IOL power.
2. Adjust for iris fixation.
3. Do not dilate the pupil.

INSTRUMENTATION AND SUPPLIES

- Wire lid speculum
- 15° sharp blade
- Keratome
- Viscosurgical device
- 0.12 forceps
- IOL folder

- IOL inserter
- Iris spatula (Barraquer sweep)
- 10-0 polypropylene suture on a long, spatulated needle (Ethicon CTC-6 or CIF-4)
- 10-0 polyglactin (Vicryl) suture
- Sinskey hook
- Acetylcholine solution
- Balanced saline solution

SURGICAL PROCEDURE

1. Anesthesia: retrobulbar injection preferred (lid block optional).
2. Prep and drape.
3. Place the lid speculum.
4. Create or enlarge a clear corneal wound with the keratome so that it is large enough to accommodate a folded IOL. A 3.5-mm incision will suffice for most IOLs.
5. Create a side port incision 180° from the corneal wound.
6. Inject acetylcholine into the anterior chamber to induce miosis. This will facilitate pupil capture.
7. Inject viscoelastic material into the anterior chamber.
8. Fold the IOL in the "moustache style" (Figure 8.1A).
9. Insert the IOL through the corneal wound, placing the haptics into the pupil, and position the optic above the plane of the iris (Figures 8.1B, 8.1C).
10. While unfolding the IOL optic above the iris plane, insert an iris spatula through the side port incision beneath the optic and unfold the lens slowly (Figure 8.1D). Make sure that the haptics are behind the iris as the IOL is unfolded. This will result in a "cat's eye" appearance of the pupil from iris capture at the haptic-optic junctions when the iris spatula and folding forceps are withdrawn (Figure 8.1E).
11. Elevate the optic with the iris spatula to outline the position of the haptics. Then pass the 10-0 polypropylene suture on the long needle through the clear cornea and iris, behind the haptic, and out through the iris and cornea on the other side of the haptic (Figure 8.2).
12. Make a new side port incision in the corneal periphery in the meridian of the apex of the haptic.
13. Using a Sinskey hook, pull the 2 ends of the suture though the side port incision (Figure 8.3).
14. Repeat Steps 11 to 13 for the second haptic.

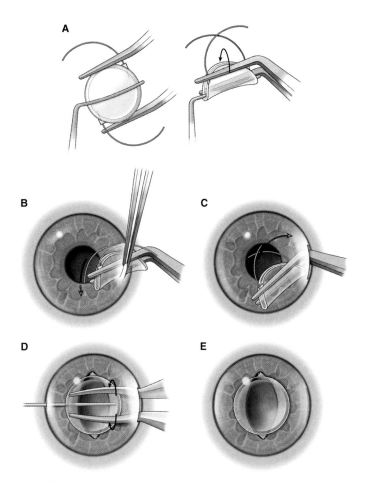

Figure 8.1. Preparation and insertion of the IOL. (A) Folding of the IOL "moustache-style." (B) Insertion of the folded IOL through the clear corneal incision. (C) Unfolding of the IOL haptics posterior to the iris. (D) Unfolding of the IOL optic anterior to the iris. (E) Capture of the IOL in the iris prior to final suturing. Note the "cat's-eye" pupil formed by the 2 haptic-optic junctions.

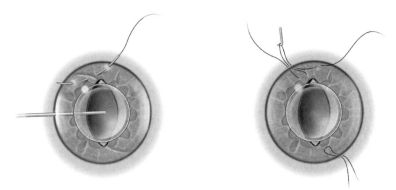

Figure 8.2. Capture of the first haptic with long polypropylene suture.

Figure 8.3. Externalization of the iris fixation suture prior to tying the knot.

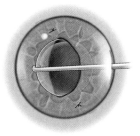
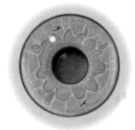

Figure 8.4. Capture of the IOL optic posterior to the iris following haptic fixation.

Figure 8.5. Final appearance of iris-sutured IOL. Note the loss of the "cat's eye" appearance of the pupil.

15. Tie the sutures. Alternatively, one may use a Siepser sliding knot to fixate the haptics.
16. Use a Sinskey hook to manipulate the optic posterior to the iris (Figure 8.4).
17. Inject acetylcholine to ensure a round, miotic pupil (Figure 8.5).
18. Remove the viscoelastic material from the anterior chamber.
19. Confirm that the anterior chamber is free of vitreous. Inject air into the anterior chamber to facilitate identification of vitreous. If vitreous is present, an iris spatula can be used to break the strands, or an anterior vitrectomy can be performed.
20. Inject balanced salt solution into the anterior chamber to bring the eye to a more normal physiologic pressure, and place a single 10-0 nylon suture in the center of the wound.
21. Test the wounds for leaks.

COMPLICATIONS

- Iris bleeding
- Difficulty capturing haptic with polypropylene suture, with subsequent IOL subluxation
- Corneal edema
- Vitreous prolapse
- Macular edema
- Endophthalmitis
- Iris irregularity

Chapter 9

Amniotic Membrane Transplantation

W. Barry Lee, MD, FACS
Ivan R. Schwab, MD, FACS

Amniotic membrane transplantation is used as an adjunct in the excision and repair of various corneal and external ocular diseases. It can be used alone to prevent further stromal degradation or in conjunction with a limbal autograft or allograft to repopulate the corneal stem cells. Amniotic membrane acts as a scaffold for ocular surface repair. Indications for surgery include the following:

- Repair of conjunctival defects, corneal pathology, or cicatricial strabismus
- Post-resection of primary and recurrent pterygia or benign or malignant conjunctival neoplasm
- Persistent epithelial defect coverage, neurotrophic corneal ulcer, or acute chemical and thermal burns
- Treatment of painful bullous keratopathy
- Reconstructions of the ocular surface
- As an adjunct in fornix reconstruction or with limbal stem cell transplant surgery

PREOPERATIVE STEPS

1. Anesthesia: retrobulbar or peribulbar block, or subconjunctival anesthesia (after topical anesthetic and antibiotic installation).
2. Be sure that amniotic membrane is available in the operating room.

INSTRUMENTATION AND SUPPLIES

- Needle driver
- Needle holder
- Marking pen or gentian violet
- Crescent blade or Grieshaber blade
- Vannas scissors
- Bipolar wet-field scleral cautery instrument
- Diamond burr corneal polisher
- Titanium tying forceps
- 0.12 forceps with typing platform
- Amniotic membrane (2 present types): fresh frozen tissue (BioTissue Services, Miami, Florida), dehydrated tissue (AmbioDry, OKTO Ophtho, Costa Mesa, California)
- 8-0, 9-0, or 10-0 monofilament suture; fibrin glue to secure tissue

SURGICAL PROCEDURES

Method to Close Conjunctival Defect With Sutures

1. Place the lid speculum.
2. Outline the area of tissue to be excised with a marking pen, including a zone of normal tissue.
3. Excise the tissue along the outline.
4. Use a crescent blade or Grieshaber blade to dissect the corneal portion of the lesion, if applicable, taking care to follow the pathologic tissue plane within the cornea and not extend into normal, deeper corneal stroma.
5. Use a diamond burr corneal polisher to lightly smooth the corneal surface and limbus and remove any surface irregularities. Apply minimal amount of polishing to leave a smooth surface.
6. Hemostasis can be achieved with scleral wet-field cautery or direct pressure from a cotton-tipped applicator. (The authors prefer to avoid or limit the use of cautery.)
7. Measure the conjunctival defect (Figure 9.1) with calipers and fashion a similar-sized amniotic graft.
8. Place the amniotic membrane graft over the conjunctival defect with the basement membrane side up (Figure 9.2). The side exposed to the air within the tissue carrier is the side that remains exposed to air

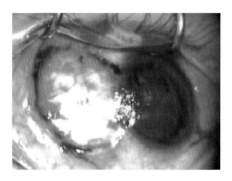

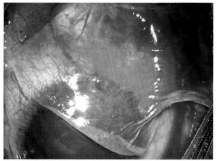

Figure 9.1. Conjunctival defect outlined with gentian violet after pterygium excision just prior to amniotic membrane placement.

Figure 9.2. Amniotic membrane placement over a conjunctival defect after pterygium excision, prior to trimming of the edges before suture placement.

when placed on the eye. The stromal side adherent to the tissue carrier should be facing down adjacent to the ocular surface.

9. Secure the tissue with interrupted sutures at each of the 4 corners, placing the first 2 sutures at the limbal corners. The first 2 limbal sutures should be anchored to the episclera.

10. Place additional interrupted sutures until no large gaps remain between the graft and host tissue, preventing underlying exposed sclera.

Method to Close a Conjunctival Defect With Fibrin Glue

1. Repeat Steps 1 to 5 in the previous section.

2. When using dehydrated amniotic membrane, place the fibrinogen component of fibrin glue on the exposed sclera within the conjunctival defect. Place the amniotic membrane graft stromal side down (oversize the graft by 1 mm on each of the 3 sides that will border conjunctiva and the same size on the limbal edge bordering the cornea). The thrombin is applied to the basement membrane surface of the amniotic membrane. When using fresh frozen amniotic membrane, apply the thrombin to the stromal side of the amniotic membrane prior to tissue placement over the conjunctival defect. Then place the tissue over the bed of fibrinogen with the stromal side down.

3. Tuck the edges of the tissue under the conjunctiva. Excess glue can be removed with Vannas scissors. Take care to flatten the graft, removing any folds or air pockets.

4. The tissue and glue are allowed to dry, holding down each quadrant with the help of an assistant for 2 to 3 minutes, taking care to avoid exposed underlying sclera.

Method to Repair Corneal Pathology

1. Remove the entire corneal epithelial surface with a Grieshaber or crescent blade, leaving Bowman's layer exposed.
2. Measure the horizontal and vertical corneal dimensions and add 2 to 3 mm in order to appropriately size the amniotic membrane tissue.
3. Place the amniotic membrane graft over the cornea with the stromal side down.
4. Secure the amniotic membrane to the limbus using 8 to 12 interrupted sutures or a continuous running suture, taking care to avoid gaps between the host conjunctiva and tissue graft. Amniotic membrane should cover the entire cornea. Some surgeons prefer to perform a 360° conjunctival peritomy with suturing of the grafted tissue to the elevated conjunctival tissue to allow better apposition between host and donor tissue; however, this is associated with more bleeding and the need for hemostasis.
5. Excess tissue can be trimmed as the sutures are passed rather than sizing the tissue prior to suture placement, depending on the surgeon's preference.

POSTOPERATIVE CARE

1. Administer subconjunctival corticosteroid injection with subconjunctival antibiotic injection or topical antibiotic. An antibiotic-corticosteroid ointment may also be applied followed by a pressure patch or eye shield.
2. Schedule a follow-up visit in 24 hours.
3. A topical antibiotic drop and a topical corticosteroid drop, along with an antibiotic-corticosteroid ointment, are often used for 4 to 6 weeks postoperatively to prevent infection and limit inflammation.

COMPLICATIONS

- Recurrence of pathology
- Pain

- Infectious keratitis or scleritis
- Conjunctival and scleral inflammation, including
    - Inflammatory scleritis
    - Episcleral injection
    - Subconjunctival hemorrhage
    - Graft dehiscence
    - Suture granuloma
    - Symblepharon formation

Chapter 10

Limbal Stem Cell Transplantation

Leejee H. Suh, MD
Roy S. Chuck, MD, PhD

The corneal limbus contains epithelial stem cells that allow for surface wound healing. Various conditions can produce limbal stem cell deficiency, including chemical and thermal burns, drug reactions (eg, Stevens-Johnson syndrome), genetic diseases (eg, aniridia), autoimmune diseases (eg, ocular pemphigoid), contact lens-induced keratopathy, cancers (eg, corneal intraepithelial neoplasia). Iatrogenic etiologies can produce limbal stem cell deficiency. A loss of limbal epithelial stem cells results in an abnormal corneal surface ("conjunctivaliza-tion") as evidenced by a fibrovascular pannus covering all or part of the entire optical axis. Conventional surgical management (eg, penetrating keratoplasty and lamellar keratoplasty) is largely unsuccessful. Limbal stem cell transplanta-tion, in the form of keratolimbal allografting (KLAL) from eye bank tissue or conjunctival limbal allografting (CLAL), usually from living related donors, or conjunctival limbal autografting (CLAU) can increase the success rate of treatment. For unilateral disease, CLAU from the contralateral eye may be the best option.

PREOPERATIVE STEPS

1. Begin systemic immunosuppression (eg, cyclosporine) 1 month pre-operatively, for allograft procedures.
2. Order donor cornea with intact limbal region, inclusive of conjunctival skirt, within 5 to 7 days (the fresher the better) of donor expiration, for

KLAL. For CLAU, obtain consent from the patient for limbal conjunctival harvest of 4 to 6 clock hours of tissue in the contralateral eye. For CLAL, obtain similar consent from the donor.

3. Obtain consent from the patient for ocular surface transplantation, as well as possible lateral tarsorrhaphy or amniotic membrane transplantation if the surgeon believes that there may be increased risk of surface inflammation and surface exposure damage. Also obtain consent for penetrating keratoplasty in case corneal perforation occurs intraoperatively.
4. Begin prednisone 1 mg/kg/day beginning 2 days preoperatively.
5. Give methylprednisolone succinate 125 mg intravenously at the start of surgery.

INSTRUMENTATION AND SUPPLIES

- Wire lid speculum
- Cautery unit
- 0.12 forceps
- Teflon block, trephine, and central cornea harvest apparatus of choice
- Crescent blade
- Calipers
- Westcott and Vannas scissors
- 10-0 nylon suture
- 8-0 polyglactin suture
- Needle driver
- Viscoelastic (sodium hyaluronate)

SURGICAL PROCEDURE

1. Anesthesia: monitored anesthesia care with intravenous sedation, topical proparacaine and 2% Xylocaine jelly, retrobulbar and modified Van Lint blocks with 1:1 mixture of 2% lidocaine and 0.75% bupivacaine, or general endotracheal anesthesia.
2. Prep and drape the patient in a sterile manner.
3. Place the lid speculum and examine the eye (Figure 10.1A).

Keratolimbal Allografting (KLAL)

1. Create a 360° conjunctival peritomy with 0.12 forceps and Wescott scissors.
2. Debride the conjunctivalized cornea and limbus using a crescent blade and Vannas scissors to remove superficial fibrovascular corneal scarring and perform manual superficial lamellar keratectomy. Lightly cauterize as necessary (Figure 10.1B).
3. Measure the diameter of healthy cornea with calipers (Figure 10.1C).
4. Place viscoelastic material and corneal protector on the recipient cornea.
5. Inspect donor cornea from the eye bank, stored in media.
6. Place the donor endothelial side up on a Teflon block mounted in the donor corneal harvesting apparatus.
7. Carefully trim the donor cornea to allow for a 2- to 3-mm circular rim of sclera and conjunctiva (Figure 10.1D).
8. Select a trephine size significantly smaller in diameter than the recipient central cornea (eg, 7.0 to 8.5 mm).
9. Use the disposable trephine blade, attached to a punch handle, to remove a central corneal button from the donor cornea.
10. Bring a doughnut-shaped donor corneoscleral graft into the surgical field.
11. With a crescent blade and Vannas scissors, perform anterior lamellar dissection to approximately one-third depth into anterior sclera and corneal stroma, taking care to remain in plane as much as possible. Make sure that the epithelium is well lubricated throughout this cumbersome manual dissection (Figure 10.1E). An assistant may be helpful to apply counter-traction during this dissection.
12. Suture the doughnut-shaped anterior corneoscleral graft onto the recipient bed with interrupted 10-0 nylon sutures. Usually 6 to 8 outer-diameter sutures are required, with secure episcleral bites. Occasionally inner diameter sutures may be required if the inner rim of the lamellar graft will not lie flat on the corneal surface (Figure 10.1F).
13. Rotate 10-0 nylon suture knots away from the cornea, and bury the knots.
14. Reapproximate conjunctiva with 8-0 polyglactin suture around the KLAL.
15. Inject subconjunctival corticosteroid and antibiotic.
16. Perform amniotic membrane graft (Chapter 9) or lateral tarsorrhaphy if deemed necessary.
17. Apply an antibiotic-corticosteroid ointment and place a cotton patch with Fox shield over the eye.

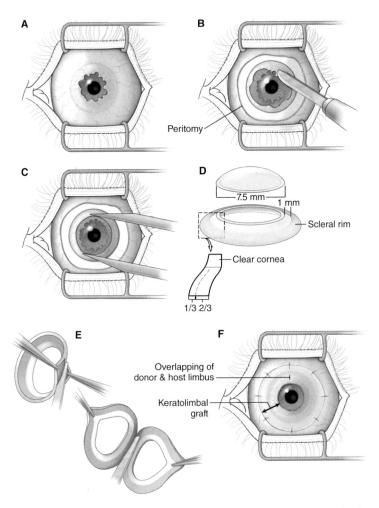

Figure 10.1. Keratolimbal allografting (KLAL). (A) Conjunctivalization of the corneal surface due to limbal stem cell deficiency. (B) Debridement of the conjunctivalized surface and superficial lamellar keratectomy. (C) Measurement of healthy cornea with calipers. (D) Preparation of the donor corneoscleral graft. (E) Anterior lamellar dissection of the corneoscleral graft. (F) Suturing of the doughnut-shaped anterior corneoscleral graft onto recipient bed.

Conjunctival Limbal Allografting (CLAL) or Autografting (CLAU)

1. Create a 360° conjunctival peritomy approximately 2 mm posterior to limbus and allow conjunctiva to recess (Figures 10.2A, 10.2B).
2. Create recipient beds of 2 to 3 clock hours at the 12 and 6 o'clock positions.
3. Remove the superficial fibrovascular corneal scarring with peeling, blunt, and sharp dissection (Figures 10.2C, 10.2D).
4. On the donor (or contralateral) eye, use a marking pen to mark 2 sectoral grafts of limbal tissue of approximately same dimensions as the

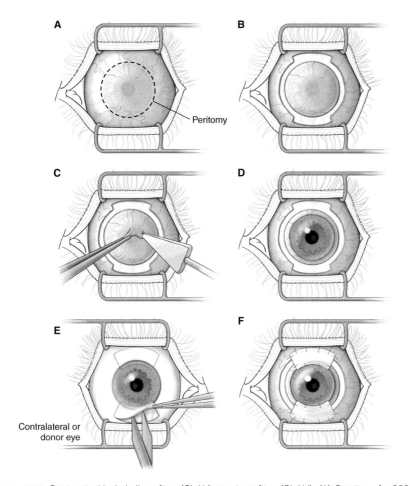

Figure 10.2. Conjunctival limbal allografting (CLAL) or autografting (CLAU). (A) Creation of a 360°
peritomy on the recipient eye. (B) Creation of recipient beds of 2 to 3 clock hours centered at 12 and
6 o'clock. (C) Removal of superficial corneal scarring. (D) Appearance of the recipient eye after removal
of scar tissue and peritomy. (E) Harvesting of 2 sectoral conjunctival limbal grafts from the donor (or
contralateral) eye. (F) Suturing of sectoral conjunctival limbal grafts to the recipient eye.

recipient beds. Each graft should be about 2 to 3 clock hours centered
at the 12 and 6 o'clock positions and should extend about 0.5 mm into
clear cornea centrally and 2 mm into bulbar conjunctiva peripherally
(Figure 10.2E).

5. Begin dissection from the conjunctival side with forceps and Westcott
scissors, and work anteriorly toward the corneal edge. Use the crescent
blade to make lamellar dissections into clear corneal edge.

6. Donor sites can remain open or they can be closed with 8-0 polyglactin suture.

7. Transfer autografts to corresponding recipient beds and secure with
10-0 nylon sutures (Figure 10.2F). Reapproximate conjunctiva with
8-0 polyglactin suture around the cornea as needed.

8. Inject subconjunctival corticosteroid and antibiotic.
9. Perform amniotic membrane graft or lateral tarsorrhaphy if necessary.
10. Apply an antibiotic-corticosteroid ointment and place a cotton patch with Fox shield over the eye.
11. Examine the patient the next operative day and then weekly until the epithelium covers the corneal surface. Often, a bandage soft contact lens is helpful if amniotic membrane grafting or lateral tarsorrhaphy is not performed.

POSTOPERATIVE CARE

1. Start on a topical corticosteroid and antibiotic 4 times daily.
2. After the epithelium heals, examine at monthly intervals. Taper the medications. If secondary penetrating keratoplasty becomes necessary, wait 3 to 6 months postoperatively.
3. CLAL patients may require immunosuppression similar to KLAL patients and tapering according to clinical response. Often lifelong systemic immunosuppression is necessary.
4. Continue systemic immunosuppression (eg, cyclosporine).
5. Examine the patient the next operative day and then weekly until the epithelium covers the corneal surface. Often a bandage soft contact lens is helpful when amniotic membrane grafting or lateral tarsorrhaphy is not done. After the epithelium heals, examine at monthly intervals. If secondary penetrating keratoplasty becomes necessary, wait 3 to 6 months postoperatively.

COMPLICATIONS

- Allo- or autograft rejection or failure
- Corneal edema and scarring
- Corneal perforation
- Uneven lamellar dissection of allograft
- Intraoperative bleeding
- Glaucoma
- Infection
- Donor eye complications, such as conjunctival scarring after removal of tissue

Chapter 11

Capsular Tension Rings

Justis P. Ehlers, MD
Robert S. Bailey Jr, MD

Loss of zonular integrity may result in lens decentration, capsular contraction, IOL dislocation, or phaco- or pseudophacodonesis. Capsular tension rings (CTRs) are designed to assist in capsular stability in cases of zonular loss or weakness in cataract surgery, thereby providing safer lens disassembly during phacoemulsification. They also assist in maintenance of IOL centration and position postoperatively. A CTR is an open polymethylmethacrylate ring with leading and trailing eyelets. Its diameter is larger than the capsular bag, providing a uniform distribution of forces throughout the equator of the capsular bag.

Causes of zonular instability include trauma (eg, penetrating or blunt injury), previous surgical intervention (eg, pars plana vitrectomy or trabeculectomy), and disease states resulting in diffuse and progressive zonular instability (eg, pseudoexfoliation syndrome, Marfan syndrome, homocystinuria, myotonic dystrophy, or uveitis). In cases of trauma or previous surgical intervention, the remaining zonules are often of normal strength and integrity, in contrast to the generally diffuse nature of the other diseases mentioned.

Indications for surgery include ≤4 clock hours of zonular loss, or pseudoexfoliation syndrome with mild zonular weakness. CTRs are particularly useful in cases of trauma.

Contraindications for surgery include noncontinuous capsulorrhexis; posterior capsular tear; or zonular loss >4 clock hours. In cases of moderate-to-severe generalized zonulopathy (eg, pseudoexfoliation syndrome with severe zonular instability), modified CTRs may be useful. CTRs help to stabilize the capsular bag in cases of mild zonulopathy. Placement of a CTR does not prevent late IOL/capsular bag dislocation from progressive zonular instability (eg, pseudoexfoliation syndrome). CTRs do not prevent postoperative capsular phimosis or contraction.

PREOPERATIVE STEPS

1. Perform a careful and thorough evaluation of zonular weakness.
   - Extent of loss
   - Location of defect
   - Type of zonulopathy (eg, trauma, pseudoexfoliation syndrome)
   - Coexisting injuries possibly complicating surgical approach (eg, vitreous prolapse or corneal scarring)
   - Signs of zonular weakness: phacodonesis, iridodonesis, anterior chamber depth (<2.5 mm in pseudoexfoliation associated with increased risk of zonular instability), lens equator visible in eccentric gaze, or crystalline lens subluxation
2. Consider the choice of CTR.
   - Multiple brands and size are available. Examples include Morcher (10/12.3 mm, 11/13 mm, FCI Ophthalmics, Pembroke, Massachusetts), Alcon Reform (10/12 mm, 11/13 mm, 12/14.5 mm, Alcon Laboratories, Fort Worth, Texas), and AMO StabilEyes (10/12 mm, 11/13 mm, Advanced Medical Optics, Santa Ana, California). Sizes represent compressed/uncompressed ring diameters. Typically, the larger size is preferred.
   - Modified CTRs may be useful in some conditions.
     - Cionni (Morcher GmbH, Germany): designed with 1 or 2 additional eyelets along the ring circumference that can be used for scleral fixation with 9-0 or 10-0 polypropylene suture. It is used in cases of zonular loss >4 clock hours or moderate to severe generalized zonular weakness.
     - Ahmed: comes in segments rather than a ring. It does not require an intact capsulorrhexis, and it is not approved by the FDA.
     - Henderson (Morcher): has 8 equally spaced indentations of 0.15 mm to improve the ease of removing nuclear and cortical material while maintaining equal expansion of the capsular bag.

INSTRUMENTATION AND SUPPLIES

- Capsular tension ring
- Geuder inserter or 2 tying forceps for manual insertion
- Ophthalmic viscoelastic device of choice

SURGICAL PROCEDURE

1. Prep and drape in the usual fashion.
2. Load the inserter. With the ring facing the injector, depress the plunger until the hook is exposed (Figure 11.1). Capture the left eyelet with the hook. Slowly release the plunger to withdraw the CTR into the injector (Figure 11.2).
3. Proceed with cataract surgery. An intact capsulorrhexis is essential. Phacoemulsification is often done most safely by first prolapsing the nucleus out of the capsular bag, so as to minimize additional stress on the zonules.
4. Consider the timing of the CTR insertion.
   - Early insertion (eg, immediately after zonular instability is noted) stabilizes the crystalline lens prior to phacoemulsification and may help prevent vitreous prolapse. Disadvantages of early insertion are that it may move posterior capsule forward, placing it at greater risk during surgery; the ring may make cortex removal more difficult by trapping it against the capsular bag.
   - Late insertion (eg, after removal of most of the cataract) does not interfere with cortical removal but may increase the risk of vitreous prolapse.
5. Place the CTR.
   - Expand the capsular bag with viscoelastic.
   - Place the injector through the main incision.

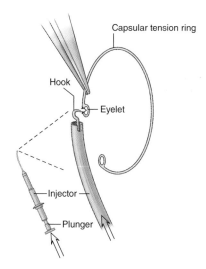

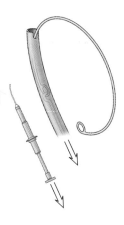

Figure 11.1. Capture of the eyelet of the CTR with the hook.

Figure 11.2. Withdrawal of the CTR into the plunger.

Figure 11.3. Injection of the CTR into the capsular bag.

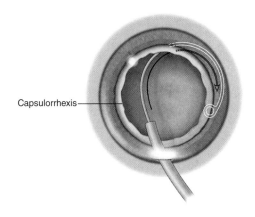

Capsulorrhexis

- Angle the opening of the plunger toward the capsular bag and the greatest area of zonular weakness (Figure 11.3). Note: injecting away from the area of weakness may result in greater zonular damage.

6. Slowly depress the plunger to carefully expose the first eyelet of the CTR.

7. Continue to depress the plunger while being sure to direct the leading eyelet under the capsulorrhexis and into the capsular bag, advancing the CTR clockwise. If resistance is encountered during insertion, slowly pull the injector away in a counter-clockwise circular motion while completing the injection.

8. Release the trailing eyelet from the hook by gently nudging the eyelet against the underside of the anterior capsule.

POSTOPERATIVE CARE

1. Provide postoperative care as for other cataract surgery procedures (eg, Chapter 1).

2. Watch for late subluxation of the IOL.

COMPLICATIONS

- Other complications of IOL surgery not prevented by CTR insertion
- Uveitis-glaucoma-hyphema syndrome from incorrect placement
- Retained lens cortex

Chapter 12

Intraoperative Pupillary Dilation

James P. Dunn, MD

Adequate pupillary dilation is essential for safe phacoemulsification and vitreo-retinal procedures. In cataract surgery, poor dilation increases the risk of an insufficiently large capsulorrhexis, the difficulty of mobilizing nuclear fragments, and the risk of capsular rupture. Inadequate visualization of peripheral retinal structures and the pars plana complicates vitreoretinal surgery. There are many causes of poor pupillary dilation, including systemic and ophthalmic medications (tamsulosin and similar alpha blockers used to treat prostatic hypertrophy, pilocarpine), mechanical scarring (posterior synechiae from uveitis), certain ocular conditions (pseudoexfoliation), and improper instillation of preoperative dilating drops. This latter cause may be overcome with additional use of cycloplegic and adrenergic drops before surgery and injection of intracameral epinephrine.

Several of the more common methods of pupillary dilation are described here. Pupils requiring only a small amount of additional dilation may require only gentle stretching with instruments. More-definitive dilation is obtained with removable iris hooks; this technique also has the advantage of stabilizing the iris (as in intraoperative floppy iris syndrome) but takes longer to perform. In either case, posterior synechiae must be broken and pupillary membranes incised or removed before pupillary dilation can be safely performed. If dilation is attempted while a ring of a pupillary membrane is present, there is a high probability of a radial iris tear. Therefore, before use of any of the techniques described here, the surgeon must remove the membrane or incise it with angled Vannas scissors in multiple meridians. Limit the incisions to the membrane itself (membranotomy) and avoid incising the iris (multiple sphincterotomies), which can cause bleeding and breakdown of the blood–iris barrier, thereby increasing the risk of uveitis and postoperative scarring.

PREOPERATIVE STEPS

1. Obtain informed consent from the patient for the main procedure as well as for mechanical pupil dilation.
2. If topical and intracameral anesthesia is planned for the main procedure (eg, cataract surgery), consider sub-Tenon's anesthesia to minimize patient discomfort.
3. Inform the nursing staff that pupillary dilation will be necessary so that the necessary instruments or hooks are immediately available.
4. Preoperative topical nonsteroidal anti-inflammatory drugs may help reduce intraoperative miosis and can be a helpful adjunct.

INSTRUMENTATION AND SUPPLIES

- Lid speculum
- 15° blade
- Disposable or reusable iris hooks (several brands)
- Lester and Kuglen hooks or similar instruments (2-handed dilation)
- Keuch (Katena Products, Denville, New Jersey) or Beehler (Rumex International, St Petersburg, Florida) dilator (1-handed dilation)
- Pupillary rings, not discussed in this chapter (eg, Perfect Pupil [Milvella, Savage, Minnesota], Graether 2000 [Eagle Vision, Memphis, Tennessee], Morcher pupil dilator [FCI Ophthalmics, Pembroke, Massachusetts]
- High molecular weight cohesive ophthalmic viscosurgical device (OVD)
- 0.12 forceps
- Tying (nontoothed) forceps (2)
- Marking pen (optional)
- Preservative-free epinephrine 1:1000
- Long-angled McPherson forceps (optional)

SURGICAL PROCEDURES

1. Prep and drape in a sterile manner.
2. Insert a lid speculum.

Removable Hooks

1. Mark the insertion sites with the marking pen. Four or five hooks are usually placed equidistant around the limbus.
   - In phacoemulsification procedures, it is generally best to perform the clear corneal phaco wound first to be sure that the side port incisions are not too close to the phacoemulsification wound, which can cause difficulty inserting the phaco probe into the anterior chamber.
   - If 2-handed phacoemulsification is planned, make an additional side port incision as usual through which the second instrument will be placed.
2. Enter the cornea posterior to the limbus so that the iris hooks will be in the plane of the iris; if the entry site is too anterior, the hooks will "tent up" the iris, reducing the surgeon's visibility and increasing the risk of postoperative cosmetic deformity. An internal corneal opening of 1 mm is adequate and will be consistently self-sealing. Fixating the eye with the 0.12 forceps placed just posterior to the limbus exactly 180° away from the planned side port incision will prevent rotation of the globe and allow controlled entry with the 15° blade.
3. Inject 0.5 mL of preservative-free epinephrine to reduce the chance of iris bleeding.
4. Fill the anterior chamber with the OVD, including a small amount posterior to the iris to reduce the risk of anterior capsular trauma. Overfilling the chamber may cause iris prolapse.
5. Lyse any posterior synechiae by inserting the tip of the viscoelastic cannula under the iris and peripheral to the synechiae (Figure 12.1A), then gently sweep centrally (Figure 12.1B).
6. In cataract procedures, one of the hooks can be placed posterior to the clear cornea phacoemulsification wound. This technique reduces the chances of subincisional iris trauma.
7. Insert 1 hook through a side port incision so that the hook is clearly visible in the anterior chamber.

A   B

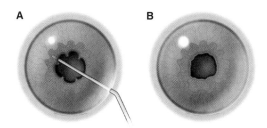

Figure 12.1. Lysis of posterior synechiae. (A) Use of a viscoelastic cannula to lyse individual synechiae. (B) The pupil usually remains small even after successful lysis of extensive posterior synechiae.

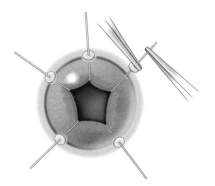

Figure 12.2. Appearance of the pupil after the initial placement of the iris hooks. Additional dilation is obtained by further pulling of each hook peripherally.

8. Stabilize the shaft near the incision with a nontoothed forceps and use a second nontoothed forceps to slide the silicone flange back so that the hook end can be inserted as far centrally as needed.

9. Advance the hook centrally, then rotate the hook down so that it can engage the pupil margin. Retract the hook slightly; use a second forceps to slide the flange centrally so that it just abuts the limbus and "locks" the hook in position.

10. Repeat Steps 7 to 9 with the other hooks. Be sure not to retract any of the hooks too far peripherally at this point, or it will decenter the pupil and make it hard to engage the pupillary border with the other hooks (Figure 12.2).

11. When all the hooks are in place, gently retract each one in sequence by grasping the end with forceps and sliding the silicone flange centrally with the other. The goal is to obtain gentle, thorough, and evenly distributed dilation with each hook.

12. Fill the anterior chamber with viscoelastic and proceed with the surgery. In phacoemulsification, it is usually possible to remove the 2 hooks immediately adjacent to the phacoemulsification wound before inserting the IOL to avoid having the leading haptic or optic edge caught on the subincisional iris.

13. Remove the remaining hooks prior to viscoelastic removal. Grasp the shaft of the hook with nontoothed forceps between the cornea and the flange, and use a second nontoothed forceps to pull the flange back.

14. Advance the hook slightly centrally to the papillary margin, rotate it 90°, then pull it out, making sure not to catch the hook on the internal lip of the side port incision.

One-Handed Dilation

1. Make the phacoemulsification incision as usual. If a pupillary membrane is present, use the Vannas scissors inserted through the

phacoemulsification wound to make a series of incisions into the membrane; in some cases, the membrane can be peeled away from the pupil with long-angled McPherson forceps.

2. Inject 0.5 mL of preservative-free epinephrine to reduce the chance of iris bleeding.

3. Fill the anterior chamber with viscoelastic, including a small amount posterior to the iris to reduce the risk of anterior capsular trauma.

4. Avoid overfilling the chamber, which can cause iris prolapse.

5. Lyse any posterior synechiae by inserting the tip of the viscoelastic cannula under the iris and peripheral to the synechiae. Then gently sweep centrally.

6. Several 1-handed pupil dilators are on the market, including the Keuch and Beehler instruments (Figure 12.3A). The former is smaller and can be inserted through a standard side port incision; however, it stretches the pupil in only 1 meridian and therefore has to be used through both the phacoemulsification incision and a side paracentesis incision. The Beehler dilator is too large to fit through a side port incision; however, it will dilate the pupil in multiple meridians when inserted through the phacoemulsification incision because its 3 hooks extend out from the main shaft. It is somewhat more difficult to use.

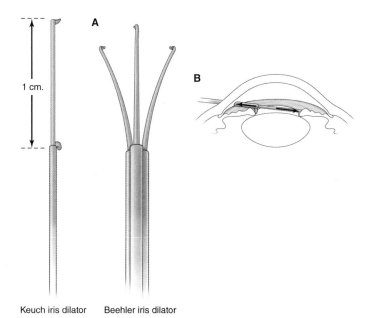

Keuch iris dilator   Beehler iris dilator

Figure 12.3. One-handed pupillary dilators. (A) Keuch (left) and Beehler (right) dilators. (B) Side view of proper orientation of 1-handed dilators within the eye.

- If the Keuch dilator is to be used, create 2 side port incisions with the 15° blade, each 90° from the phacoemulsification wound.
- If the Beehler dilator is to be used, create a side port incision as usual for 2-handed phacoemulsification.
- The side port incisions must be at least 1 mm wide internally.

7. Both instruments have a retractable hook or series of hooks that extend along the shaft for approximately 1 cm. A hook on the under-surface of the shaft engages the subincisional iris, and the retractable end is extended outward until the concave hook at the end engages the iris on the opposite side (Figure 12.3B). The hook (Keuch) or hooks (Beehler) is/are advanced by means of the thumb-controlled knob on the shaft.

8. Apply gentle but sustained pressure for 15 to 20 seconds to dilate the pupil. Avoid overstretching the pupil, which can cause radial iris tears (Figure 12.4) and bleeding.

9. After removing the instruments, refill the anterior chamber with viscoelastic to confirm adequate dilation and proceed with surgery as usual.

10. Depending on whether the surgeon is left- or right-handed, either side port incision can be used for the second instrument during phacoemulsification.

Two-Handed Dilation

1. Repeat Steps 1 to 4 as for 1-handed dilation.
2. Create 2 side port incisions with the 15° blade, each 90° from the phacoemulsification wound. The internal wound must be at least 1 mm wide to allow easy entry of the instruments.
3. Insert a Lester or Kuglen hook through each side port incision and engage the iris. Turning the hook at a 45° angle provides good visualization of the entire hook so the surgeon can be sure the anterior lens capsule is not touched.

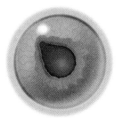

Figure 12.4. Permanently peaked pupil due to overaggressive stretching of iris in 1 meridian.

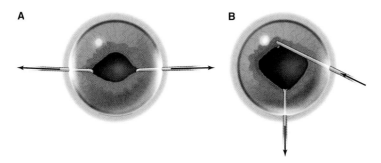

Figure 12.5. Two-handed dilation. Gentle stretching in the meridian of the side port incisions (A) and the phaco wound (B).

4. Apply gentle, sustained stretching for 15 to 20 seconds in the meridian of the side port incisions (Figure 12.5A).
5. Remove a hook and re-insert it through the phacoemulsification wound so that it engages the pupil margin subincisionally. Reposition the second hook already in the eye so that it engages the pupil margin 180° from the phaco wound. Apply gentle, sustained stretching for 15 to 20 seconds in the meridian of the phaco wound (Figure 12.5B).
6. Remove each hook carefully, taking care not to traumatize the side port incision architecture.
7. After removing the instruments, refill the anterior chamber with viscoelastic to confirm adequate dilation and proceed with surgery as usual.
8. Depending on whether the surgeon is left- or right-handed, either side port incision can be used for the second instrument during phacoemulsification.

COMPLICATIONS

- Inadvertent tear of the anterior capsule
- Infection
- Iris trauma or bleeding
- Subconjunctival hemorrhage
- Lens trauma in phakic vitreoretinal patients
- Cosmetic deformity from overaggressive mechanical stretching
- Glare from persistently dilated pupil

Chapter 13

Extracapsular Cataract Extraction

Emily Graubart, MD
Geoffrey Broocker, MD

Extracapsular cataract extraction (ECCE) is defined as the removal of the central anterior lens capsule and extraction of the lens nucleus and cortex, while the peripheral anterior lens capsule, posterior capsule, and zonular attachments remain intact. Planned ECCE typically refers to the removal of the intact lens nucleus through a large incision (greater than 6 to 8 mm). A strict definition of the procedure would also include phacoemulsification as a form of ECCE.

Although the vast majority of cataract surgeries performed in the United States use phacoemulsification to remove the crystalline lens, understanding the principles of planned ECCE is important so that cataract surgery can be completed when phaco equipment fails. Other indications for ECCE include significant endothelial failure precluding the visualization required for phacoemulsification, lens density precluding phacoemulsification, and intraoperative complications requiring conversion from phacoemulsification. There are many different ways in which to perform ECCE, including self-sealing-incision ECCE. This chapter describes the classic ECCE procedure with a 10.5-mm incision.

PREOPERATIVE STEPS

1. Ensure the appropriate IOL is available (consider both capsular and sulcus fixation).
2. Evaluate the operative eye carefully for irido/phacodonesis indicating poor zonular support that can complicate planned ECCE.

3. In addition to topical mydriatic agents, some surgeons use topical nonsteroidal anti-inflammatory drugs to help maintain intraoperative mydriasis.

INSTRUMENTATION AND SUPPLIES

- Lid speculum
- 0.12 forceps
- 0.3 forceps
- No. 66 or No. 69 Beaver blade (crescent, straight, and angled)
- No. 75 Beaver blade or equivalent (stab or paracentesis blade)
- High molecular weight viscoelastic
- Cystotome or 25-gauge needle with a bend at the tip
- Angled forceps (eg, Kelman-McPherson)
- Calipers
- Corneoscleral scissors
- Sinskey hook
- Irrigating lens loop
- Manual aspirating device (eg, Simcoe cannula) or automated irrigation/ aspiration (I/A) tip
- Blunt Westcott scissors
- Vannas scissors
- 10-0 nylon suture
- 8-0 polyglactin suture (if necessary, to close conjunctiva)
- 4-0 silk suture with tapered needle (if superior rectus bridle suture is needed)
- Needle driver
- Hemostat
- Eraser-tip cautery unit
- Smooth tying forceps
- Corneal light shield

SURGICAL PROCEDURE

1. Anesthesia: monitored anesthesia care with intravenous sedation and retrobulbar or sub-Tenon's block. A modified Van Lint lid block may also be useful. A sub-Tenon's block with a blunt, curved (eg, Greenbaum) cannula is helpful in patients with bleeding concerns.

2. Reduce vitreous volume with a Honan balloon (set to 30 mm Hg), manual compression, or a mercury bag for a minimum of 10 minutes (use caution in patients with zonular instability). Pressure and vitreous volume may also be reduced with intravenous mannitol 25 to 50 mg/kg, 15 to 20 minutes preoperatively.

3. Prep and drape.

4. Place the lid speculum.

5. Place bridle suture if there is not adequate exposure of the superior limbus and sclera. Rotate the globe inferiorly with a muscle hook in the inferior cul-de-sac, or grasp the superior limbus with 0.12 forceps. Then, with the opposite hand, grasp the superior rectus (SR) with 0.3 toothed forceps approximately 10 mm posterior to the limbus and lift the tendon off the globe. Pass a 4-0 silk suture with a tapered needle under the SR tendon (Figure 13.1). The needle should be parallel to the globe to avoid penetration. Cut off the needle and clamp the suture to the drape with a hemostat to rotate the globe down. This suture should be released when the wound is opened to prevent viscoelastic prolapse and anterior chamber collapse.

6. Create a conjunctival peritomy using blunt Wescott scissors to make a radial incision at the 10 o'clock position (for a right-handed surgeon), 2 mm posterior to the limbus (Figure 13.2). Assure exposure of bare sclera for the extent of the wound. The conjunctival peritomy should measure approximately 12 mm.

7. Use cautery as needed to obtain hemostasis. Use a sweeping motion over the sclera and start posteriorly, approximately 2 to 3 mm from the limbus to prevent scleral shrinkage.

8. Measure the length of the desired wound by marking the sclera with the caliper tips set at 10.5 mm.

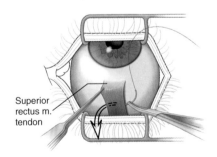
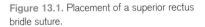

Figure 13.1. Placement of a superior rectus bridle suture.

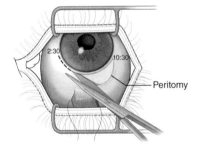

Figure 13.2. Making the conjunctival peritomy.

9. Create the incision by using 0.12 forceps to grasp sclera at approximately the 2 o'clock position to stabilize the globe (for a right-handed surgeon). Hold the No. 66 blade handle perpendicular to the globe and make the incision from left to right, approximately 1 mm posterior to the blue line (Figure 13.3). Consider making the groove more anterior when the sclera is thin to prevent early entry and iris prolapse. The depth of the groove should be approximately one-half to one-third scleral depth. The length of the groove should be 10.5 mm, beginning at the 10:30 clock-hour position and ending at approximately the 2:30 clock-hour position. Attempt to make the groove in a continuous motion by rotating the blade.

10. Tunnel into clear cornea using either a No. 66 or No. 69 (crescent) blade (Figure 13.4). Use a sweeping, circular motion with the blade to

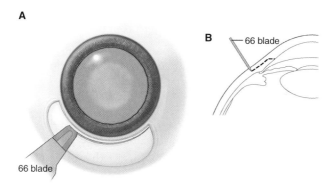

Figure 13.3. Creation of the vertical scleral tunnel incision. (A) External view. (B) Side view.

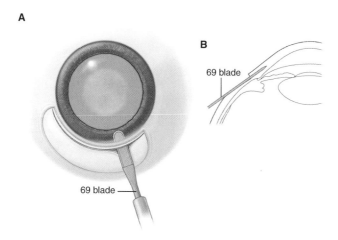

Figure 13.4. Extension of the scleral tunnel incision into clear cornea. (A) External view. (B) Side view.

enlarge the tunnel for the entire length of the groove. Do not lift the blade to avoid "dog-earring" the flap. The anterior extent of the flap should be at least 1 to 1.5 mm to avoid entering too posteriorly (over the iris root) and risking iris prolapse.

11. Enter the anterior chamber by elevating the anterior lip of the wound with the 0.12 forceps, exposing the apex of the flap, and enter the anterior chamber with the No. 75 blade parallel to the iris plane (Figure 13.5). Make a 3-mm incision either to the right side of the wound (right-handed surgeon) or to the left (left-handed surgeon). Take care not to lift the flap with the forceps sufficiently to cause anterior chamber collapse.

12. Inject viscoelastic into the anterior chamber (fill from inferior anterior chamber toward the wound).

13. Create a can-opener capsulotomy by holding the cystotome in a way to provide stabilization and penetrate the anterior capsule at the 6 o'clock position and sweep gently to the right side. Continue making multiple small punctures circumferentially to complete a 6- to 7-mm capsulotomy (Figure 13.6).
    • With each puncture, the surgeon will sweep to the right while going up the left side and to the left while going up the right side.
    • With each puncture, the surgeon will sweep the cystotome toward the previous puncture in order to connect the tears.

14. Remove the anterior capsule using angled forceps to grasp the central anterior capsule (Figure 13.7). Ensure that the anterior capsule is free from the peripheral capsule by pulling the capsule gently in all

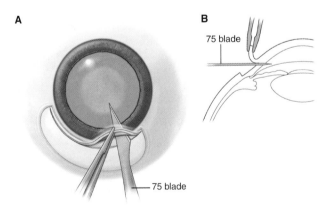

Figure 13.5. Entry into the anterior chamber. (A) External view. (B) Side view.

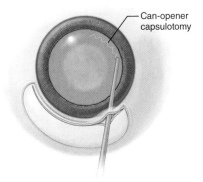

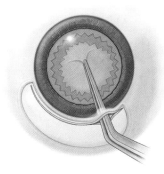

Figure 13.6. Initiation of the can-opener capsulorrhexis.

Figure 13.7. Removal of the anterior capsular remnant.

directions, and then slowly remove the anterior capsule from the eye. Persistent attachments may require cutting with Vannas scissors.

15. Separate corticocapsular adhesions by gently tilting or "rocking" the nucleus in different directions using a Sinskey hook (Figure 13.8) or the cystotome attached to the viscoelastic cannula.

16. Enlarge the wound with corneoscleral scissors, enter the anterior chamber with the lower jaw of the scissors, and cut toward the opposite side of the wound. Push gently toward the 6 o'clock position as you cut to ensure that you enlarge the wound at the most anterior aspect of the tunnel. Maintain scissor blades in the groove and keep blades parallel to the iris plane (Figure 13.9).

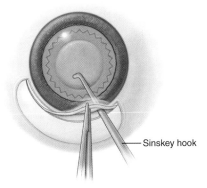

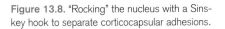

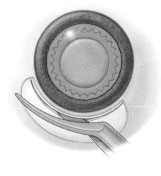

Figure 13.8. "Rocking" the nucleus with a Sinskey hook to separate corticocapsular adhesions.

Figure 13.9. Enlargement of the corneoscleral wound with scissors.

17. Remove nucleus with either manual expression or lifting the nucleus out of the bag by rotation/hydrodissection.
    - Manual expression is achieved by applying external, posterior pressure with forceps or the irrigating lens loop 2 mm posterior to the limbus at the 12 o'clock position and using an assistant to elevate the anterior lip of the wound. When the nucleus begins to prolapse, counter-pressure is applied with a muscle hook at the 6 o'clock position to facilitate removal of the lens (Figure 13.10). Once the nucleus is partially out of the eye, any pointed instrument may be used to rotate the remainder of the lens out of the eye.
    - Hydrodissection or manual rotation should be performed to elevate the lens at the 12 o'clock position into the anterior chamber. To manually rotate the nucleus, use a Sinskey hook, cannula, or cystotome to gently rock the lens in a dialing/circumferential manner, and then lift and rotate. Once the superior portion of the lens is elevated, an irrigating lens loop may be inserted under the lens. Care is taken to gently glide the lens loop over the iris in a sweeping fashion to engage the lens. The irrigating lens loop is then flattened parallel to the iris plane, lifted toward the cornea, and removed from the eye with the nucleus.
18. Place 2 or 3 10-0 nylon sutures at the 10, 12, and 2 o'clock positions to help maintain the anterior chamber during cortical clean-up (Figure 13.11). If the iris is light-colored or there is a tendency for iris prolapse, additional sutures may be placed. It may be possible to avoid this step and perform "open sky" irrigation/aspiration if the eye is soft and the chamber stays deep with the wound open.
19. Remove cortex with a manual aspirating device (eg, Simcoe) or an automated I/A system. Take care not to accidentally grasp the anterior capsular leaflets. Strip the cortex toward the center of the pupil and

Figure 13.10. Manual expression of the lens.

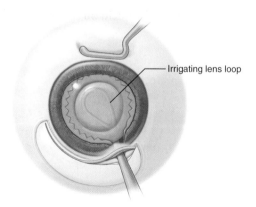

Irrigating lens loop

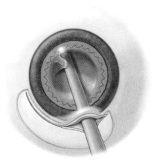

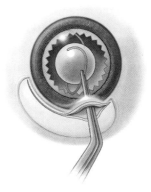

Figure 13.11. Aspiration of lens cortex.

Figure 13.12. Insertion of the IOL into the capsular bag.

aspirate more aggressively (above the iris plane) only when the port is fully occluded with cortex.

20. Reform the capsular bag with viscoelastic prior to implanting the IOL.

21. Remove 1 or 2 previously placed sutures in order to insert the lens.

22. Insert the lens by grasping the lens approximately one-half to one-third onto the optic of the IOL (polymethylmethacrylate or unfolded acrylic or silicone) with long-angled forceps. Hold the anterior lip of the wound and ease the IOL into the bag by tilting the lens down and pushing the leading haptic into the 6 o'clock position. When the majority of the IOL is in the capsular bag, the anterior wound is released and the trailing haptic is grasped to prevent extrusion of the IOL when the haptic is released (Figure 13.12). Tap the IOL further into the bag with closed angled forceps until the optic is completely behind the pupil. Place directly or rotate the trailing haptic into the capsular bag with the Sinskey hook. Assure centration.

23. Place a light shield on the cornea. Close the wound with interrupted 10-0 nylon sutures. With proper wound construction, 4 or 5 sutures should be adequate. Rotate sutures to bury knots.

24. Remove viscoelastic by leaving a suture untied to allow entry with the automated or manual I/A instrument to completely remove the viscoelastic. Tapping posteriorly on the anterior surface of the IOL (while aspirating) will facilitate removal of the viscoelastic retained behind the IOL.

25. Inject intracameral acetylcholine or carbachol to reduce the risk of optic-iris capture postoperatively.

26. Fill the anterior chamber with balanced salt solution and check to make sure wound is watertight. Close the conjunctival wound using cautery or, if necessary, 2 to 3 interrupted polyglactin sutures.

27. Inject subconjunctival antibiotics and corticosteroids (eg, cefazolin, dexamethasone), if necessary.

28. Apply an antibiotic-corticosteroid ointment to the eye, then patch and shield.

POSTOPERATIVE CARE

1. See the patient the next postoperative day. Carefully examine the wound for leakage or a postoperative bleb. The postoperative care for the ECCE patient is similar to that for phacoemulsification (topical corticosteroid and antibiotic drops 4 to 6 times a day and an antibiotic-corticosteroid ointment at bedtime). Consider use of topical nonsteroidal anti-inflammatory drugs to avoid postoperative cystoid macular edema.

2. Manage postoperative astigmatism created by tight sutures by cutting sutures when adequate wound closure has been achieved (wait at least 4 weeks after surgery).

COMPLICATIONS

- Hyphema
- Choroidal hemorrhage
- Iridodialysis
- Endophthalmitis
- Wound leak/bleb formation with hypotony
- Corneal edema
- Posterior capsular tear/zonular dehiscence
- Vitreous loss
- Cystoid macular edema
- Posterior capsule opacification
- Persistent or severe uveitis
- Glaucoma
- Retinal tear or detachment
- IOL decentration or dislocation

Chapter 14

Manual Small Incision Cataract Surgery

Venkatesh Prajna, MD
Rengaraj Venkatesh, MD

Manual small incision cataract surgery (MSICS) offers the use of a smaller incision compared to traditional extracapsular cataract surgery (ECCE), resulting in faster visual rehabilitation, less astigmatism, and better postoperative vision without spectacles compared to traditional ECCE. Recent studies have also shown that MSICS is more cost-effective than conventional ECCE. Indications for these procedures are similar, including mature cataracts, phacolytic glaucoma, and hypermature cataracts with liquefied cortex and hard nuclei. As with traditional ECCE, MSICS can be performed without the expensive or automated equipment required with phacoemulsification. Finally, MSICS is useful as a transition step in learning how to perform phacoemulsification.

PREOPERATIVE STEPS

1. Plan for a temporal approach if there is more than 1 D of against-the-rule astigmatism.
2. Obtain IOL calculations.

INSTRUMENTATION AND SUPPLIES

- Wire lid speculum
- 0.12 forceps

- 0.3 toothed forceps
- No. 66 or No. 69 Beaver blade (crescent, straight, and angled)
- 15° blade (stab or paracentesis blade)
- Cystotome or 25-gauge needle with a bend at tip
- High molecular weight viscoelastic
- Angled forceps (eg, Kelman-McPherson)
- Calipers
- Metal 3.2-mm keratome (bent)
- Sinskey hook
- Irrigating lens loop or vectis
- Manual aspirating device (eg, Simcoe cannula) or automated irrigation/aspiration (I/A) tip
- Blunt Westcott scissors
- Vannas scissors
- 10-0 nylon suture
- 8-0 polyglactin suture (if necessary, to close conjunctiva)
- 4-0 silk suture with tapered needle (if superior rectus bridle suture is needed)
- Needle driver
- Hemostat
- Eraser-tip cautery unit
- Smooth tying forceps
- Corneal light shield

SURGICAL PROCEDURE

1. Anesthesia: monitored anesthesia care with intravenous sedation and local anesthetic block (sub-Tenon's block with a blunt, curved [eg, Greenbaum] cannula or retrobulbar or peribulbar injection with Atkinson needle [1.25- to 1.5-inch/23- to 25-gauge/flat], using approximately 3 to 4 mL of a 1:1 mixture of 2% lidocaine and 0.75% bupivacaine [+/- hyaluronidase 150 units]). A modified Van Lint lid block may also be useful.
2. Reduce vitreous volume with a Honan balloon (set to 30 mm Hg), manual compression, or a mercury bag for a minimum of 10 minutes (use caution in patients with zonular instability).
3. Prep and drape.
4. Place the lid speculum.
5. Place superior rectus bridle suture if there is not adequate exposure of the superior limbus and sclera.

6. Rotate the globe inferiorly with a muscle hook in the inferior cul-de-sac or grasp the superior limbus with 0.12 forceps. Then, with the opposite hand, grasp the superior rectus (SR) with 0.3 toothed forceps approximately 10 mm posterior to the limbus and lift the tendon off the globe.

7. Pass a 4-0 silk suture with a tapered needle under the SR tendon. The needle should be parallel to the globe to avoid penetration. Cut off the needle, and clamp the suture to the drape with a hemostat to rotate the globe down. This suture should be released when the wound is opened to prevent the prolapse of viscoelastic and chamber collapse. (In cases of a temporal approach, a lateral rectus bridle suture can be used in a similar fashion.)

8. Make a fornix-based conjunctival flap of approximately 6.5 mm.

9. After dissecting Tenon's capsule, apply light cautery.

10. A one-third to one-half-thickness external scleral groove, 6 to 6.5 mm in width, is made 2 to 3 mm from the surgical limbus. It may be circumferential, linear, or frown-shaped, but frown-shaped incisions are commonly preferred because they are more likely to seal. The actual tunneling is done by a gentle wriggling and swiping movement of the bevel-up crescent blade along the tunnel. It should be uniform in thickness and extended up to 1.5 mm into the clear cornea along the entire width of the incision. This maneuver will prevent the tearing of the wound lips during tunneling forward; one should raise the tip and depress the heel of the blade to prevent premature entry into the anterior chamber.

11. Create a side port entry using a 15° blade 1 to 2 clock hours clockwise from the scleral tunnel incision (right-handed surgeon) or counterclockwise (left-handed surgeon).

12. Inject viscoelastic to fill the anterior chamber.

13. Enter the scleral tunnel incision with the bent keratome.

14. While continuous curvilinear capsulorrhexis may be preferable for good centration of the IOL, manual small incision cataract surgery may be safely performed using a can-opener capsulotomy; in cases of dense nuclear sclerosis, a can-opener capsulotomy is preferred, since it facilitates an easy prolapse of the hard nucleus into the anterior chamber. Multiple small tears (approximately 15 to 20 punctures per quadrant) are preferred to avoid capsular tags. If a continuous curvilinear capsulorrhexis is used, it should be at least 6 to 6.5 mm in diameter.

15. Perform hydrodissection using a 27-gauge, bent-tipped or flat-tipped hydrodissection cannula attached to a syringe filled with balanced salt solution. In the presence of a capsulorrhexis, this procedure is completed in one smooth step by injecting the fluid beneath the anterior capsular rim. In the presence of a can-opener capsulotomy, small

amounts of fluid can be injected in multiple areas so as to "unshackle" the nucleus from the confines of the cortical hug. At the end of a successful hydrodissection, the nucleus should be freely mobile within the capsular bag.

16. Prolapse the nucleus into the anterior chamber.
    - If one pole of the nucleus has prolapsed into the anterior chamber along with the fluid wave, further hydrodissection can be stopped; and the rest of the nucleus can be brought out by rotating the prolapsed pole with a Sinskey hook (Figure 14.1).
    - If there is no prolapse of the nucleus following hydrodissection, a moderate amount of viscoelastic is used to partially fill the anterior chamber. A Sinskey hook is introduced into the anterior chamber, and the tip is placed on the surface of the lens just under the plane of the anterior capsule. It is best to hook the nucleus between 1 to 3 clock-hours from the central incision so that manipulation is easy. After a part of the nucleus is prolapsed, the rest can slowly be wriggled into the anterior chamber by rotating the edges of the prolapsed part.

17. Sandwich the nucleus with viscoelastic.

18. Extraction of the nucleus through the scleral tunnel can be performed various ways, but the most common is the *irrigating vectis technique*. An irrigating vectis is necessary for this procedure. This vectis is 8 mm long and 4 mm wide; the anterior surface has a slight concavity. There are 3 small irrigating ports, each 0.3 mm in size, at the leading edge. The bridle suture is held loosely by the assistant. After the patency of the ports is checked, the vectis is inserted under the nucleus with its concave side up. As the superior rectus bridle suture is pulled tight, the irrigating vectis is slowly withdrawn, without irrigating, until the superior pole of the nucleus is engaged in the tunnel. Irrigation is then

Figure 14.1. Prolapse of nucleus into the anterior chamber with a Sinskey hook.

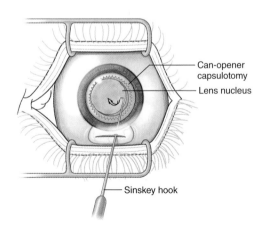

Can-opener capsulotomy

Lens nucleus

Sinskey hook

started, and the vectis is slowly withdrawn, while pressing down the posterior scleral lip. The force of irrigation has to be reduced when the maximum diameter of the nucleus just crosses the inner lip of the tunnel (Figures 14.2A, 14.2B, 14.3). This maneuver keeps the nucleus from

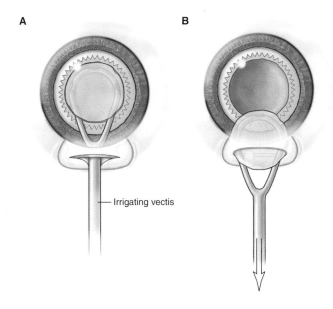

Figure 14.2. Nucleus delivery by irrigating vectis. (A) Placement of vectis under the nucleus. (B) Withdrawal of nucleus into the scleral tunnel incision.

Figure 14.3. Removal of nucleus through the scleral tunnel incision; the tight wound and hydrostatic forces from the irrigating vectis keep the anterior chamber formed.

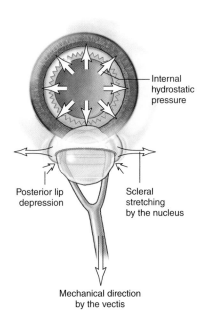

being expelled out forcefully with consequent sudden decompression and shallowing of the anterior chamber. If the wound is placed temporally, a pull on the nasal conjunctiva by the assistant will aid in nucleus extraction since the bridle effect of the lateral rectus is not sufficient.

- In a *phaco sandwich modification*, a Sinskey hook can be used in conjunction with the irrigating vectis. Once the vectis is in position, the Sinskey hook is carefully introduced and placed on top of the nucleus, sandwiching it between the vectis and the Sinskey hook (Figure 14.4A). The tip of the Sinskey hook is placed beyond the central portion of the lens to get a better grip using a 2-handed technique. With the Sinskey hook in the dominant hand and the vectis in the other, the nucleus is sandwiched and extracted (Figure 14.4B).

- In the *phaco fracture modification*, a bisector or a trisector can be used to cleave its way through the nuclear substance. Steady and constant pressure on the bisector or the trisector, and gentle lifting pressure with the vectis, will split the nucleus. The split entities can then be removed one by one, using the irrigating vectis (Figures 14.5A, 14.5B, 14.6A, 14.6B).

A   B

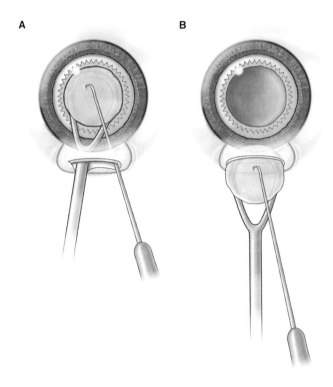

Figure 14.4. Nucleus delivery by the sandwich technique. (A) Positioning of nucleus between irrigating vectis posteriorly and Sinskey hook anteriorly. (B) Withdrawal of nucleus through the scleral tunnel incision.

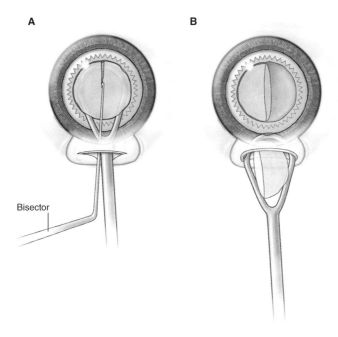

Figure 14.5. Nucleus delivery by the phaco fracture technique. (A) Positioning of nucleus between ir-rigating vectis posteriorly and nucleus bisector anteriorly prior to fracturing. (B) Removal of 1 heminucleus through the scleral tunnel incision using irrigating vectis.

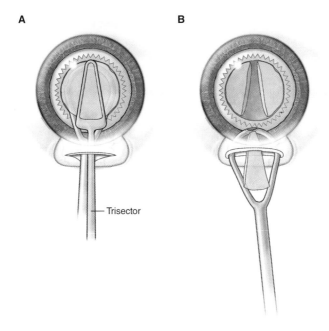

Figure 14.6. Nucleus delivery by the trisector technique. (A) Positioning of nucleus trisector around nucleus prior to fracturing. (B) Removal of the middle fragment of nucleus using irrigating vectis.

19. After the extraction of endonucleus from the anterior chamber, a mixture of epinucleus and viscoelastic materials remains in the anterior chamber. This mixture is easier to remove with the help of an irrigating vectis, by either of the following methods.
    • It can be flipped out of the bag by introducing the Simcoe cannula under the anterior capsular rim and lifting out the epinucleus into the anterior chamber. The prolapsed epinucleus can then be extracted by depressing the inferior scleral lip with the Simcoe cannula and pulling the superior rectus bridle suture at the same time.
    • Viscoelastic material is injected under the capsular rim, between the capsule and cortex, lifted out of the bag into the anterior chamber, and extracted through the tunnel. The rest of the cortical matter can then be aspirated using a Simcoe cannula. As the size of the wound is larger than 6 mm, it is preferable to place a 6-mm, rigid, polymethylmethacrylate IOL if a can-opener capsulotomy has been made. If a capsulorrhexis has been performed, then a foldable lens can be implanted in the bag as well.
20. The anterior chamber is formed by injecting balanced salt solution through the side port.
21. In cases of temporal incisions, and in the presence of a watertight wound, no sutures are necessary. However, in cases of superior tunnel, an interrupted or horizontal mattress 10-0 nylon suture can help against astigmatic decay.
22. Remove the lid speculum after applying a drop of topical antibiotic.

POSTOPERATIVE CARE

1. See patient the first postoperative day. Carefully examine the wound for leakage or an inadvertent bleb.
2. The postoperative care for the MSICS patient is similar to that for phacoemulsification (eg, topical corticosteroid drops 4 to 6 times a day, antibiotic drops 4 times a day, and an antibiotic-corticosteroid ointment at bedtime).
3. Some surgeons recommend the use of topical nonsteroidal anti-inflammatory drugs to reduce the risk of cystoid macular edema.

COMPLICATIONS

- Trapped nucleus
- Corneal edema
- Wound leak
- Iris trauma
- Posterior capsular rupture
- Macular edema
- Astigmatism
- Iris dialysis

Chapter 15

Microincision Phacoemulsification and Posterior Chamber Lens Implantation

Anat Galor, MD
Sonia H. Yoo, MD

Microincision phacoemulsification is a technique that separates the irrigation instrument from the phaco tip, thereby allowing surgery to be performed through 2 small incisions. Advantages over traditional phacoemulsification include a more stable anterior chamber during capsulorrhexis and hydrodissection because of the small incisions, enhanced "followability" of nuclear fragments because the irrigation and aspiration are separated, and better access to subincisional cortex because the instruments are interchangeable. Disadvantages include the need to enlarge the small incision for intraocular lens (IOL) insertion, the possibility of corneal wound burn because the phaco tip has no protective irrigating sleeve, and decreased infusion capacity because of the smaller irrigating tip.

PREOPERATIVE STEPS

1. Per surgeon preference, start antibiotics a few days to a few hours prior to surgery.

INSTRUMENTATION AND SUPPLIES

- Side port incision blade (several varieties available)
- Viscoelastic
- Cystotome/micro-capsulorrhexis forceps
- Hydrodissection cannula

- Balanced salt solution
- Phacoemulsification unit (all types compatible)
- 19- or 20-gauge irrigating instrument (chopper or manipulator)
- Nonsleeved phaco tip with irrigation port capped
- 20-gauge aspirating instrument
- Diamond or metal keratome (for wound enlargement)
- IOL

SURGICAL PROCEDURE

1. The procedure is usually done under topical or intracameral anesthetic, although retrobulbar, peribulbar, or subconjunctival anesthesia may be used.
2. Prep and drape.
3. Place the lid speculum in the operative eye.
4. Make a clear corneal incision (<1.5 mm) in the infero- and superotemporal quadrant (for a temporal approach) with the side port incision blade.
5. Make the width of the incision slightly larger than the phaco tip and irrigating instrument so fluid can circulate around the instruments. This will help prevent wound burns.
6. Inject viscoelastic into the anterior chamber.
7. Start the capsulorrhexis with a cystotome and continue either with the cystotome or with microforceps made specifically for the bimanual procedure.
8. Hydrodissect and hydrodelineate the lens.
9. For right-handed surgeons, insert the irrigating instrument through an incision using the left hand and the phaco tip through the other incision using the right hand (Figure 15.1).

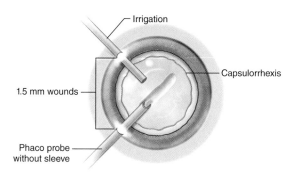

Irrigation

Capsulorrhexis

1.5 mm wounds

Phaco probe without sleeve

Figure 15.1. Microincision phacoemulsification of the lens performed through 2 small corneal incisions.

10. Remove the lens using the preferred technique (typically horizontal and vertical chop). Prefer advanced phacoemulsification technology to limit the ultrasound energy (eg, Infiniti, Alcon, Ft Worth, Texas; Stellaris, Bausch and Lomb, Tampa, Florida; Sonic Wave, Staar Surgical, Monrovia, California; WhiteStar, AMO, Santa Ana, California). Use the irrigating handpiece to direct lens fragments into the phaco tip.

11. Due to the smaller irrigating tip, the anterior chamber may become unstable when high vacuum is used. Therefore, when compared to coaxial phaco, use a higher bottle height and lower vacuum, aspiration flow rate, and ultrasound energy.

12. Insert the 20-gauge irrigating instrument with the left hand and the aspirating instrument with the right hand.

13. Remove cortex with bimanual irrigation/aspiration handpieces. Instrument positions may be switched to remove subincisional cortex.

14. Create a 2.4- to 2.8-mm incision between the 2 paracentesis incisions or enlarge one of the previous incisions.

15. Fill the capsular bag with viscoelastic.

16. Inject the IOL into the capsular bag (Figure 15.2) and ensure a good position.

17. Remove residual viscoelastic.

18. Hydrate all wounds with balanced salt solution.

19. Inject subconjunctival antibiotic and corticosteroid (if retro/peribulbar anesthesia has been used).

20. Apply antibiotic-corticosteroid ointment.

21. Place patch and shield.

Figure 15.2. Insertion of the intraocular lens into the capsular bag through a 2.4- to 2.8-mm incision.

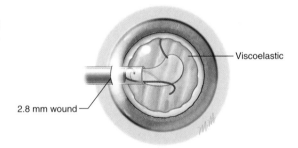

Viscoelastic

2.8 mm wound

POSTOPERATIVE CARE

1. The patch may be left in place overnight, although some surgeons ask patients to remove it several hours after surgery if only topical/intracameral anesthesia has been used.

2. Start antibiotic and corticosteroid drops 4 times daily following removal of the patch. Patients should be seen 1 day after surgery. The topical antibiotic is typically continued for 1 week; topical corticosteroids are typically tapered over 1 month, depending on clinical response. Some surgeons use a topical nonsteroidal anti-inflammatory drug to decrease the risk of cystoid macular edema.

3. A final refraction is usually performed about a month after uncomplicated surgery.

COMPLICATIONS

Complications are similar to those possible with coaxial phacoemulsification (Chapters 1 and 2).

Chapter 16

Staining of the Anterior Capsule in Cataract Surgery

Mark D. Mifflin, MD
Krista Kinard, MD

Capsular staining is often used in complicated or difficult cases of cataract surgery and may be a planned or unplanned adjunct to a surgeon's normal routine. Since the first use of vital stains in cataract surgery in the early 1990s, the variety of stains and indications has broadened. The United States Food and Drug Administration approved trypan blue for capsular staining in ocular surgery in December 2004. It is marketed in the United States as VisionBlue (trypan blue 0.06%, DORC International, The Netherlands). The American Academy of Ophthalmology Ophthalmic Technology Assessment committee concluded that data support the use of dye when poor visualization of the capsule may compromise the outcome in cataract surgery. The panel also reviewed the substantial body of literature on safety and recommended further studies on toxicity. The rationale for use of capsular staining in cataract surgery is to improve visualization, thereby optimizing capsulorrhexis and maintenance of capsular integrity throughout the case. The use of capsular staining may justify the use of the 66982 (complicated cataract) billing code, but this code should not be used when the dye is used only to facilitate the capsulorrhexis for the beginning surgeon. One vial of trypan blue costs about $80.

Indications for the procedure include the following:

- Poor red reflex: mature, white, or other very dense cataract; inadequate dilation of the pupil; or corneal opacification
- More difficult or less-predictable capsulorrhexis: traumatic cataract or pediatric cataract

- Expectation of complex surgical maneuvers: capsular tension ring; suturing of IOL or ring; or endocapsular iris prosthesis
- Inexperienced surgeon/teaching situation

INSTRUMENTATION AND SUPPLIES

- Capsular stain: trypan blue 0.06% (recommended) or indocyanine green (ICG) 0.125% to 0.5% (off-label use; must be reconstituted)
- Ophthalmic viscoelastic device (OVD) of surgeon's preference
- 27-gauge cannula on a 3-mL syringe (air, balanced salt solution)
- 30-gauge cannula for trypan blue
- 15° or similar blade for paracentesis

SURGICAL PROCEDURE

1. For experienced surgeons, sub-Tenon's or topical and intracameral anesthesia may be preferred as this helps limit posterior pressure and facilitates patient cooperation. Regional block (retrobulbar or peribulbar) or general anesthesia may be indicated in certain cases.
2. Create a side port (paracentesis) incision as usual.
3. Inject a small amount OVD just inside the paracentesis to help prevent escape of air.
4. Fill the anterior chamber with air, using a 27-gauge cannula on a 3-mL syringe.
5. Use 30-gauge cannula to place 2 or 3 drops of trypan blue 0.06% on anterior capsule. Avoid using large amounts of dye, which may increase the risk of endothelial toxicity.
6. Allow contact for 15 to 30 seconds, then gently rinse anterior chamber with balanced salt solution.
7. Inject the OVD of choice.
8. Perform surgery as usual. Note that staining might not be readily visible until the capsulorrhexis is started (Figures 16.1, 16.2, 16.3).

Variations in Technique

1. Direct staining. Dye is directly injected into the anterior chamber and then rinsed with BSS or OVD. This technique allows more contact with the iris and corneal endothelium and therefore is not preferred by the authors.

Figure 16.1. Initiation of the capsulorrhexis after staining. Note the difference between the anterior capsule (stained blue) and the underlying white cataract.

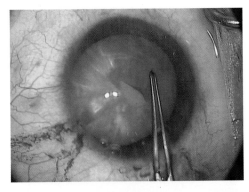

Figure 16.2. Capsulorrhexis extended through 270°. The capsular staining makes it easy to identify the leading edge of the capsulorrhexis tear.

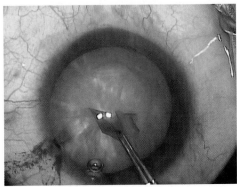

Figure 16.3. Completion of the continuous capsulorrhexis. The edges of the anterior capsule are now visible for 360° in preparation for hydrodissection of the lens.

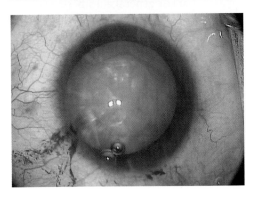

2. Use of viscoelastic. OVD is injected prior to staining to fill the anterior chamber. The syringe with dye and a 30-gauge cannula is placed over the lens, and a "windshield-wiper" technique is used to sweep an area on the anterior lens surface. While continuing to sweep, a small amount of dye is injected, which tracks along the cannula edge and stains the capsule. This technique protects the endothelium and saves time, but may not provide as intense a capsular stain as the air technique.

3. Blocking spread of dye. In cases of known compromise of capsule, zonules, or iris, it may be necessary to block spread of the dye to the posterior segment. This may be done by injecting OVD (usually a higher molecular weight, cohesive type) selectively in the area of the defect before the dye is introduced.

4. Use of cohesive and dispersive viscoelastic. The chamber may be filled with a cohesive viscoelastic and then a dispersive viscoelastic is injected posterior to it, forcing the cohesive viscoelastic against the endothelium. Through the larger incision, the irrigation/aspiration handpiece is used to remove the posterior viscoelastic, leaving the endothelium protected. Viscoelastic is left at the entrance to the paracentesis to trap the air. The dye is then injected and left for 30 to 60 seconds. The irrigation/aspiration handpiece is then used to remove the dye, and the chamber is refilled with viscoelastic for the capsulorrhexis.

COMPLICATIONS

- Corneal toxicity
- Unwanted staining of other ocular structures (eg, elimination of red reflex due to extension of dye into the vitreous cavity)
- Potential retinal toxicity

Corneal decompensation necessitating corneal transplantation has been reported by the inadvertent use of methylene blue 1% instead of trypan blue.

Chapter 17

Corneal Transplantation With Phaco and IOL

Robert S. Weinberg, MD

When both cataract surgery and corneal transplantation are indicated, and the cornea is clear enough to provide adequate visualization for phacoemulsification, the procedures may be done sequentially during a single operative procedure. By decreasing the time during which the eye is at zero pressure, compared to open-sky cataract extraction through a keratoplasty incision, sequential phacoemulsification and keratoplasty may add safety and decrease the risk of hypotony-induced choroidal hemorrhage.

PREOPERATIVE STEPS

1. Calculate the IOL power. The surgeon will need to decide whether to use the patient's actual keratometry measurements or empirical keratometry numbers based on the individual surgeon's expected post-keratoplasty keratometry.
2. Order corneal tissue from the eye bank several weeks before the procedure; confirm the adequacy of tissue with the eye bank (serologies, endothelial count, overall quality, time from death to enucleation) when it becomes available and check for obvious abnormalities prior to starting surgery.

INSTRUMENTATION AND SUPPLIES

- Appropriately sized corneal trephines
- Scleral support (Flieringa) rings
- McNeill-Goldman blepharostat (integrated lid speculum, Figure 17.1)
- Phacoemulsification instrumentation
- 10-0 nylon suture
- 5-0 Mersilene suture on spatulated needle
- Schiøtz tonometer
- Needle driver
- 0.12 forceps
- Pierse-Colibri forceps
- Preservative-free acetylcholine or carbachol
- Viscoelastic (sodium hyaluronate)
- Corneal cutting blocks
- Paton spatula

SURGICAL PROCEDURE

1. Anesthesia: local; sub-Tenon's, retrobulbar, or peribulbar block preferred. General anesthesia may be used if necessary.
2. Decrease intraocular pressure (IOP) with massage or external compression. Intravenous mannitol may be necessary if IOP is elevated.
3. Prep and drape.
4. Insert the scleral support ring (McNeill-Goldman blepharostat) between the lids.

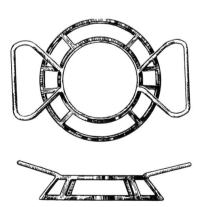

Figure 17.1. McNeill-Goldman blepharostat (scleral support ring with integrated lid speculum).

5. Check IOP with a sterile Schiøtz tonometer and lower intraocular pressure with ocular massage or intravenous mannitol.

6. Suture the scleral support ring to episclera with 4 interrupted 5-0 Mersilene (or other 5-0 to 8-0) sutures at 7:30, 4:30, 1:30, and 10:30 clock hours.

7. Proceed with phacoemulsification of cataract using the standard approach (Chapters 1 and 2). Steps include the side port incision, viscoelastic injection, creation of peripheral clear corneal or scleral tunnel incision with diamond knife or keratome, standard capsulorrhexis, phacoemulsification of the lens nucleus, irrigation and aspiration of lens cortex, and insertion of the intraocular lens. The clear corneal incision should begin peripherally and not extend to the location of the keratoplasty incision (Figure 17.2).

8. It is not necessary to remove viscoelastic material prior to proceeding with keratoplasty.

9. Inject 0.5 to 2 mL of acetylcholine or 1:100 solution of carbachol into the anterior chamber to constrict the pupil.

10. Suture the clear corneal incision with a single 10-0 nylon suture and bury the knot. Additional 10-0 nylon sutures may be necessary to ensure a watertight closure.

11. Mark the corneal epithelium centrally with a trephine, centering the trephine over the pupil after drying the cornea with a cellulose spear. If using Castroviejo trephines, set the marking depth to 0.2 mm. The diameter of the trephine should be at least 7 mm but small enough not to extend to the distal end of the clear corneal phacoemulsification incision. The anterior chamber should not be entered until the donor cornea is prepared.

12. Prepare the donor cornea, using a trephine blade diameter 0.5 mm larger than that used on the host cornea, cutting from endothelial to epithelial surface on a Teflon cutting block. The donor corneal button

Figure 17.2. Clear corneal incision (a) stopping peripheral to the keratoplasty (b) incision.

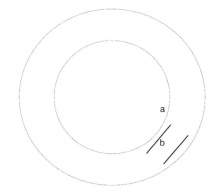

may be prepared freehand with a Castroviejo trephine or with a trephination system with a guiding shaft.

13. Deepen the initial trephine mark in the host cornea by creating a groove with a Castroviejo trephine set at a depth of 0.4 mm.

14. Enter the anterior chamber using a sharp blade at the 9 o'clock position if right-handed or at the 3 o'clock position if left-handed, making an opening large enough to insert 1 blade of a curved corneal scissors.

15. Add additional viscoelastic and acetylcholine if necessary.

16. Excise the corneal button with curved corneal scissors extending from the 9 o'clock position to the 2:30 position (if right-handed), stabilizing the corneal button with a toothed forceps, and maintaining the same scissors angle throughout the incision.

17. Continue excising the corneal button with curved corneal scissors extending from the 9 o'clock position to the 2:30 position.

18. Remove the corneal button.

19. Transfer the donor corneal button on a Teflon cutting block to the operative field, with the Teflon block in the surgeon's left hand (right-handed surgeon).

20. Elevate the donor corneal button with a Paton spatula in the surgeon's right hand (right-handed surgeon).

21. Grasp the donor corneal button with a Pierse-Colibri forceps in the surgeon's left hand and pass a 10-0 nylon suture through the donor and host cornea to the level of Descemet's membrane, at the 12:00 position, and tie the suture in place.

22. Continue with 10-0 nylon suture placement at 3, 6, and 9 o'clock positions, tying each suture before placing the next one.

23. Continue with additional 10-0 nylon suture placement, either individual sutures or a continuous suture, or both, depending on surgeon preference. Depending on the number of individual sutures used, remove viscoelastic material from the anterior chamber through the 10:30 site with the irrigation/aspiration instrument of the phacoemulsification machine prior to placing the 10:30 suture. Alternatively, viscoelastic could be removed from the anterior chamber through the clear corneal incision after removing the suture that had been placed there prior to keratoplasty.

24. Inject balanced salt solution into the anterior chamber through the side port phacoemulsification incision site to normalize IOP.

25. Test the side port incision, the clear corneal phacoemulsification incision, and the keratoplasty incision for leaks, adding additional 10-0 nylon sutures if necessary.

POSTOPERATIVE CARE

1. Administer subconjunctival corticosteroid injection with subconjunctival antibiotic injection or topical antibiotic. An antibiotic-corticosteroid ointment may also be applied followed by a pressure patch or eye shield.
2. Schedule a follow-up visit in 24 hours.
3. A topical antibiotic drop and a topical corticosteroid drop, along with an antibiotic-corticosteroid ointment, are often used for 4 to 6 weeks postoperatively to prevent infection and limit inflammation.
4. Begin selective suture cutting at 3 months.

COMPLICATIONS

- Posterior capsule opening
- Vitreous loss
- IOL dislocation
- Wound leak
- Macular edema
- Postoperative glaucoma—retained viscoelastic
- Endophthalmitis
- Failure of graft to re-epithelialize
- Corneal astigmatism
- Graft failure
- Graft rejection

Chapter 18

Limbal Relaxing Incisions or Peripheral Corneal Relaxing Incisions

Pankaj C. Gupta, MD
Roberto Pineda II, MD

Corneal astigmatism can lead to a decrease in best spectacle-corrected visual acuity when even regular astigmatism is greater than 0.50 D. Limbal relaxing incisions (LRIs), more properly called *peripheral corneal relaxing incisions* (PCRIs), are performed during cataract surgery or as a separate procedure to improve undercorrected visual acuity in patients who are intolerant of rigid gas-permeable contact lenses or astigmatic (toric) soft contact lenses or who prefer spectacle independence. This procedure can be performed without intra-operative pachymetry or a diamond blade micrometer. It can be done before, during, or after cataract surgery.

Arcuate keratotomy (AK) is similar to LRI/PCRI except that the incisions are deeper, transverse rather than circumferential, and made in the corneal mid-periphery. AK will correct greater astigmatism than LRI/PCRI but is more likely to result in irregular astigmatism, glare, and aberrations.

PREOPERATIVE STEPS

1. Incisions are best limited to patients with regular astigmatism.
2. Exclusion criteria include pterygium, anterior basement membrane dystrophy, Salzmann nodular degeneration, keratoconus, pellucid marginal degeneration, Terrien marginal degeneration, or contact lens warpage. Manual keratometry and a Placido disk image can help delineate the amount and axis of astigmatism.

3. Many surgeons recommend corneal topography to determine irregular astigmatism or early pathology that may not be recognized on other testing.

4. Review other treatment options with the patient: glasses after surgery, astigmatic (toric) contact lenses, on-axis cataract incisions, laser vision correction, or toric IOLs.

INSTRUMENTATION AND SUPPLIES

- Marking pen
- Wire lid speculum
- LRI reference marker (Figure 18.1)
- LRI axis marker (Figure 18.2)
- LRI blade (depends on surgeon's preference). Metal preset blade (0.5, 0.55, 0.6 mm): inexpensive, single-use disposable, but has more tissue resistance (not as smooth). Gem preset blades (sapphire, crystal): reusable for hundreds to thousands of cases, less tissue resistance than metal blade, and less expensive than diamond blade. Diamond blade (preset or adjustable): most expensive, reusable for thousands of cases, and has least tissue resistance. Mechanized systems are also available.

SURGICAL PROCEDURE

1. Mark the cornea, with the patient seated upright, using an LRI reference marker inked with marking pen prior to anesthesia.

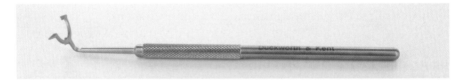

Figure 18.1. Example of a 3-point reference marker (Cionni) used when the patient is sitting upright.

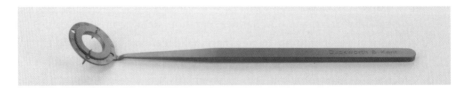

Figure 18.2. Example of an axis marker (Cionni) used when the patient is lying down.

2. Anesthesia: monitored anesthesia care with intravenous sedation, topical proparacaine and 2% Xylocaine jelly, retrobulbar and modified Van Lint blocks with 50/50 mixture of 2% lidocaine and 0.75% bupivacaine, or general endotracheal anesthesia.
3. Prep and drape.
4. Place the lid speculum.
5. Mark the axis with the LRI axis marker, using preoperative reference marks.
6. On-axis cataract incisions are optional:
   - They are placed on a steep meridian using a keratome blade; there is greater flattening with a Langerman hinge incision. Smaller incisions less than 3 mm have minimal effect.
   - They can be used as supplementation with LRIs and toric IOLs.
   - The phacoemulsification incision should never be allowed to intersect the LRI/PCRI.
   - A sutureless, astigmatically neutral phacoemulsification wound is essential.
7. Complete standard cataract surgery (Chapters 1 and 2).
8. Preset the blade to 500 to 600 μm and place 1 mm inside the limbus. The blade should be held perpendicular to corneal surface.
9. Base the incisions on length or degrees centered at the steep meridian.
   - In general, paired incisions (coupling) in circumferential LRIs/PCRIs allow for correction of astigmatism without inducing a substantial hyperopic shift of the spherical equivalent of the preoperative refraction.
   - Length (modified Gills nomogram). One 6-mm incision corrects 1 D (Figure 18.3A). Paired 6-mm incisions correct 2 D (Figure 18.3B). Paired 8-mm incisions correct 3 D (Figure 18.3C). Paired 10-mm incisions correct 4 D (Figure 18.3D).

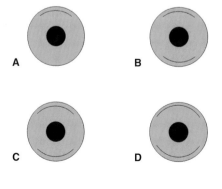

A   B

C   D

Figure 18.3. Modified Gills nomogram (blade 1 mm inside limbus). (A) One 6-mm incision, 1 D. (B) Paired 6-mm incisions, 2 D. (C) Paired 8-mm incisions, 3 D. (D) Paired 10-mm incisions, 4 D.

- Koch's with-the-rule astigmatic nomogram uses PRCIs based on degrees: marks 45° (4.5 mm), 60° (6.0 mm), and 80° (8.0 mm) with incisions 10.5 mm apart.
- Age less than 65: 0.75 to 1.00 D, two 45° incisions or one 60° incision; to 1.50 D, two 60° incisions; or >1.50 D, two 80° incisions.
- Age greater than 65: 0.75 to 1.00 D, one 45° incision; to 1.50 D, two 45° incisions or one 60° incision; or >1.50 D, two 60° incisions.

10. Consider key points.
- Rule out corneal pathology prior to performing LRIs/PCRIs.
- Make reference marks in the upright position (corneal pachymetry not necessary) to avoid errors due to cyclorotation in supine patient.
- Place the blade 1 mm inside the limbus.
- Hold the blade perpendicular to the corneal surface for maximum effect.
- Never allow LRIs/PCRIs to intersect with other corneal incisions, such as a new or previously made phacoemulsification wound, which can result in persistent epithelial defects and wound instability.

POSTOPERATIVE CARE

1. Apply an antibiotic-corticosteroid ointment and place a cotton patch with Fox shield over the eye.
2. Examine the patient the next operative day.
3. Start topical corticosteroid and antibiotic 4 times daily on the first postoperative day.
4. Follow the patient during the first postoperative week.
5. If visual acuity is undercorrected, continue corticosteroids for 1 to 3 months to enhance the effect.
6. If overcorrected, begin a rapid corticosteroid taper to minimize the effect and add hypertonic saline ointment (NaCl 5%), topical nonsteroidal anti-inflammatory drug, or both, 4 times daily for 1 to 3 months.
7. Overcorrection may require resuturing of the incision.
8. Confirm that the epithelium is intact prior to discontinuing antibiotics.

COMPLICATIONS

- Incision along the incorrect axis
- Wound gape
- Persistent nonepithelialization (especially common if LRIs/PCRIs intersect other corneal incisions)
- Corneal perforation
- Overcorrection
- Undercorrection
- Infection
- Pain and discomfort

Chapter 19

Corneal Endothelial Cell Replacement Techniques

Walter Camacho, MD
Ashley Behrens, MD

Endothelial dysfunction remains the leading indication for penetrating kerato-plasty (PK) in the United States. More than half of the nearly 40,000 corneal transplants performed each year are to treat either Fuchs corneal endothelial dystrophy or pseudophakic bullous keratopathy. In the past, endothelial re-placement was solely accomplished by PK. Although PK enjoys a high ana-tomic success rate, visual rehabilitation is often slow due to delayed stromal wound healing, surgically induced astigmatism, suture-related complications, and anisometropia associated with unexpected changes in the postoperative corneal power. In contrast, posterior lamellar corneal surgery allows for selec-tive replacement of diseased host endothelium, avoiding several of the former complications.

Selective endothelial replacement surgery offers several significant advan-tages over PK: improved surface topography with the elimination or reduction of irregular astigmatism, improved predictability of postoperative corneal re-fractive power with better intraocular lens (IOL) calculations, and retention of good donor endothelial cell densities and function. Faster visual rehabilitation, improved surface topography, rapid wound healing, and better intraocular lens calculation have been reported.

Of the different techniques used in endothelial cell replacement, the most widely used are posterior lamellar keratoplasty (PLK), also known in the United States as deep lamellar endothelial keratoplasty (DLEK); Descemet's stripping endothelial keratoplasty (DSEK); and Descemet's stripping automated endothelial keratoplasty (DSAEK).

PREOPERATIVE STEPS

1. Order donor tissue from the eye bank.
2. Determine if other anterior segment procedures are to be done prior to endothelial replacement (eg, IOL removal or repositioning, phacoemulsification).

INSTRUMENTATION AND SUPPLIES

- Wire lid speculum
- 0.12 forceps
- Artificial anterior chamber
- Microkeratome (optional)
- 9-mm diameter suction recipient trephine
- Crescent blade and dissecting instruments
- Donor punch block
- Keratome
- Calipers
- Transfer (insertion) spatula or spoon-shaped glide
- Lamellar dissection spatula (for DLEK)
- Interlamellar scissors
- DSEK/DSAEK graft forceps (nonopposing)
- Sinskey hook
- 15° or similar blade
- LASIK roller (for DSEK/DSAEK)
- Irrigation/aspiration (I/A) handpiece
- 10-0 nylon suture
- Needle driver
- Viscoelastic (methylcellulose or sodium hyaluronate)
- Air syringe with filter
- Gentian violet

SURGICAL PROCEDURES

Most surgeons have chosen topical monitored anesthesia to perform endothelial keratoplasty, specially DLEK and DSEK procedures. Topical anesthesia permits recognition of early postoperative pressure elevation from pupillary block because the patient is able to notice and report discomfort. Other anesthesia can be used according to the surgeon's experience and the technique employed, including monitored anesthesia care with intravenous sedation, topical proparacaine and 2% lidocaine jelly, sub-Tenon's or retrobulbar and modified Van Lint blocks with 50/50 mixture of 2% lidocaine and 0.75% bupivacaine, or even general endotracheal anesthesia.

The concerns with donor preparation techniques lie in ensuring endothelial cell survival, technical ease, and visual outcomes. Use of the microkeratome is associated with faster visual recovery at 1 month and provides better depth control. However, long-term results seem to be comparable to manual dissection techniques.

Manual Dissection

1. Mount the donor corneoscleral cap in an artificial anterior chamber with viscoelastic on the endothelial side, and inject air to pressurize the artificial chamber.
2. Apply a suction recipient trephine, 9 mm in diameter, to the surface of the donor cornea and engage suction. Carry out trephination to approximately 75% depth, and remove the trephine.
3. Use the crescent blade and dissecting instruments to excise sharply and carefully the anterior stromal 9-mm diameter lamellar cap, removing all but the posterior 150 μm of tissue. Extend the dissection depth limbus-to-limbus by undermining the peripheral tissue edges.
4. Remove the donor tissue from the artificial anterior chamber and mount it, endothelial side up, on a donor punch block. Use a donor trephine with the same diameter as the recipient bed to punch out the posterior donor disc.
5. Separate the healthy endothelium donor disc with 150 μm of posterior stroma from the rest of the anterior donor button, and place the disc endothelium side down onto a viscoelastic substance-coated insertion spatula.

Microkeratome Dissection

Microkeratomes have been enhanced, and optical properties of corneal flaps have greatly improved. Compared with manual dissection, microkeratomes create a smoother donor-recipient interface and more uniform depth than manual dissection.

1. Position the donor corneoscleral shell with the endothelial side down and carefully center it on an artificial chamber. The donor shell must be at least 15 mm in diameter to achieve a tight seal. Pressurize the

chamber with either air from a locking syringe or balanced salt solution from a source bottle hung at least 100 cm above the chamber to achieve a pressure of 70 mm Hg.

2. Remove the epithelium with a methylcellulose sponge to avoid irregular surfaces, and then measure the cornea with ultrasound pachymeter to guide the choice of the microkeratome head. Corneas thicker than 570 μm require a 350 μm head, and thinner corneas require a 300 μm head. The thickness of the residual bed, containing stroma, Descemet's membrane, and endothelium, should be 100 to 150 μm. This ensures enough rigidity for manipulation and flexibility for insertion into the anterior chamber through a small incision.

3. Mark the corneoscleral button, inscribing a small "s" on the stromal surface of the donor cornea with gentian violet to be used as further orientation during surgery. It is then removed from the chamber with careful attention to avoid collapse of the cornea and damage to the endothelial cell layer in the time that the artificial chamber is disassembled.

4. Place the button with the endothelial side up in a Teflon cutting block and carefully center and trephine it, using a trephine between 7 and 9 mm in diameter to match to recipient bed.

5. Maintain the donor button endothelial side up in the concavity of the cutting block with the endothelium covered with viscoelastic or preservation medium.

DLEK Procedure

1. Through a side port incision, completely fill the anterior chamber with air.

2. Make a temporal or 12 o'clock curvilinear incision (9 or 5 mm), one-third-depth incision into the sclera, 1 mm away from and parallel to the limbus.

3. Use a lamellar dissection spatula to dissect from this incision into the stroma to a corneal depth of about 75% to 80% so as to create a lamellar pocket, considering the air-to-endothelium interface as a reference plane for dissection depth. Once the desired depth is reached, use a crescent blade and dissection spatula to extend this lamellar plane over the entire (limbus-to-limbus) cornea.

4. Insert a 7- to 8-mm interlamellar trephine into the lamellar pocket and inject viscoelastic substance into the anterior chamber to provide back-pressure for the trephination, to excise the lamellar disc (posterior stroma, Descemet's membrane, and endothelium) from the posterior cornea.

5. Once the trephine slightly enters the anterior chamber, withdraw it from the lamellar plane and insert interlamellar scissors to complete

the trephination to a full 360°, then remove the recipient's posterior corneal lamellar disc from the eye through the incision.

6. Take great care to completely remove all of the viscoelastic material in the anterior chamber, using standard irrigation/aspiration techniques, to allow for later donor attachment.

7. Measure the resultant recipient bed diameter with external calipers (7 to 8 mm).

8. Insufflate air into the anterior chamber through a 0.5 mm limbal side port incision at the 2 o'clock position. The air functions to create a fluid free working space for careful insertion and manipulation of the donor tissue and to enhance self-adherence of the donor tissue to that of the recipient.

9. Fold the donor disc either in a taco-like fashion with 60% of the button on one side of the fold and 40% on the other (endothelial side inside), or place it endothelial side down on a transfer spatula or spoon-shaped glide (decision depends on the size of the scleral incision). Insert the disc and lift it anteriorly until the donor and recipient bed stromal surfaces are approximated within the host anterior chamber through the scleral incision. It is important to place viscoelastic material on the endothelial side to protect that layer.

10. Position the donor disc into the recipient's posterior corneal defect using the transfer spatula/forceps. Minor adjustments to further fit the donor into the recipient bed can then be made with a Sinskey hook through the 2 o'clock limbal stab wound.

11. Close the scleral incision with 10-0 monofilament nylon sutures. An air bubble, with a diameter of 75% of the graft diameter, is left in place temporarily to support the donor tissue.

DSEK/DSAEK Procedure

Descemet's stripping with endothelial keratoplasty (DSEK) produces a smooth recipient surface that can decrease the interface haze that has occurred with DLEK. DSEK creates a smoother surface on the recipient cornea and is a faster procedure that does not require a lamellar pocket dissection through the entire cornea as in DLEK.

1. Prepare the donor cornea, as described above.

2. Make 2 side port incisions near the 3 and 9 o'clock positions. Fill the anterior chamber with balanced salt solution, which is used to maintain anterior chamber pressure throughout the procedure.

3. Mark a small, superior clear corneal or scleral tunnel incision (approximately 3 to 4 mm) with calipers and a keratome blade. The internal opening of the incision should be no further than 1 mm central to limbus to avoid contact with the outer edge of the graft.

4. Mark a circle on the recipient corneal epithelium with a 7- to 9-mm trephine densely coated with gentian violet. Use a bent needle or custom instrument to score the Descemet's membrane on the posterior side of the cornea along the circle marked on the anterior cornea.

5. Strip the Descemet's membrane and endothelium using a custom Descemet's stripper or an irrigation/aspiration handpiece. Laying the Descemet's membrane on the anterior surface of the eye after dissection helps to verify that all of the desired tissue has been removed. Injecting trypan blue into the anterior chamber also aids in the visualization of any remaining Descemet's membrane.

6. Apply a dispersive viscoelastic material to the endothelial surface of the donor button. Fold the button in a taco-like fashion so that the endothelium is on the inside, with 60% of the button on one side of the fold (top and facing to the cornea when inserted) and 40% on the other (bottom and facing the iris), Figure 19.1. Take care not to apply excess pressure to the graft with forceps to prevent damage to the endothelium.

7. Gently grasp the folded graft with a specially designed DSEK graft forceps (the distal edges of the platforms do not appose completely) and introduce the graft into the recipient anterior chamber through

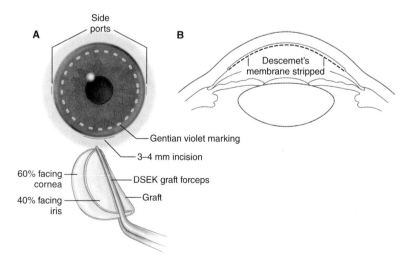

Figure 19.1. Donor disc prior to its insertion in the anterior chamber. (A) The 60% semicircle faces up toward the posterior surface of the cornea, whereas the 40% remaining semicircle facing down faces down toward the iris. (B) Side view of the anterior chamber with Descemet's membrane removed.

the 3- to 4-mm incision. Remove the forceps once the graft is disengaged from it (Figure 19.2).

8. Gently inject air using a cannula to unfold the graft. Center the graft by engaging the edge with the cannula. The entire recipient stroma should be covered by donor tissue, because areas of bare stroma might produce postoperative edema.

9. Use a LASIK roller device to move residual fluid trapped in the interface toward the periphery. Four small fenestrations can be placed in the mid-peripheral recipient cornea either before or after donor insertion to help provide pathways for fluid to exit from the interface. A 30-gauge needle can also be used in the periphery to drain trapped fluid. Alternatively, the surface of the cornea may be dried with air to promote stromal dehydration and donor disc adherence (Figure 19.3).

10. Fill the anterior chamber with air to achieve moderate tactile tension, and allow the air to remain for 10 minutes. The bubble holds the graft in place until it has adhered to the recipient stroma. After 10 minutes, remove approximately 40% of the bubble and replace it with balanced salt solution.

11. Test the incision for leakage. If necessary, close the wound with 10-0 nylon suture.

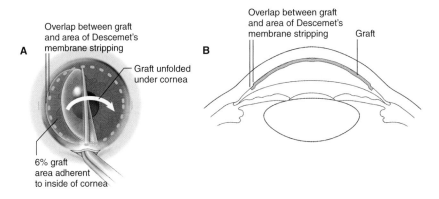

Figure 19.2. Insertion of the donor into the anterior chamber. (A) The larger part of the "taco" is ideally adhered to the posterior surface of the cornea while the transplant is still folded due to the surface tension of the viscoelastic material on the endothelial surface. The graft is then unfolded. (B) Side view of the graft after complete unfolding.

Figure 19.3. Adherence of the graft to the host cornea due to dehydration.

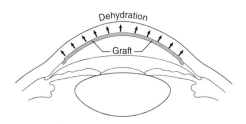

Combined Procedures

When patients require both corneal endothelial replacement and cataract removal, the cataract surgery is performed prior to the insertion of the donor tissue. This procedure creates a deeper anterior chamber and avoids the risk of damaging the endothelium of the donor graft. If the corneal surface is too edematous, the surgeon can clear the view for phacoemulsification surgery by placing sterile hypertonic glycerin drops on the epithelium to dehydrate the microcysts or bullae or scraping off the corneal surface epithelium.

It is important to have an anterior chamber clear of any viscoelastic substance that can interfere with the adhesion between the donor button and the recipient stroma, especially when a dispersive viscoelastic substance is used. Some surgeons have also performed Nd:YAG laser peripheral iridotomy prior to surgery to reduce the risk of pupillary block postoperatively, especially in phakic procedures.

POSTOPERATIVE CARE

1. Have the patient remain supine for approximately 1 hour after surgery to lower the risk of graft dislocation.
2. One hour after surgery, examine the eye with a slit-lamp biomicroscope and check the IOP.
3. In order to avoid pupillary block, keep the pupil dilated if a peripheral iridectomy was not completed. Air can also be released from the anterior chamber through a side port incision at the slit lamp to clear the inferior pupillary border. Patients may use a regimen of topical corticosteroids and antibiotics comparable to that prescribed after traditional PK.

COMPLICATIONS

- Allo- or autograft rejection or failure
- Dislocation of donor tissue
- Corneal edema and scarring
- Corneal perforation
- Irregular astigmatism
- Intraoperative bleeding
- Glaucoma
- Infection

Chapter 20

Pterygium Excision With Conjunctival Autograft Transplantation

Irina Bykhovskaya Ganelis, MD
Albert Jun, MD, PhD

A pterygium is a wing-shaped fold of conjunctiva and fibrovascular tissue that invades the superficial cornea, typically in the interpalpebral fissure. Indications for surgery include the following:

- Chronic inflammation not responding to medical therapy
- Enlargement causing threat of visual loss
- Impairment of visual acuity by growth across the visual axis or by induction of astigmatism
- Restriction of eye movement
- Atypical appearance
- Intolerable cosmetic appearance
- Ocular discomfort or irritation unresponsive to conservative therapy

While various techniques for pterygium excision are used, any variation that does not involve closure of the bare sclera following excision is associated with a high risk of recurrence. The use of rotational or sliding flaps from adjacent conjunctiva results in somewhat better outcomes, but the most commonly used technique involves coverage of exposed sclera with an autologous free graft from the same or fellow eye.

PREOPERATIVE STEPS

1. Perform a thorough ocular examination, including refraction, gonioscopy, and assessment of superior conjunctiva and optic nerve.
2. Take photographs to document any growth over time.

INSTRUMENTATION AND SUPPLIES

- Wire lid speculum
- Povidone-iodine 5% solution
- Calipers
- Crescent blade
- 0.12-mm forceps
- Conjunctival (smooth, nontoothed) forceps
- Tying forceps
- Muscle hook
- Marking pen or gentian violet
- 3-cc syringe with 27- or 30-gauge needle
- Blunt Westcott scissors
- 8-0 silk suture on a cutting needle
- 8-0 or 10-0 polyglactin suture
- Eraser-tip cautery unit (optional)

SURGICAL PROCEDURE

1. Anesthesia: sub-Tenon's or retrobulbar injection of 2% lidocaine and 0.75% bupivacaine.
2. Disinfect with povidone-iodine and drape.
3. Place the lid speculum.
4. Place an 8-0 silk traction suture in clear cornea just anterior to the 12 o'clock limbus.
5. With surgical marking pen or gentian violet, outline the edge of the pterygium to be excised (Figure 20.1A). Avoid the plica semilunaris and caruncle.
6. Use local anesthesia (lidocaine 1% to 2%) in a 27- or 30-gauge needle to balloon the pterygium, separating it from sclera. The landmarks of the pterygium will be lost but the pen marks will remain visible.

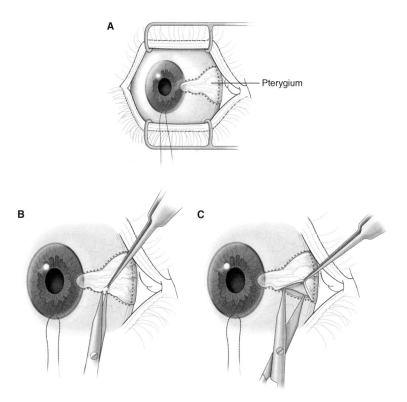

Figure 20.1. Initial marking and preparation of the surgical site. (A) The edges of the lesion are marked with gentian violet. (B) Initial incision of the pterygium edge with Westcott scissors. (C) Undermining of the pterygium with scissors.

7. Following the pen marks, use Westcott scissors and forceps to incise the conjunctival portion of the pterygium (Figure 20.1B).

8. Dissect the conjunctival and subconjunctival portions of the pterygium off bare sclera to the limbus (Figure 20.1C). Be careful not to cut the medial or lateral rectus muscle. A muscle hook placed under the insertion of the rectus muscle can be helpful here.

9. To remove the corneal portion of the pterygium, grasp the excised, conjunctival portion of the pterygium with a nontoothed, ridged forceps, such as a fine-smooth forceps (Figure 20.2A). Begin pulling the excised portion toward the central cornea slowly and allow either the inferior or the superior edge of the corneal portion of the pterygium to separate from the underlying corneal stroma. Once this edge is raised, continue pulling in the same direction to strip this entire edge of the pterygium off the cornea. As the separation reaches the most anterior (central) extent of the pterygium head, continue stripping

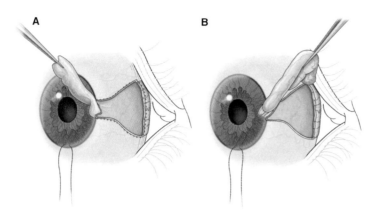

Figure 20.2. Removal of the pterygium. (A) The conjunctival aspect of the pterygium is separated from the sclera. (B) The head (corneal extension) of the pterygium is grasped with a forceps and pulled peripherally to remove the lesion completely.

around the anterior aspect of the pterygium and turn back toward the limbus until the entire corneal portion of the pterygium is freed (Figure 20.2B). Try to keep the entire corneal portion of the pterygium in a single piece as stripping is performed.

10. Place the excised pterygium flat on a firm platform, such as a piece of Whatman filter paper or cardboard from the suture package, fix in formalin, and send for pathologic examination.

11. Dissect any remaining large, adherent portions of the pterygium in a lamellar fashion with 0.12 forceps and an angled crescent blade.

12. Using a fine-smooth forceps and Westcott scissors, bluntly dissect conjunctiva from underlying Tenon's capsule along the entire superior, inferior, and posterior edges of the conjunctival defect to allow a clear conjunctival edge into which the graft can be sewn. Some surgeons apply light cautery at this point for any prominent episcleral bleeding.

13. Unravel any rolled edges of the conjunctival defect with forceps and measure the defect with calipers.

14. With the limbal traction suture, rotate the globe downward to expose the superior bulbar conjunctiva.

15. With surgical pen, mark the 4 corners and edges of the conjunctival graft, measured with calipers, to be 0.5 to 1 mm larger than the conjunctival defect to be filled.

16. From a site outside the marked graft area, inject 1% or 2% lidocaine to balloon the conjunctiva, separating it from the underlying Tenon's capsule (Figure 20.3A).

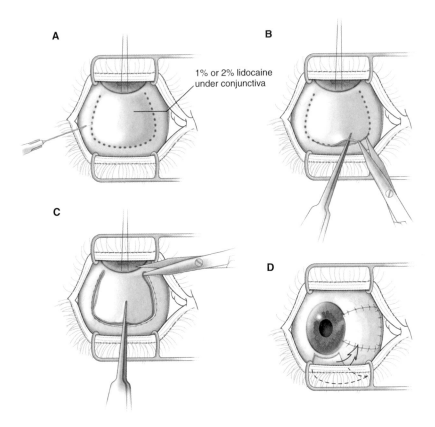

Figure 20.3. Placement of the autologous conjunctival graft. (A) Using the superior limbal traction suture to infraduct the eye, the outline of the free graft is marked with gentian violet and the tissue ballooned up with an anesthetic injection. (B) Scissors are used to initiate the dissection. (C) The conjunctival graft is dissected freely on 3 sides, leaving the adherent limbal tissue until last. (D) The autologous graft is placed over the primary excision site, maintaining the limbal orientation of the graft at the limbal border of the pterygium site, then secured with sutures (or in some cases with tissue glue).

17. With Westcott scissors and a fine-smooth forceps, incise the conjunctiva along on an entire radial edge of the marked graft (Figure 20.3B). Try to incise only conjunctiva elevated by the lidocaine injection and not Tenon's capsule. Perform blunt or sharp dissection as necessary to free the graft from underlying Tenon's capsule without buttonholes. Cut the posterior and both radial edges of the conjunctival graft before carefully cutting the anterior edge (Figure 20.3C). Be careful to leave the freed graft flat and avoid allowing it to curl on itself.

18. With the nontoothed conjunctival forceps, gently slide the conjunctival graft along the surface of the globe to its new location, keeping the epithelial side up and the limbal edge oriented properly (Figure 20.3D).

19. Suture the graft at the 4 corners with absorbable (8-0 or 10-0 polyglactin) sutures and tying forceps. Position the first 2 sutures through the 2 limbal corners of the graft, into episclera, and then into conjunctiva. The next 2 sutures secure the posterior corners of the graft to the bulbar conjunctiva. Then place additional interrupted sutures approximately 2 mm apart to close the wound edges. Suture any large buttonholes with suture material on a tapered (non-cutting) needle.
20. Use subconjunctival corticosteroids and an antibiotic-corticosteroid ointment followed by a sterile pad (shield optional).

POSTOPERATIVE CARE

1. Place a pressure patch over the eye for 24 hours.
2. Prescribe topical corticosteroid and antibiotic drops or ointment 4 to 6 times a day. Corticosteroid drops are used to control inflammation as needed but can be reduced if epithelialization is slow.
3. Reassess the patient at 1 day, 1 to 2 weeks, 1 month, 3 to 6 months, and 1 year after surgery. Optimum follow-up time to identify recurrence is 1 year.

COMPLICATIONS

- Edema
- Corneal infiltrate or ulceration
- Poor healing
- Other complications

Edema of the conjunctival graft should resolve with continued use of corticosteroids.

Corneal infiltrate or ulceration in the area of the pterygium excision should be scraped for smears and cultures and treated with antibiotics.

Poor healing of the conjunctival graft can be provoked by large buttonholes, poor wound apposition, or excessive tension on the graft.

Other complications include recurrent corneal erosions, corneal scarring, dislocation of the autograft, pyogenic granuloma, avascular scleral necrosis, corneal delle, corneoscleral thinning, astigmatism, restriction of eye movements causing diplopia, and pterygium recurrence with conjunctival cicatrization.

ADJUNCTIVE THERAPY

Therapy to reduce the rate of pterygium recurrences includes the following:

- Postoperative beta irradiation: 15 Gy in either single or divided doses. Complications: scleromalacia, corneal ulceration, endophthalmitis, glaucoma, ptosis, symblepharon, dry eye, iris atrophy, or cataract.
- Postoperative thiotepa: 1:2000 thiotepa drops given up to every 3 hours for 6 weeks. Complications: conjunctival allergic reactions, permanent focal depigmentation of the eyelids.
- Preoperative mitomycin: subconjunctival injection into the head of the pterygium of 0.1 mL of 0.15 mg/mL mitomycin C.
- Intraoperative mitomycin C: 0.2 mg/mL applied for 3 to 5 minutes intraoperatively prior to suturing conjunctival autograft. Complications: severe pain, scleral necrosis, iridocyclitis, or glaucoma.
- Postoperative mitomycin C: 0.2 mg/mL 1 drop twice a day for 14 days. Complications: corneal and scleral necrosis, iridocyclitis, or glaucoma.
- Postoperative argon laser: spot size of 50 μm at the limbus in a pattern of 4 rows, including treatment of all neovascular fronds, applied in the first to second month postoperatively. Complications: conjunctival epithelial burn or shrinkage.

Chapter 21

Corneal Biopsy

Agnieszka Trzcinka, MD
Shahzad I. Mian, MD

Organisms such as atypical mycobacteria, acanthamoeba, and fungi may cause chronic keratitis. Such infections are initially evaluated with corneal scraping; however, laboratory evaluation may not yield the organism. The infected tissue may also be located deep within the stroma covered by the unaffected corneal layer. If clinical evaluation indicates an ongoing infection despite treatment, corneal biopsy is recommended to identify the organism. This procedure may also assist in the diagnosis of corneal degenerative or dystrophic diseases and systemic conditions with specific corneal findings. In most cases, partial-thickness biopsy is sufficient. The tissue sample with diameter of at least 1 to 2 mm should provide sufficient specimen for evaluation via cultures and histopathologic examination. The biopsy sample should include the affected tissue with a fragment of adjacent healthy corneal tissue. If possible, the biopsy should be performed in an area of cornea outside of the visual axis.

PREOPERATIVE STEPS

1. Consider obtaining pachymetry measurements, which may be particularly useful when the pathology is in thin corneal tissue. The corneal thickness will aid in a conservative approach to obtain optimal sample thickness and prevent corneal perforation. Anterior segment optical coherence tomography may also provide further visualization and assessment of depth of the corneal lesion.

2. Consider consulting a microbiologist and pathologist about proper specimen division, storage, and transport.

3. Consider these media and staining techniques based on specific suspected organisms:
   - *Acanthamoeba*: place in sterile medium, such as saline. Transfer to non-nutrient agar with *E coli.* Stains: calcofluor white or Giemsa.
   - Fungus: Sabouraud agar. Stains: calcofluor white stain, methenamine-silver, acridine orange, periodic acid-Schiff, or Giemsa.
   - Bacteria: blood agar, chocolate agar, thioglycolate broth (anaerobes), or Löwenstein-Jensen medium (mycobacteria). Stains: Gram, Giemsa, or acid fast (mycobacteria).
   - Herpes virus: specific viral medium.

INSTRUMENTATION AND SUPPLIES

- Slit lamp or microscope in the operating room
- Sterile trephine 2 to 3 mm in diameter
- 0.12 forceps
- No. 66 or No. 69 Beaver blade
- Calipers
- Westcott scissors
- Vannas scissors
- 9-0 nylon suture
- Needle holders
- Sterile dish with preservative-free saline
- Culture plates

SURGICAL PROCEDURES

1. Topical tetracaine or proparacaine is used. Sub-Tenon's or retrobulbar anesthesia may be used if the patient is unable to tolerate the procedure under topical anesthetic.
2. Prep and drape.
3. Place the lid speculum.
4. Assess the location and size of the area to be biopsied (Figure 21.1A).
5. Make an incision in the cornea, using the corneal trephine with an approximate depth of 0.2 to 0.3 mm (Figure 21.1B). A diamond knife may also be used with depth set at 0.2 to 0.3 mm to achieve desired penetration with subsequent use of a corneal trephine.

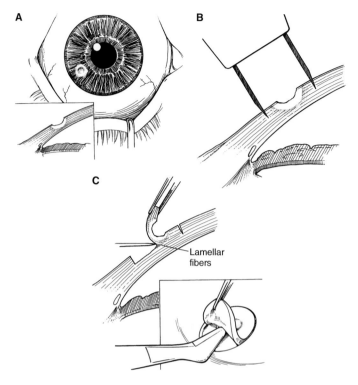

Figure 21.1. Schematic drawing of corneal biopsy technique. (A) Site of corneal pathology. (B) The incision is made using a corneal trephine with an approximated depth of 0.2 to 0.3 mm. The sample includes the affected area with a fragment of neighboring healthy corneal tissue. (C) A lamellar dissection is performed with the blade parallel to the corneal surface. (Originally published in *Principles and Practice of Ophthalmology,* 2nd ed, vol 2, Albert DM, Jakobiec FA, eds, Fungal Keratitis, page 909, copyright Elsevier © 1999.)

6. If possible, ensure that the sample includes the entire affected area with a fragment of neighboring healthy corneal tissue.
7. Lift the edge of the biopsy sample with 0.12 forceps.
8. Perform dissection using an angled or straight blade. Hold the blade parallel to the corneal surface to ensure horizontal dissection through one tissue plane (Figure 21.1C). Alternatively, straight or angled (Vannas) scissors may be used for dissection using a similar technique.
9. Consider placing a suture through the sample before the excision to prevent the loss of a small tissue sample.
10. Put the tissue sample on a sterile surface, such as a Petri dish.
11. Divide the specimen according to recommendations of pathology and microbiology laboratories.
12. Unless otherwise instructed by a microbiologist, send one specimen fragment in preservative-free saline for evaluation via cultures.

13. Send the second specimen fragment in appropriate medium to pathology for histopathologic examination. If adequate sample size is obtained, one fragment may be evaluated by electron microscopy.

14. Consider obtaining additional tissue sample by swabs and curettage of the base of the biopsy site. These samples may be sent for routine smears and culture.

15. Consider application of a cycloplegic agent for pain control.

16. Apply antibiotic ointment.

17. A bandage lens or pressure patch may be placed over the eye.

18. Place a shield over the eye.

Alternative Procedures

- In noninfectious cases, consider placement of a lamellar patch graft in corneal areas with stromal deficiency.
- A full-thickness biopsy should be considered for a very deep infiltrate that cannot adequately be sampled with a partial-thickness biopsy. This procedure requires a penetrating keratoplasty.
- If a deep infiltrate is covered by an unaffected tissue layer, consider putting a silk suture through that area and send it for microbiologic evaluation. The yield may not be adequate to identify the organism.

POSTOPERATIVE CARE

1. Examine the patient on the first postoperative day with further follow-up based on the clinical diagnosis.

2. Prescribe use of topical antibiotics and corticosteroids until epithelial healing has taken place.

COMPLICATIONS

- Corneal scarring
- Persistent corneal epithelial defect
- Intraoperative bleeding
- Astigmatism
- Infection
- Corneal perforation

For small corneal perforations that are less than 1.5 mm in diameter without prolapse of uvea or vitreous, consider use of cyanoacrylate tissue adhesive. Otherwise, use donor tissue to cover the biopsy site if the cornea is perforated.

Chapter 22

Anterior Chamber Paracentesis

James P. Dunn, MD

The diagnosis of many ocular inflammatory diseases may be confirmed by tests of aqueous humor. The widespread availability of polymerase chain reaction (PCR) testing for small amounts of fluid may enable the clinician to distinguish among viral infections (eg, cytomegalovirus versus herpes simplex or varicella zoster) that may have different treatments. In the near future, rapid PCR testing will likely be available for other pathogens, such as toxoplasmosis, bacteria, and fungi. Anterior chamber paracentesis can also be critical in the diagnosis of some uveitis masquerade syndromes, such as metastatic tumors, pseudoendophthalmitis, and phacolytic glaucoma.

As with many diagnostic tests, it is critical that the specimen be handled appropriately. Consultation with the laboratory prior to obtaining the specimen will confirm that the proper test is being performed. The fluid should be brought promptly to the laboratory; and all necessary paperwork filled out, including any clinical information that might be of use to the microbiologist or pathologist.

PREOPERATIVE STEPS

1. Have all necessary storage containers present.
2. An assistant is necessary for this procedure.

INSTRUMENTATION AND SUPPLIES

- Slit lamp or operating microscope
- 25- or 27-gauge needle on a 1-cc tuberculin syringe
- Cotton-tipped swabs
- Sterile specimen containers
- Glass slides if stains are to be performed
- Proparacaine 0.5% solution
- 5% povidone-iodine solution
- Wire lid speculum
- Culture plates if bacterial or fungal cultures are to be obtained

SURGICAL PROCEDURE

1. Anterior chamber paracentesis is usually performed at the slit lamp but may be done under a microscope in a minor procedure or operating room in children or anxious, uncooperative, or tremulous adults. If possible, the pupil should be undilated so as to reduce the risk of lens trauma during the procedure. The surgeon should choose the site of entry that will permit adequate support for the hand holding the syringe. A slight rotation of the patient's head may provide better access. A 30-gauge needle lacks the rigidity to penetrate the cornea easily and a 23-gauge needle is usually too large; hence, a 25- or 27-gauge is typically best.
2. Instill proparacaine. Retrobulbar anesthesia may be required if the patient is not cooperative. A cellulose sponge or cotton-tipped applicator soaked with the anesthetic is then applied over the planned site of entry for approximately 30 seconds.
3. Instill several drops of povidone-iodine.
4. Place the lid speculum.
5. Remove the plunger from the syringe and give it to the assistant. The plunger must remain sterile.
6. Place the needle securely on the syringe.
7. Engage the peripheral cornea with the needle tip and confirm that the patient will be cooperative.
8. Advance the needle horizontally (parallel to the plane of the iris), Figure 22.1A, using a combination of gentle radial pressure and rotatory movements of the syringe (Figure 22.1B).

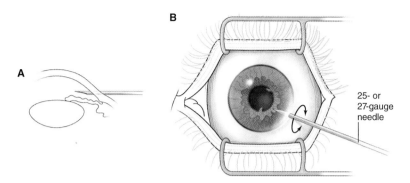

Figure 22.1. Anterior chamber paracentesis. (A) Side view of the needle in the anterior chamber. Note the orientation in the iris plane and the bevel facing posteriorly. (B) Surgeon's view of the needle entry into the anterior chamber. Both radial and rotatory forces are used to enter the eye in a controlled fashion.

9. As the needle tip penetrates into the anterior chamber, there will be a drop in resistance to forward advancement and the tip will be seen more clearly through the slit-lamp oculars.

10. Advance the needle with the bevel facing posteriorly; this reduces the chance of inadvertently engaging the iris with the tip. The aqueous humor will start to flow slowly into the syringe.

11. Ask the assistant to monitor flow of aqueous humor into the syringe. Usually no more than 0.2 mL is necessary for diagnostic purposes.

12. Withdraw the needle and confirm that the anterior chamber is formed and that there is no bleeding.

13. Insert the syringe with the needle in the bottom of the specimen container, insert the plunger, and gently inject the fluid into the container. Do not attempt to place the plunger in the syringe and expel air before putting the needle in the specimen container, as valuable fluid may be lost.

14. If cultures are to be obtained, place a single drop onto the center of each culture plate and on as many glass slides as necessary.

15. Remove the lid speculum.

16. Instill an additional drop of povidone-iodine on the eye.

17. Have the patient use a topical antibiotic (eg, moxifloxacin 0.5%, gatifloxacin 0.3%) 4 times daily for 2 to 3 days.

Optional Techniques

1. When plating samples, consider these media and staining techniques based on specific suspected organisms:
    - Fungus: Sabouraud agar. Stains: calcofluor white, methenamine-silver, acridine orange, periodic acid-Schiff, or Giemsa.
    - Bacteria: blood agar, chocolate agar, thioglycolate broth (for suspected anaerobic organism), or Löwenstein-Jensen medium (for suspected mycobacteria). Stains: Gram, Giemsa, or acid-fast (for suspected mycobacteria).

COMPLICATIONS

- Pain
- Infection
- Iris trauma or bleeding
- Cataract

Part II

Refractive Surgery

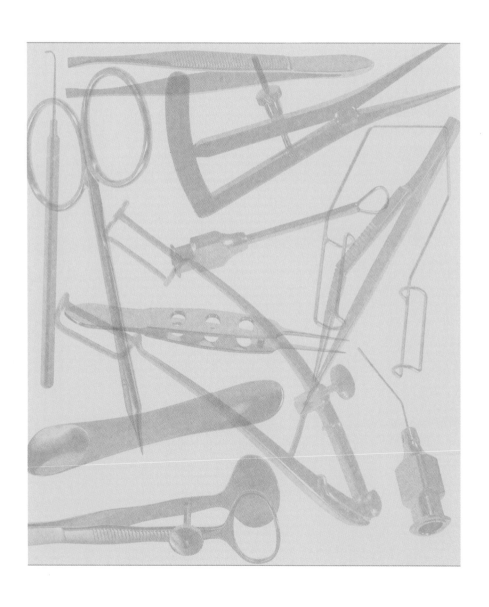

Chapter 23

Phototherapeutic Keratectomy

Holly B. Hindman, MD
Scott M. MacRae, MD

Because of its precision, the excimer laser can be used to remove superficial corneal opacities and to smooth irregular surfaces. In this setting, the aim of phototherapeutic keratectomy (PTK) is not to correct refractive errors, but is to treat anterior corneal dystrophies and degenerations, recurrent epithelial erosions, and superficial corneal scars (typically less than 100 μm deep). It can also be used to smooth superficial irregularities in the corneal surface, such as those that occur with corneal dystrophies or following trauma or penetrating keratoplasty (Figure 23.1). PTK minimizes the amount of tissue removed and induces less surgical trauma. It can be used instead of or as a supplement to mechanical debridement. A smoother corneal surface leads to improved corneal clarity, better epithelial adhesion, and less postoperative scarring and haze.

Possible indications for PTK include surface irregularities or scars caused by the following:

- Recurrent corneal erosions
- Anterior basement membrane dystrophy
- Superficial scars from trauma, surgery, or healed viral or bacterial infections
- Haze after photorefractive keratectomy
- Corneal dystrophies
- Band keratopathy
- Salzmann nodular degeneration

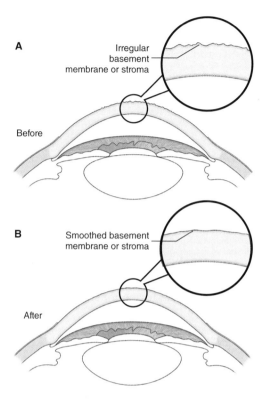

Figure 23.1. Smoothing of the corneal surface with phototherapeutic keratectomy. (A) Before surgery, surface irregularities or opacities can limit visual acuity. (B) After phototherapeutic keratectomy, the surface is smoothed and the opacities are reduced.

- Apical elevation or scarring precluding contact lens wear in keratoconus
- Button-hole LASIK flaps

Contraindications include the following:

- Severe inflammatory ocular disorders
- Uncontrolled or severe conjunctival, corneal, or lid disease
- Systemic conditions that could alter wound healing (severe collagen vascular disease, immunosuppression, severe dry eye, and pregnancy)

PREOPERATIVE STEPS

1. Set realistic expectations: help the patient to understand the benefits and limitations of PTK.
2. Inform patients of the possible off-label uses of supplemental medications (eg, mitomycin C to reduce stromal haze).

3. Inform patients that the pathology may recur after PTK (eg, stromal dystrophies).
4. Provide a description of the procedure with orientation to the variable course of postoperative discomfort (usually 3 to 4 days) and visual recovery (usually 1 to 3 weeks).

INSTRUMENTATION AND SUPPLIES

- Wire lid speculum
- Broad beam laser approved for PTK
- Anesthetic drops (proparacaine 0.5%)
- 5% to 10% povidone-iodine antiseptic solution
- Antibiotic drops (moxifloxacin 0.5% or gatifloxacin 0.3%)
- Oral anxiolytic (eg, diazepam, 5 to 10 mg) as needed
- Occluder for nonoperative eye
- 5-cc syringe
- Disposable cannula
- Cellulose sponges
- Timer
- No. 64 blade
- Balanced salt solution
- PRK spatula (eg, Maloney spatula)
- Ultrasound pachymeter
- Mitomycin C 0.02% (for treatment of haze, as needed)
- 8-mm cellulose sponge
- Topical nonsteroidal anti-inflammatory drug
- Bandage soft contact lens
- Masking agent: a combination of medium- and high-viscosity preservative-free artificial tears, such as a 2:1 mixture of Cellufresh and Celluvisc (Allergan, Irvine, California)

SURGICAL PROCEDURE

1. Describe the operative procedure in detail to the patient, and orient the patient to the sights and sounds of the laser.
2. Place anesthetic and antibiotic in the operative eye(s).
3. Cleanse lids and lashes with povidone-iodine (5% to 10% solution).
4. Carefully review the designed treatment plan. The ablation profile should be set to minimize changes in refraction and depth of ablation.

5. If the appropriate plane for laser ablation is difficult to identify (eg, Salzmann nodular degeneration, band keratopathy, and certain scars), a superficial keratectomy, performed at the slit lamp or under the operating microscope, can be performed to debulk the lesion. Start adjacent to the lesion in normal tissue to identify Bowman's layer and the appropriate tissue plane then debride toward the nodule. The following mechanical debridement laser can be used to smooth the corneal surface.

Intraoperative

1. Calibrate the laser according to the manufacturer's specifications.
2. Occlude the nonoperative eye.
3. Apply additional anesthetic drops to the operative eye(s).
4. Place the lid speculum and center the eye under the laser microscope.
5. If the appropriate plane is readily identifiable, consider removing the epithelium manually with a PRK spatula. Irregularities of the surface may be smoothed prior to laser ablation using a No. 64 blade. In cases where the appropriate plane is difficult to identify, consider prior superficial keratectomy performed at the slit lamp as described above.
6. In cases where there are stromal depressions (eg, healed ulcers), consider leaving the epithelium intact and ablating on the epithelial surface to minimize unnecessary tissue removal and using the epithelium as a masking agent. One can also use a liquid masking agent to further smooth the surface once the epithelium is removed.
7. In most cases, the eye tracker is not necessary. For a centered treatment, however, adjust the infrared eye tracker into the appropriate position.
8. Dry the cornea with a cellulose sponge or apply masking agent to help smooth out elevated areas. Masking agents will fill the depressions in the cornea while the laser hits the peaks, thereby smoothing the surface.
9. Start the laser treatment and interrupt as needed to ensure patient fixation and laser centration. We perform a central ablation followed by overlapping peripheral radial treatments. The circular mid peripheral series of laser spots (ranging from 2 to 6 mm in diameter) can be placed to (1) minimize hyperopic shift (in deep treatments >50 μm, using the 2 mm diameter spot); (2) blend the midperipheral transition zone; and (3) lightly treat anterior basement membrane irregularities in anterior basement membrane dystrophies and recurrent erosion (in

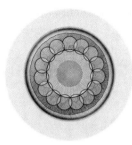

Figure 23.2. To minimize hyperopic shift, a central ablation can be performed, followed by overlapping peripheral radial treatments.

superficial treatments, using the larger diameters 5- to 6-mm diameter spots), Figure 23.2. Alternatively, myopic or hyperopic treatment profiles can be added.

10. Encourage and reassure the patient throughout the treatment. It can also be helpful to examine the patient at the slit lamp one or more times during the PTK procedure to make sure the treatment is adequate but not excessive.

11. Measure the residual stromal bed thickness with pachymetry at the conclusion of the laser treatment.

12. If indicated, dry the cornea again and apply an 8-mm cellulose sponge soaked in mitomycin C 0.02% for 30 to 120 seconds, absorb the residual mitomycin C with a cellulose sponge, and then flush the cornea generously with balanced salt solution.

13. Place a contact lens on the cornea and ensure there is no debris under the lens. In some cases, a pressure patch may be preferred.

14. Place a topical antibiotic (moxifloxacin 0.5% or gatifloxacin 0.3%) and nonsteroidal anti-inflammatory drop on the operative eye.

15. Remove the lid speculum from the eye.

POSTOPERATIVE STEPS

1. Examine the patient at the slit lamp and confirm proper positioning of the contact lens.

2. Review postoperative instructions with the patient.

3. Review medications:
   - Antibiotic drop 4 times daily in operative eye(s) as long as the contact lens is in place (usually 5 to 6 days)
   - Topical corticosteroid drop 4 times daily in operative eye(s) to relieve inflammation

- Nonpreserved artificial tears every 30 to 60 minutes in operative eye(s) (keep chilled in refrigerator between drops)
- Use of oral analgesics (acetaminophen or ibuprofen if possible)
- Ice packs applied gently over closed lids for ~10 minutes to reduce postoperative pain

4. Review postoperative appointments including:
   - Postoperative day 1: assess for status of epithelial healing, inflammation, and infection.
   - Postoperative day 6: remove bandage lens if fully re-epithelialized and assess inflammation.
   - Additional postoperative visits: schedule as needed.

COMPLICATIONS

- Pain
- Glare, halos, or starburst aberrations
- Corneal haze or scarring
- Reduced vision
- Hyperopic shift (greater with greater depths of treatment)
- Recurrence of pathology (stromal dystrophies tend to recur)
- Dryness for the first 2 to 3 months
- Temporary decreased corneal sensitivity
- Visual fluctuations for first few weeks
- Recurrent erosions
- Bacterial keratitis

To reduce hyperopic shift, it has been recommended that the minimal amount of PTK that reduces a scar or irregularity (though it may not completely eliminate it) is preferable, because aggressive tissue removal may result in unanticipated central corneal flattening and hyperopia. Less tissue removal is preferable to more; one can re-treat the patient later but one cannot add tissue once it has been removed. The use of transition zone settings and masking agents may also reduce hyperopic shifts.

Chapter 24

Photorefractive Keratectomy

Holly B. Hindman, MD
Scott M. MacRae, MD

Laser refractive surgery is intended to adjust the corneal curvature, thereby correcting refractive error and reducing dependence on glasses and contact lenses. In photorefractive keratectomy (PRK), the corneal epithelium is removed and the anterior stromal surface is ablated and reshaped with an excimer laser.

Variants of PRK include transepithelial PRK, in which the epithelium is removed by ablation with the excimer laser; laser epithelial keratomileusis (LASEK), in which the corneal epithelium is loosened by a dilute alcohol soaking (Figure 24.1); and epi laser in situ keratomileusis (Epi-LASIK), in which a microkeratome is used to separate the epithelium from Bowman's layer (Figure 24.2). In both LASEK and Epi-LASIK, the loosened epithelium is retracted, and the laser treatment is performed on the anterior stroma. After the laser ablation, the epithelium is either removed or repositioned depending on surgeon preference, and a soft contact lens is applied.

Indications include the following:

- PRK can be used in the treatment of mild to moderate myopia (typically up to −10 D), astigmatism (up to 6 D), and hyperopia (up to +4 to +5 D). PRK is the laser refractive procedure of choice in patients in whom tissue conservation is important, such as those with thin corneas; because no stromal flap is created in PRK, a thicker residual stromal bed is possible compared with LASIK.

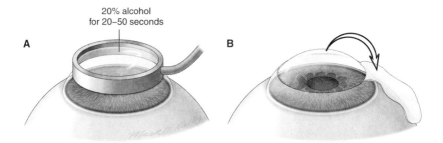

Figure 24.1. LASEK. (A) The corneal epithelium is first loosened by soaking it in dilute alcohol. A well is placed on the cornea centering over the visual axis and 20% alcohol is placed into the well for 20 to 50 seconds. (B) The epithelium can then be easily retracted with a cellulose sponge.

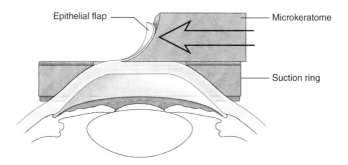

Figure 24.2. Epi-LASIK. A suction ring is applied to the cornea and a microkeratome is used to separate the epithelium from the underlying Bowman's layer.

- PRK may also be the procedure of choice when the patient has a steep cornea (>48 D) or flat cornea (<40 D), as these corneas are at increased risk of flap complications such as buttonholes or free flaps when cut with the microkeratome or the femtosecond laser
- Because PRK tends to aggravate dry eye conditions less than LASIK, it may also be preferred in patients with a history of dry eye. Other advantages of PRK over LASIK include elimination of the risks associated with creation and healing of the stromal flap and the ability to simultaneously treat other conditions of the superficial cornea such as anterior basement membrane dystrophy or recurrent erosion. The disadvantages of PRK compared to LASIK include longer visual recovery time and more discomfort.

Ideal candidates should meet the following requirements:

- Stable refractive error for 1 to 2 years. If needed, bring the patient back to recheck the refractive error.

- No contact lens warpage. The patient should discontinue soft contact lenses 1 to 3 weeks and gas-permeable lenses 6 to 12 weeks before measurements, and stability of corneal topography over time should be confirmed.
- Good ocular health.

Contraindications include the following:

- Severe inflammatory ocular disorders
- Ectatic diseases of the cornea such as keratoconus, forme fruste keratoconus, or pellucid marginal degeneration
- Uncontrolled or severe conjunctival, corneal, or lid disease
- Systemic conditions that could alter wound healing (severe collagen vascular disease, immunosuppression, severe dry eye, and pregnancy)

PREOPERATIVE STEPS

1. Help the patient understand the benefits and limitations of laser refractive procedures and ensure that he or she has realistic expectations.
2. For the patient who does not select monovision, inform him or her that surgery does not eliminate presbyopia, and the need for reading glasses in patients over 40 will persist.
3. Inform the patient about the possible off-label uses of medications or laser treatments (eg, mitomycin C to reduce stromal haze, treatments outside approved ranges, or PRK using a laser FDA-approved for LASIK).
4. Provide a description of the procedure with orientation to the variable course of postoperative discomfort (usually 3 to 4 days) and visual recovery (usually 1 to 2 weeks).

INSTRUMENTATION AND SUPPLIES

- Wire lid speculum
- Broad beam or scanning laser
- Anesthetic drops (proparacaine 0.5%)
- 5% to 10% povidone-iodine antiseptic solution
- Topical antibiotics (povidone-iodine 5%, moxifloxacin 0.5%, or gatifloxacin 0.3%)

- Topical nonsteroidal anti-inflammatory drug
- Oral anxiolytic (eg, diazepam 5 to 10 mg)
- Sterile marking pen
- Occluder for nonoperative eye
- LASEK Well or Epi-LASIK microkeratome (7.5 to 9 mm)
- 20% alcohol (for LASEK)
- 5-cc syringe
- Disposable cannula
- Cellulose sponges
- Timer
- Balanced salt solution (BSS)
- Maloney spatula
- Ultrasound pachymeter
- Frozen BSS-soaked cellulose sponges
- Mitomycin C 0.02% (for high myopia, as needed)
- 8-mm cellulose sponge
- Bandage soft contact lens

SURGICAL PROCEDURE

1. Describe the operative procedure in detail and orient the patient to the sights and sounds of the laser.
2. Place anesthetic and antibiotic in the operative eye(s).
3. Cleanse lids and lashes with povidone-iodine solution.
4. Carefully review the designed treatment plan.
5. Mark the cornea at the 6 o'clock position, using a sterile marker to avoid cyclorotation-induced errors when the patient goes from sitting to a supine position.

Intraoperative

1. Calibrate the laser per the manufacturer's specifications.
2. Occlude the nonoperative eye.
3. Apply additional anesthetic drops to the operative eye(s).
4. Place the lid speculum and center the eye under the laser microscope.
5. Remove the epithelium in preparation for anterior stromal ablation.
   - For LASEK, center the trephine over the pupil and gently press to demarcate the edge of treatment. Then center the LASEK well into the previously made depression and fill it with 20% alcohol for 20 to 50 seconds (Figure 24.1A). Absorb the alcohol with a cellulose

sponge, fill the well with BSS to dilute the residual alcohol, and then remove the well and flush generously with BSS. Peel back the epithelium (Figure 24.1B).

- For Epi-LASIK, apply the suction ring and microkeratome, perform a pass of the microkeratome, and peel back the epithelium (Figure 24.2).
- For PRK, debride the epithelium manually with a cellulose sponge or other instrument.

6. Clean the edges of the treatment zone with a PRK spatula.
7. Hydrate the cornea with BSS and adjust the infrared eye tracker into the appropriate position.
8. Dry the cornea with a cellulose sponge.
9. Start the laser treatment and interrupt as needed to ensure patient fixation and laser centration.
10. Encourage and reassure the patient throughout the treatment.
11. Measure the residual stromal bed thickness with pachymetry at the conclusion of the laser treatment.
12. Place a cellulose sponge that has been soaked in BSS, and then frozen, on the cornea for 20 seconds. This cools the cornea and decreases inflammation.
13. If indicated, dry the cornea again and apply for 12 to 120 seconds an 8-mm cellulose sponge that has been soaked in mitomycin C 0.02%. Then remove the mitomycin C soaked cellulose sponge and flush the cornea generously with BSS. (Use mitomycin C 0.02% to reduce stromal haze in cases where it can be predicted such as in the correction of high myopia.)
14. Replace the epithelial flap if Epi-LASIK or LASEK was performed. Alternatively, if the surgeon prefers, the epithelial flap can be removed and discarded.
15. Place a contact lens on the cornea, and ensure there is no debris under the lens.
16. Place an antibiotic (moxifloxacin 0.5% or gatifloxacin 0.3%) and non-steroidal anti-inflammatory drug on the operative eye.
17. Remove the lid speculum from the eye.

POSTOPERATIVE CARE

1. Examine the patient at the slit lamp and confirm proper positioning of the contact lens.
2. Review postoperative instructions with the patient.

3. Review medications:
   - Antibiotic drop (moxifloxacin 0.5% or gatifloxacin 0.3%) 4 times daily in operative eye(s) as long as the contact lens is in place (usually 5 to 6 days)
   - Nonpreserved artificial tears every 30 to 60 minutes in operative eye(s) (keep chilled in refrigerator between eye drops)
   - Variable courses of topical corticosteroid drops to reduce postoperative inflammation and haze
   - Use of oral analgesics (acetaminophen or ibuprofen if possible)
   - Ice packs applied gently over closed lids for ~10 minutes to reduce postoperative pain
4. Review postoperative appointments including:
   - Postoperative day 1: assess for status of epithelial healing, inflammation, and infection.
   - Postoperative day 6: remove bandage lens if fully re-epithelialized. Assess inflammation.
   - Additional postoperative visits: schedule as needed.
5. If re-treatments are considered, they should not be performed until stability of vision and refractive error is confirmed (usually 3 to 6 months).

COMPLICATIONS

- Pain
- Glare, halos, or starburst aberrations (warn patients they will have glare and halos at night for 1 to 2 months)
- Under- or overcorrection
- Corneal haze
- Scarring
- Reduced vision
- Dryness for first 2 to 3 months
- Variable vision for first few weeks
- Infection

Chapter 25

Laser In Situ Keratomileusis (LASIK)

Parag Parekh, MD, MPA
Elizabeth Davis, MD

Laser in situ keratomileusis (LASIK) is an elective corneal refractive procedure for patients who want to decrease their dependence on contact lenses and glasses. This chapter is written based on the commonly used IntraLase femtosecond laser (Advanced Medical Optics [AMO], Santa Ana, California), the Hansatome microkeratome (Bausch & Lomb, Rochester, New York), and the VISX S4-IR excimer laser (AMO).

As of the writing of this chapter, the United States Food and Drug Administration has approved wavefront-guided LASIK for the following degrees of refractive error:

- Low myopia (6 D sphere and 3 D cylinder)
- Hyperopia (3 D sphere and 2 D cylinder)
- Mixed astigmatism (1.5 D)
- High myopia (11 D sphere and 3 D cylinder)

Conventional LASIK (ie, non-wavefront) has been approved for:

- Low myopia (14 D sphere and 5 D cylinder)
- Hyperopia (5 D sphere and 3 D cylinder)
- Mixed astigmatism (6 D)

Ideal candidates should meet the following requirements:

- Stable refractive error for 1 to 2 years. If needed, bring the patient back to recheck the refractive error.
- No contact lens–related corneal warpage. The patient should discontinue soft contact lenses 1 to 3 weeks and gas-permeable lenses 6 to 12 weeks before measurements, and stability of corneal topography over time should be confirmed.
- Good ocular health.

Contraindications include the following:

- Severe inflammatory ocular disorders
- Ectatic diseases of the cornea such as keratoconus, forme fruste keratoconus, or pellucid marginal degeneration
- Uncontrolled or severe conjunctival, corneal, or lid disease
- Systemic conditions that could alter wound healing (severe collagen vascular disease, immunosuppression, severe dry eye, and pregnancy)
- Use of amiodarone or isotretinoin

Relative contraindications include diabetes, history of herpes simplex or varicella zoster virus keratitis, anterior basement membrane dystrophy (do PRK instead), or deep-set eyes (difficult to achieve suction).

A residual stromal bed thickness of greater than 250 μm is desirable following a primary treatment in case an enhancement needs to be done. A very rough estimate is that 1 D of correction requires 15 to 20 μm of ablation. Based on the thickness of the flap (110 μm on the IntraLase, ~160 μm on the Hansatome), an estimation of the residual bed thickness can be made. If the residual stromal bed will be too thin after LASIK, consider photorefractive keratectomy (PRK) instead (Chapter 24).

PREOPERATIVE STEPS

1. Counsel the patient about presbyopia: set appropriate expectations; explain that the goal is to reduce dependence on glasses, not eliminate the need altogether.
2. Explain that most patients have dry eye for at least 6 months.
3. Obtain informed consent: include discussion about loss of vision, especially from ectasia or infection; explain diffuse lamellar keratitis

(DLK), possible need for enhancement(s), cancelling the procedure for an imperfect flap, glare, and halos.

4. Recheck the measurements. The surgeon must also double check that the desired treatment has been correctly programmed into the excimer laser, including any nomogram adjustments. Surgeons generally create a nomogram after retrospectively reviewing their treatment outcomes (usually at least 50 eyes). The nomogram adjustment allows up to a 10% change of the entire WaveScan ablation, in the hopes of achieving emmetropia. Nomograms are generally dependent on room temperature, humidity, and whether the surgeon prefers to keep the stromal bed dry or moist during treatment (see below), and based on patient age and the amount of correction. The physician adjustment allows the surgeon to change the refractive goal away from emmetropia (eg, monovision in a patient with presbyopia).

INSTRUMENTATION AND SUPPLIES

- Wire lid speculum
- Flap elevator (many types of forceps or spatulas are available)
- Irrigating cannula
- Broad beam or scanning laser
- Anesthetic drops (proparacaine 0.5%)
- Topical antibiotics (povidone-iodine 5%, moxifloxacin 0.5%, or gatifloxacin 0.3%)
- Topical nonsteroidal anti-inflammatory drug
- Oral anxiolytic (eg, diazepam 5 to 10 mg)
- Sterile marking pen
- Occluder for nonoperative eye
- 5-cc syringe
- Disposable cannula
- Cellulose sponges
- Timer
- Balanced salt solution (BSS)
- Maloney spatula
- Ultrasound pachymeter
- Mitomycin C 0.02% (for high myopia, as needed)
- 8-mm cellulose sponge
- Bandage soft contact lens

SURGICAL PROCEDURE

1. Prep and drape. After a drop of topical anesthetic, the lids should be prepped with a povidone-iodine solution. Topical anesthetics are toxic to the cornea and should be used judiciously. The eyelashes must be out of the surgical field and can be sequestered using an adhesive sterile drape, a Steri-Strip, or medical tape.
2. Occlude the contralateral eye.
3. Position the head so that the cornea is in the center of the interpalpebral fissure.
4. Create the flap. When using the IntraLase, place the lid speculum after the flaps have been made, but before lifting. When using the microkeratome, place the lid speculum before placing the Hansatome ring. An asymmetrical ink mark is sometimes placed, so that if the flap is amputated, the marks will help the surgeon reorient the flap correctly. The marks also help with repositioning the flap at the end of the case.
5. Pupil tracker/iris registration: tell the patient to look at the amber light. Adjust the illumination to help with iris registration. A lower illumination will help keep the patient comfortable and help achieve iris registration. If necessary, dim the room lights. Typically, the pupil needs to be between 4 to 6 mm for registration (as close as possible to the WaveScan pupil diameter). The pupil tracker helps minimize the effect of X-Y movements so that the treatment remains well centered. It will not compensate for large movements and, in fact, can be fooled by them. Iris registration identifies the patient's unique iris pattern and compensates for the few degrees of cyclorotation that naturally occurs when a patient goes from the upright/sitting position to the supine position and for small shifts in pupillary centration with constriction.
6. Once iris registration has been engaged, the patient's head should not be repositioned. If there is movement, iris registration should be restarted. Light settings should not be changed once the pupil tracker and iris registration are activated.
7. If the microkeratome is to be used, the iris registration can be performed before or after creation of the flap. It can also be activated once the flap has been lifted; however, in this case, it must be done rapidly to prevent excessive dehydration of the stromal bed. For IntraLase cases, it is typically done after the IntraLase portion of the case, and immediately before lifting the flap. Again, it can also be activated once the flap has been lifted, but this must be done rapidly to prevent excessive dehydration of the stromal bed.

8. Create the flap.
    • When using the Hansatome (Figure 25.1):
        – In myopic patients, an 8.5-mm ring is used for steep corneas (greater than 45 to 46 diopters) and the 9.5-mm ring for flatter corneas. For a hyperopic treatment, a 9.5-mm ring is generally used if possible.
        – After placing the speculum, place the ring on the eye, with sufficient downward pressure using one hand temporally and the other nasally to apply an evenly distributed force, and ask the technician to turn on suction. Occasionally, the surgeon may need to put pressure on the speculum to push the globe anteriorly, allowing for better exposure and proper suction. As suction builds, ask the patient if his or her vision is getting dimmer, and reassure the patient that dimming is normal and expected. The surgeon will also note pupillary dilation at this point.
        – Once suction is achieved, the surgeon's hands can assume a more neutral force (ie, decrease the downward pressure on the globe). At this point, some surgeons will check the intraocular pressure (>65 mm Hg) using a Barraquer tonometer.
        – Place the keratome and a drop of artificial tear, warn the patient about a loud buzzing sound, and make the microkeratome pass.
        – Once the pass is complete, press the "reverse" foot pedal. Once the reverse pass is complete, ask the technician to turn suction off. Once the technician confirms that suction is off, the ring can be removed.
        – If the microkeratome suddenly stops moving midway through the forward pass, check for any obstacles to its progress (eg, lid speculum edge) and then tap the foot pedal through the area of difficulty. If forward progress is not possible, reverse the keratome and turn suction off. Never back up and go forward again.

Stromal bed   Microkeratome flap

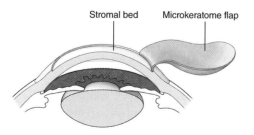

Figure 25.1. Appearance of the microkeratome flap.

Figure 25.2. Use of the femtosecond laser (IntraLase) to create the flap.

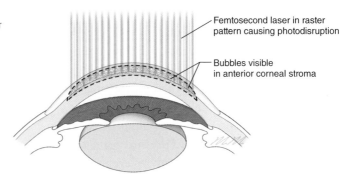

Femtosecond laser in raster pattern causing photodisruption

Bubbles visible in anterior corneal stroma

- When using the IntraLase (Figure 25.2):
  - The patient interface suction device is often placed without a lid speculum, either under the excimer laser microscope on low magnification, or without the use of a microscope. Some surgeons prefer not to use the attached clip.
  - With sufficient downward pressure, using one hand nasally and one hand temporally to apply an evenly distributed force, ask the technician to turn suction on. Reassure the patient that dimming is normal and expected. The surgeon will also note pupillary dilation at this point.
  - Once suction is achieved, the surgeon no longer needs to hold the interface device; the patient be should be rotated into position under the IntraLase laser and docking with the cone should commence. The handles of the patient interface device must be squeezed to allow docking. Many surgeons use the computer screen instead of the oculars to assure the eye is centered as applanation is achieved. The patient is told to anticipate a pressure sensation and to hold steady; the laser is then started by pressing the foot pedal.
  - It usually takes approximately 30 seconds to create the flap. Once complete, the technician should turn suction off. Only after this is confirmed can the joystick be used to move the cone and patient interface away from the patient. Many surgeons make the flaps in each eye first before performing the excimer ablation; others do the flap and excimer ablation sequentially in each eye.
9. Dry the fornices with a sponge then inspect and lift the flap using a forceps or spatula. The IntraLase flap requires a few extra maneuvers, such as lifting the edge of the flap to find the correct plane, using the spatula to open the area closest to the "pocket" first (the slightly

deeper area closest to the hinge), and breaking the remaining adhesions in several smooth motions. Once the flap is lifted, it should be positioned in the fornix or on the lid speculum. It should not be crinkled or folded on itself in order to prevent any wrinkles.

10. Dry the stromal bed with a cellulose sponge. Note: either a "dry bed" or a "moist bed" technique can be used. As long as the surgeon is consistent and the nomogram is adjusted to the technique, either method can work well. A drier bed results in more effect from the excimer laser. If peripheral corneal blood vessels are bleeding at this point, a sponge should be used to dry the blood. Excessive bleeding responds well to a drop or a sponge soaked in apraclonidine 0.5%. Recall that a hyperopic treatment steepens the peripheral cornea and therefore control of bleeding is most important in this setting. Work swiftly in order to minimize the time between lifting the flap and starting the ablation.

11. Center the patient's eye under the laser and focus on the corneal surface, leaving the pupil and iris details slightly out of focus. The iris registration may be activated at this point, if not already done (see above). Ablation begins once the surgeon presses the foot pedal.

12. The pupil tracker can be fooled by large eye movements, resulting in a decentered treatment, so do not be hesitant about stopping the treatment. In such a situation, redirect the patient to look at the amber light and restart the treatment.

13. Reposition the flap. Once it is on the stromal bed, the irrigating cannula is used to irrigate BSS beneath the flap from the hinge outward, in a smooth, efficient technique to remove any debris (eg, meibum, lint, or heme). The cannula can also be used to physically remove any debris adherent to the stroma. Excessive irrigation can lead to stromal and flap edema; it can also stir up more meibum and debris from the fornices.

14. Check flap alignment and adhesion. The flap may take a few moments to adhere to the stromal bed. A slightly moistened cellulose sponge should be used to dry the flap surface and to stroke the flap in a motion away from the hinge to ensure it is in good position and without striae. Look to see that the corneal markings are aligned and that the edges of the flap ("gutters") are symmetric. Some surgeons allow up to 3 to 5 minutes for drying. As a final check, examine both flaps under the excimer laser's microscope.

15. Place 1 drop each of a corticosteroid, an antibiotic, and a nonsteroidal anti-inflammatory drug on the eye. A drop of viscous artificial tears

can also be placed to reduce friction during blinking. If the second eye will be treated immediately, the tape is removed from the second eye and placed over the first eye. Once both eyes are treated, the procedure is complete.

POSTOPERATIVE CARE

1. It is imperative that the patient go home and take at least a 1-hour nap. The patient is also told that significant burning and tearing may begin within a few minutes, as the topical anesthetic wears off.
2. Topical corticosteroid and antibiotic regimens vary among refractive surgeons. Some surgeons recommend preservative-free, nonsteroidal anti-inflammatory drugs.
3. Examine the patient on the first postoperative day; if there is any sign of DLK, increase the topical corticosteroid dose to hourly and see the patient again on or before the third postoperative day. Lifting of the flap and irrigation of the bed may be necessary for more severe cases.

COMPLICATIONS

- Pain
- Fluctuations in vision
- Infection (beware of atypical mycobacterial keratitis)
- Dry eye
- Flap dislocation (striae)
- Amputation of the flap
- Deep lamellar keratitis
- Glare, halos, starbursts
- Halos
- Over- or undercorrection of refractive error
- Need for enhancement to reduce higher-order aberrations
- Corneal ectasia
- Scarring

Part III

Glaucoma

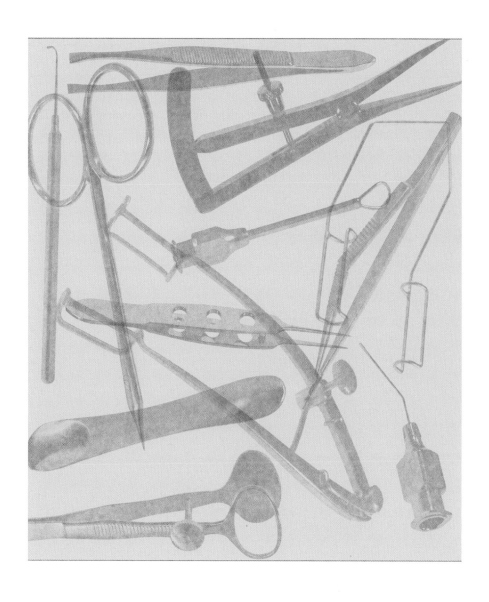

Chapter 26

Cyclodestructive Procedures

Camille Hylton, MD

Cyclodestruction, or deliberate ablation of ciliary tissues that produce aqueous humor, may be helpful in eyes with uncontrolled glaucoma refractory to conventional surgical and medical therapy. Eyes with limited visual potential (eg, severe neovascular glaucoma), severely scarred conjunctiva precluding trabeculectomy or shunt surgery, or pain from bullous keratopathy, and patients who are poor surgical candidates, from a medical standpoint, may benefit from cyclodestructive procedures. Types of cyclodestructive procedures include cyclocryotherapy, Nd:YAG laser cyclophotocoagulation (CPC), diode laser cyclophotocoagulation (CPC), and endocyclophotocoagulation (ECP).

PREOPERATIVE STEPS

1. Carefully review the goals of surgery with the patient and discuss other options. In most cases, the use of cyclodestructive procedures is limited to eyes with minimal or no visual potential in which improvement in pain is achieved through reduction of IOP and severity of bullous keratopathy.

INSTRUMENTATION AND SUPPLIES

- Cryotherapy procedure: cryotherapy system and probe
- CPC: transscleral Nd:YAG laser and probe (+/- contact lens)
- CPC: contact transscleral diode laser and probe

- Limbal approach: endoprobe, 2.5 mm microkeratome, viscoelastic, and 10-0 nylon suture
- Pars plana approach: endoprobe with standard instrumentation and MVR blade

SURGICAL PROCEDURES

1. Anesthesia: administer a retrobulbar or peribulbar block, as significant discomfort occurs with this procedure.
2. Sterile preparation for cyclocryotherapy, Nd:YAG laser CPC, and diode laser CPC is not necessary. For ECP, a retrobulbar or peribulbar block should be followed by sterile preparation and draping of the operative eye.
3. Place an eyelid speculum in the operative eye.

Cyclocryotherapy

1. Confirm the settings and placement of the cryotherapy system and probe. Temperature: -80°C. Duration: each application should last 50 to 60 seconds. Number of applications: one per clock hour. Cryoprobe placement: (transscleral): 1 to 2 mm posterior to the limbus.
2. Apply the probe (with moderate pressure) using a single application at each clock hour for 180° for 50 to 60 seconds (Figure 26.1). An iceball should be visible, emanating from the probe tip (Figure 26.2).

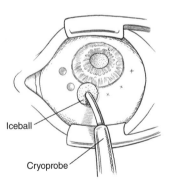

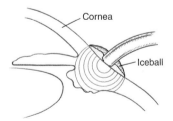

Figure 26.1. Cryoprobe for glaucoma cyclocryotherapy with the tip 2 mm posterior to the limbus. (Reproduced, with permission, from Weinreb RN, Mills RP, eds. *Glaucoma Surgery: Principles and Techniques.* 2nd ed. Ophthalmology Monograph 4. San Francisco: American Academy of Ophthalmology; 1998:159.)

Figure 26.2. Cross-sectional view of cryoprobe 2 mm behind the limbus, showing scleral uveal iceball. (Reproduced, with permission, from Weinreb RN, Mills RP, eds. *Glaucoma Surgery: Principles and Techniques.* 2nd ed. Ophthalmology Monograph 4. San Francisco: American Academy of Ophthalmology; 1998:159.)

Nd:YAG Laser Cyclophotocoagulation (CPC)

1. Review the settings and placement of the Nd:YAG laser and probe (+/- contact lens). Power: 7 to 9 W (heavily pigmented eyes may require less power) for contact mode. Energy: 4 to 8 J for noncontact mode. Duration: 0.8 to 0.9 seconds. Number of applications: 16 to 32 (contact mode) (Figure 26.3); 30 to 40 (noncontact mode). Laser probe placement: transscleral, 1.5 mm posterior to the limbus.
2. Apply the sapphire tip of the probe (with moderate pressure) using single applications for 360° (avoiding the 3 and 9 o'clock positions, as this can cause pain from damage to the long posterior ciliary nerves).
3. If 2 or more popping sounds are heard during a single application, decrease the power.

Diode Laser Cyclophotocoagulation (CPC)

1. Confirm the settings and placement of the diode laser and probe (Figure 26.4). Power: 1250 to 2000 mW (contact mode); 1200 to 1500 mW (noncontact mode). Duration: 1 to 4 seconds (contact mode); 1 second (noncontact mode). Spot size: 100 to 400 μm (noncontact mode). Number of applications: 17 to 19 (for 270°); 22 to 24 (for 360°). Laser probe placement: transscleral, 1 to 1.5 mm posterior to limbus.

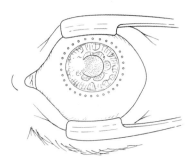

Figure 26.3. Immediate postoperative view of Nd:YAG laser cyclophotocoagulation showing sites of 32 applications over 360°. (Reproduced, with permission, from Weinreb RN, Mills RP, eds. *Glaucoma Surgery: Principles and Techniques.* 2nd ed. Ophthalmology Monograph 4. San Francisco: American Academy of Ophthalmology; 1998:163.)

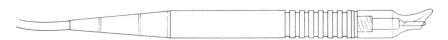

Figure 26.4. Contact handpiece of semiconductor diode laser. (Reproduced, with permission, from Weinreb RN, Mills RP, eds. *Glaucoma Surgery: Principles and Techniques.* 2nd ed. Ophthalmology Monograph 4. San Francisco: American Academy of Ophthalmology; 1998:163.)

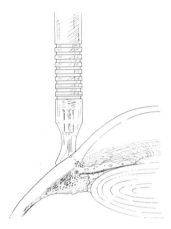

Figure 26.5. Probe handpiece attachment, which facilitates orientation parallel to visual axis. (Reproduced, with permission, from Weinreb RN, Mills RP, eds. *Glaucoma Surgery: Principles and Techniques.* 2nd ed. Ophthalmology Monograph 4. San Francisco: American Academy of Ophthalmology; 1998:165. G-Probe handpiece courtesy of IRIDEX Corporation.)

2. Apply the probe to the limbus (with the footplate of the probe tip directed away from the cornea) for 270° to 360° (Figure 26.5).
3. If 2 or more popping sounds are heard during a single application, decrease the power. Settings of lower power and longer duration (eg, 1250 mW for 4 seconds or 1500 mW for 3.5 seconds) may cause more effective tissue coagulation and less tissue destruction.

Endocyclophotocoagulation (ECP)

1. Confirm the settings and placement of the endoprobe. Power: 0.3 to 0.8 W. Duration: set to continuous wave. Number of applications: multiple for 360°.
2. For the limbal approach, follow these steps:
   - Make two 2.5 mm corneal incisions 180° apart.
   - Inject viscoelastic into the posterior chamber to lift the iris and expose the ciliary processes.
   - Place the endoprobe into the anterior chamber posterior to the iris.
   - Use the video monitor to visualize and guide treatment to the ciliary processes. Whitening and shrinkage of the ciliary processes occurs with treatment. Popping sounds and gas bubble formation occur with overtreatment.
   - Close the incisions with 10-0 nylon suture.

3. For the pars plana approach, follow these steps:
   - Place the endoprobe through the vitrectomy ports.
   - Use the video monitor to visualize and guide treatment to the ciliary processes. Whitening and shrinkage of the ciliary processes occurs with treatment. Popping sounds and gas bubble formation occur with overtreatment.
   - Close sclerotomies and conjunctiva in the usual fashion.

POSTOPERATIVE CARE

1. Use sub-Tenon's corticosteroid injection and topical corticosteroid drops (eg, prednisolone acetate 1%) as needed to control inflammation. Cycloplegic agents and an antibiotic-corticosteroid ointment may also be helpful.
2. For procedures that involve intraocular probes, topical antibiotics are appropriate.

COMPLICATIONS

- Pain
- Failure to control intraocular pressure
- Loss of vision
- Hypotony
- Corneal edema
- Hyphema
- Uveitis
- Hypopyon
- Vitreous hemorrhage
- Choroidal hemorrhage
- Retinal detachment
- Endophthalmitis
- Sympathetic ophthalmia
- Phthisis

Chapter 27

Laser Trabeculoplasty:
Argon Laser Trabeculoplasty (ALT) and
Selective Laser Trabeculoplasty (SLT)

Gail Schwartz, MD

Laser trabeculoplasty can be employed for reduction of intraocular pressure (IOP) in patients with open-angle glaucoma, or, when medically appropriate, in selected patients with ocular hypertension or who are glaucoma suspects.

Argon laser trabeculoplasty (ALT) works best in patients with highly pigmented trabecular meshwork, including pigmentary glaucoma and pseudoexfoliation. ALT success is best in patients over 60 years, has intermediate success between ages 40 to 60 years, and is least successful in patients under age 40. Success of selective laser trabeculoplasty (SLT) appears to be more independent of the level of pigment or age of the patient.

Contraindications include the following:

- Angle-closure glaucoma
- Neovascular glaucoma
- Uveitic glaucoma
- Angle-recession glaucoma
- Children with congenital or developmental glaucoma

PREOPERATIVE STEPS

1. Measure the IOP.
2. Pre-treat 30 to 60 minutes before the procedure with an alpha$_2$ adrenergic agonist (apraclonidine 0.5% or 1%; brimonidine 0. 1%, 0.15%, or 0.2%)
3. Confirm proper setup of the laser and a clean laser lens.

INSTRUMENTATION AND SUPPLIES

- Proparacaine 0.5%
- Argon laser trabeculoplasty or Latina (SLT) lens
- Gonioscopic solution (methylcellulose)

SURGICAL PROCEDURES

ALT Procedure

1. Seat the patient comfortably at the laser.
2. Confirm the eye to be treated.
3. Instill topical anesthetic.
4. Place gonioscopic (methylcellulose) solution on the trabeculoplasty lens (avoid bubbles).
5. Check the settings. Duration: 0.1 seconds. Spot size: 50 μm (Figure 27.1). Power: most frequently referenced starting energies are in the range of 600 to 1000 mW; however, this may be specific to the model of the argon laser, and starting with much lower power may be appropriate. The heavier the pigment in the trabecular meshwork, the lower the energy needed.

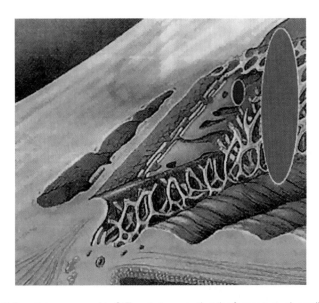

Figure 27.1. ALT spot size compared to SLT spot size; note that the former is much smaller. (Rhee D, *Color Atlas & Synopsis of Clinical Ophthalmology: Glaucoma*, Copyright © 2003, McGraw-Hill Education. Reproduced with permission of The McGraw-Hill Companies.)

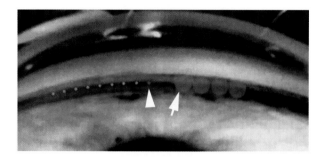

Figure 27.2. ALT compared to SLT treatment. The arrowhead on the left shows the smaller ALT laser; the arrow on the right shows the larger SLT spots. (Rhee D, *Color Atlas & Synopsis of Clinical Ophthalmology: Glaucoma*, Copyright © 2003, McGraw-Hill Education. Reproduced with permission of The McGraw-Hill Companies.)

6. Place the lens on the correct eye.

7. Apply laser energy over the anterior portion of the pigmented trabecular meshwork (Figure 27.2) for a total of 180° to 360°, aiming for approximately 50 spots over 180° or 80 to 100 spots over 360°.

8. Adjust the laser power to obtain slight blanching and small-bubble formation (Figure 27.3 illustrates treatment responses).

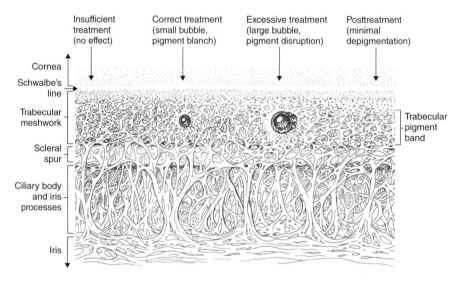

Figure 27.3. Treatment responses in trabecular meshwork to light, optimal, and excessive argon laser applications. (Reproduced, with permission, from Weinreb RN, Mills RP, eds. *Glaucoma Surgery: Principles and Techniques*. 2nd ed. Ophthalmology Monograph 4. San Francisco: American Academy of Ophthalmology; 1998:182.)

SLT Procedure

1. Repeat Steps 1 to 2 in the ALT procedure.
2. Place gonioscopic (methylcellulose) solution on the Latina lens (avoid bubbles).
3. Check the settings. Power: 0.8 mJ (start). Spot size: 400 μm (see Figure 27.1); this is a fixed size.
4. Place the lens on the correct eye.
5. Apply laser energy over the trabecular meshwork (see Figure 27.2) for a total of 180° to 360°, aiming for approximately 50 spots over 180° and 80 to 100 spots over 360°.
6. Adjust the power to produce fine "champagne bubbles" in the treated area. The heavier the pigment in the trabecular meshwork, the lower the power needed, but do not lower power below 0.6 mJ.

POSTOPERATIVE CARE

1. Check the IOP 30 to 60 minutes following the procedure.
2. Prescribe the following regimen:
   • ALT: topical corticosteroid 4 times daily for 4 to 7 days (if there is a history of corticosteroid-induced IOP increase, a topical nonsteroidal anti-inflammatory drug can be used instead)
   • SLT: topical nonsteroidal anti-inflammatory drug or topical corticosteroid 4 times daily for 4 to 7 days
3. Perform a follow-up examination within 2 weeks after the procedure, then 4 to 8 weeks after the procedure.

COMPLICATIONS

• IOP spike at 30 to 60 minutes or at the first follow-up visit
• Inflammation
• Corneal abrasion from the lens
• Failure to control IOP adequately

Chapter 28

Tube Shunt Surgery

Steven J. Gedde, MD

Reduction of intraocular pressure (IOP) is the goal of glaucoma therapy. When medical therapy or laser trabeculoplasty (Chapter 27) has failed or is not feasible, surgical approaches are indicated. Several "filtration" techniques are commonly utilized. These are usually more likely to control IOP than less-invasive techniques but have significantly greater risk. Tube shunts involve placement of a tube into the anterior chamber (or, less commonly, through the pars plana in vitrectomized eyes). The tube is attached to an end plate or sutured to the sclera and covered by conjunctiva. The tube shunt may be valved or nonvalved and the limbal portion of the tube is usually covered with tissue such as pericardium, banked sclera, or dura to help prevent erosion.

Tube shunt surgery is generally used when conventional filtering surgery (Chapter 29) has failed or is likely to fail. Indications include the following:

- Neovascular glaucoma
- Uveitic glaucoma
- Congenital glaucoma
- Fibrous or epithelial downgrowth
- Iridocorneal endothelial (ICE) syndrome
- Prior failed glaucoma filtering surgery
- Aphakia or pseudophakia
- Prior penetrating keratoplasty
- Prior retinal surgery (scleral buckling or pars plana vitrectomy)
- Conjunctival scarring

PREOPERATIVE STEPS

1. Note ocular motility, status and mobility of the conjunctiva, and health of the sclera at the anticipated tube and end plate sites.
2. Perform gonioscopy, looking for peripheral or anterior synechiae near the possible tube insertion site. Note whether there is any vitreous prolapse.

INSTRUMENTATION AND SUPPLIES

- Implant (valved [Ahmed or Krupin] or nonvalved [Baerveldt or Molteno])
- Patch graft (sclera, cornea, pericardium, dura mater, or fascia lata)
- Balanced salt solution
- 7-0 polyglactin (Vicryl) suture
- 9-0 nylon or polypropylene suture
- 30-gauge cannula
- 23-gauge needle
- Lid speculum
- Blunt Westcott scissors
- Serrated tissue forceps
- 0.12-mm toothed forceps
- Needle holder
- Eraser-tip cautery unit
- Suture scissors
- Muscle hooks
- Tying forceps

SURGICAL PROCEDURE

1. Anesthesia: administer retrobulbar anesthesia.
2. Prep and drape in a sterile manner.
3. Place the lid speculum.
4. Place a 7-0 polyglactin traction suture through the peripheral cornea to improve exposure (Figure 28.1).
5. Dissect a fornix-based conjunctival flap with blunt Westcott scissors and serrated tissue forceps. Make a radial relaxing incision at the inferior extent of the peritomy (Figure 28.2). Alternately, a limbus-based flap may be used without the relaxing incision.

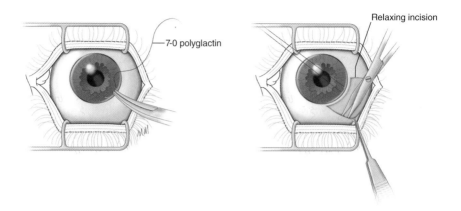

Figure 28.1. Placement of a 7-0 polyglactin traction suture through the peripheral cornea to improve exposure.

Figure 28.2. Fornix-based conjunctival flap with relaxing incision inferiorly.

6. Cauterize bleeding vessels.

7. Dissect posteriorly between the rectus muscles.

8. When using valved implants, prime the device by irrigating balanced salt solution through the tube using a 30-gauge cannula.

9. Identify adjacent rectus muscles and insert the end plate between the muscles (Figure 28.3).

10. Suture the anterior edge of the end plate to sclera approximately 10 mm from the limbus using an 8-0 or 9-0 nylon or polypropylene suture. Knots should be buried to prevent erosion through the conjunctiva (Figure 28.4).

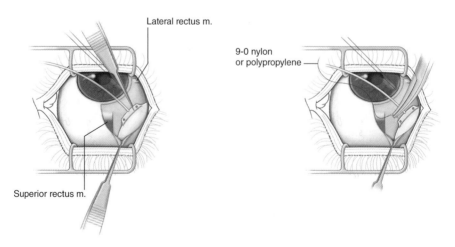

Figure 28.3. Placement of the end plate between recti muscles.

Figure 28.4. Suturing of the anterior edge of the end plate to the sclera.

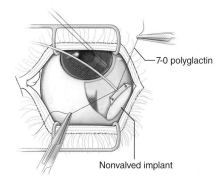

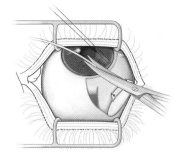

Figure 28.5. Temporary ligation of the nonvalved tube with absorbable suture.

Figure 28.6. Trimming of the tube prior to insertion into the anterior chamber.

11. When using nonvalved implants, temporarily occlude the tube by ligating it with a 7-0 polyglactin suture near the tube-plate junction (Figure 28.5). Confirm complete occlusion of the tube by attempting to irrigate balanced salt solution through the tube with a 30-gauge cannula.

12. Trim the tube with a bevel facing anteriorly to extend 2 to 3 mm into the anterior chamber (Figure 28.6).

13. Create an entry incision into the anterior chamber using a 23-gauge needle. The anterior chamber should be entered just anterior to the iris insertion (Figure 28.7A) and be directed parallel to the iris plane (Figure 28.7B).

14. Insert the tube through the needle track using nontoothed forceps or a specially designed tube insertion forceps.

15. Cover the limbal portion of the tube with a donor patch graft to prevent erosion of the tube through the overlying conjunctiva (Figure 28.8).

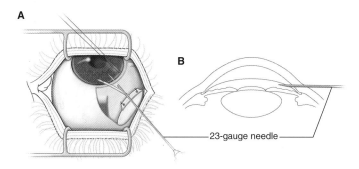

Figure 28.7. Entry into the anterior chamber. (A) A track is created with a 23-gauge needle. (B) Note the orientation of the needle parallel to the iris plane.

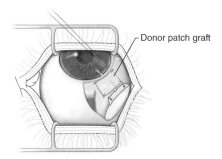

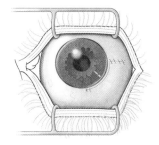

Figure 28.8. Placement of the donor patch graft over the limbal portion of the tube.

Figure 28.9. Closure of the fornix-based conjunctival flap.

16. Reapproximate the conjunctiva to the limbus with a 7-0 polyglactin mattress suture and a running closure of the radial relaxing incision (Figure 28.9). If a limbus-based flap has been used, close the conjunctiva and Tenon's capsule with a continuous suture of 8-0 polyglactin.

COMPLICATIONS

- Scleral perforation
- Hyphema
- Hypotony
- Tube obstruction
- Choroidal effusion
- Suprachoroidal hemorrhage
- Aqueous misdirection
- Cystoid macular edema
- Bleb encapsulation
- Diplopia
- Endophthalmitis
- Corneal edema
- Tube or implant erosion
- Cataract

Chapter 29

Trabeculectomy

Kathryn E. Bollinger, MD, PhD
Scott D. Smith, MD, MPH

Trabeculectomy is performed with the goal of lowering intraocular pressure (IOP) in patients with glaucoma. The procedure is indicated when testing reveals that the optic nerve has been damaged or is threatened because the IOP is too high despite maximal medical and laser therapy. This procedure may be combined with cataract surgery at the same site or at a separate site, depending on the surgeon's preference.

PREOPERATIVE STEPS

1. Note ocular motility, status and mobility of the conjunctiva, and health of the sclera at the anticipated trabeculectomy site.
2. Perform gonioscopy, and look for peripheral anterior synechiae near the planned opening of the internal ostium of the trabeculectomy.

INSTRUMENTATION AND SUPPLIES

- Castroviejo 0.12 or Colibri forceps, and smooth or serrated conjunctival forceps
- 7-0 polyglactin (Vicryl) suture (cutting needle), 10-0 nylon, and 9-0 or 10-0 polyglactin or monofilament suture (tapered needle)
- Straight hemostat
- Blunt Westcott scissors

- 15° microsurgical blade
- 18- and 23-gauge cautery
- No. 57 Beaver blade or similar blade
- Kelly punch
- Vannas scissors
- Iris scissors
- Balanced salt solution in a 3-mL syringe with 30-gauge cannula
- Needle holder
- Viscoelastic (optional)
- Antifibrotic agents, optional (mitomycin C or 5-fluorouracil)

SURGICAL PROCEDURE

1. Anesthesia: monitored anesthesia care with intravenous sedation, retro- or peribulbar block with 50/50 mixture of 2% lidocaine and 0.75% Marcaine. Subconjunctival anesthesia or topical lidocaine 4% or lidocaine 2% gel may suffice in some patients, in which case intracameral preservative-free lidocaine 1% is recommended to anesthetize the iris and ciliary muscle.
2. Exposure: place the lid speculum and adjust it to keep pressure off the globe. If greater exposure is necessary (as with limbus-based flaps), place a clear corneal traction suture using 7-0 polyglactin and infra-duct the eye to expose the superior limbus and bulbar conjunctiva.
3. Conjunctival flap: the flap should be made within either superior quadrant, leaving the adjacent quadrant available for further surgery, if required.
    - Fornix-based flap: incise the conjunctiva and Tenon's capsule inser-tion at the limbus (Figure 29.1). Avoid posterior radial incisions. The arc length of the incision should be approximately 6 to 7 mm. Preservation of a thin rim of tissue (<1 mm) at the limbus will facilitate suturing at the end of the surgery (see Step 8). Bluntly

Figure 29.1. Creation of a fornix-based conjunctival flap.

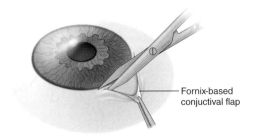

Fornix-based conjuctival flap

dissect between Tenon's capsule and episclera posteriorly toward the superior fornix. Gently retract the conjunctiva with smooth conjunctival forceps.

- Limbus-based flap: incise the conjunctiva and Tenon's capsule 8 to 10 mm posterior to the limbus while carefully avoiding trauma to the tendon of the superior rectus muscle. The circumferential incision should be long enough to allow good access to the area of the planned scleral flap. Bluntly dissect anteriorly to the superior limbus.

4. Scleral flap: flap designs vary and may be rectangular, trapezoidal, or triangular in shape (Figure 29.2), but the base of the flap should be 3 to 4 mm wide. Gently cauterize the area of the planned flap and several millimeters surrounding the site. If antifibrotic agents are to be used (see Step 9), apply them at this time. Outline the margins of the flap to one-half to two-thirds scleral thickness using the 15° blade. Dissect the flap anteriorly into clear cornea with the No. 57 Beaver blade or equivalent blade until approximately 1 mm of the blue-gray zone is exposed.

5. Side port incision: a paracentesis is performed to allow control of the anterior chamber and intraoperative testing of the patency of the filtration site.

6. Sclerostomy: enter the anterior chamber with a knife just behind the hinge of the scleral flap. Create the sclerostomy with a Kelly punch (Figure 29.3) or using sharp dissection. A small amount of tissue (approximately 0.5 mm) should remain at the margins of the sclerostomy to provide partial resistance to outflow.

7. Peripheral iridectomy: a peripheral iridectomy is generally recommended in order to prevent the iris from occluding the sclerostomy. Avoid cutting ciliary processes, zonular fibers, or the hyaloid face. In pseudophakic eyes with deep anterior chambers, some surgeons do not routinely perform a peripheral iridectomy. A small knuckle of peripheral iris is grasped with the 0.12 forceps, externalized through the sclerostomy, and then excised with the iris scissors (Figure 29.4).

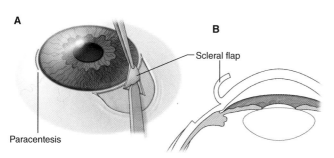

A

Paracentesis

B

Scleral flap

Figure 29.2. Creation of a triangular scleral flap. (A) Use of No. 57 Beaver blade to dissect the flap anteriorly. (B) Side view of flap dissection into clear cornea.

Figure 29.3. Use of Kelly punch to create sclerostomy (removal tissue from posterior lip of internal incision). (A) Surgeon's view. (B) Side view.

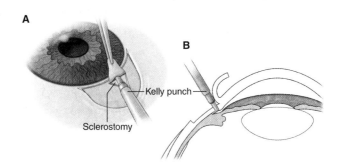

Figure 29.4. Creation of peripheral iridectomy. (A) Surgeon's view. (B) Side view.

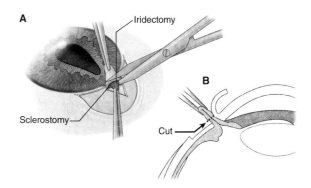

The iris is then reposited into the anterior chamber with balanced salt solution (BSS); injection of viscoelastic may be useful for this step, as it facilitates suturing of the flap.

8. Closure of the scleral flap: approximate the flap to its scleral margins with interrupted 10-0 nylon sutures (Figure 29.5). Closure should achieve mild to moderate resistance to aqueous flow with maintenance of the anterior chamber depth. Adjust leakage around the flap intraoperatively by placement of additional sutures or removal of sutures and adjustment of the suture tension. Inject BSS through the side port

Figure 29.5. Closure of scleral flap with 10-0 nylon sutures.

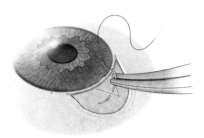

incision into the anterior chamber in order to test the scleral flap for adequate resistance to aqueous outflow.

9. A releasable 10-0 nylon suture can be used to close the scleral flap and allow selective postoperative removal to titrate the IOP. Injection of viscoelastic into the anterior chamber facilitates this step. A 2 to 3 mm clear corneal bite is made, entering the cornea about 1 mm anterior to the edge of the flap. A short bite is then taken immediately adjacent and carried radially through the anterior flap (do not close the sclerostomy) and out through the undersurface of the flap 1 to 2 mm from its base. Pass the suture over the edge of the flap and through the sclera. Take another bite on the opposite side of the flap. Pull a slight loop of the 10-0 nylon over the flap and tie this down with a triple or quadruple throw, adjusting to the amount of tension desired. In most cases, a similar releasable suture is placed on the opposite side.

10. Closure of conjunctiva: watertight closure of the conjunctival flap is critical. Use a fine absorbable suture, such as 9-0 or 10-0 polyglactin on a tapered needle. A running horizontal mattress suture can be used for fornix-based flaps if a small (1 mm) edge of conjunctiva is preserved at the limbus. Fornix-based flaps can also be closed with interrupted sutures placed at both flap ends. Limbus-based flaps should be closed with a running suture so that the conjunctiva does not leak when BSS is introduced through the side port incision, elevating the conjunctiva.

11. Use of antifibrotic agents:
    - Mitomycin C: intraoperatively, prior to sclerostomy creation, place a mitomycin C-soaked sponge (concentration 0.2 to 0.5mg/mL) within the subconjunctival space in contact with the sclera for 1 to 4 minutes. Intracameral exposure must be avoided. Irrigate ocular tissues thoroughly with BSS after removing the sponge.
    - 5-fluorouracil: if used intraoperatively, apply a soaked sponge (50 mg/mL) to the surgical site for 5 minutes.

POSTOPERATIVE CARE

1. Consider a regimen of topical prednisolone acetate 1%, 4 to 8 times daily; topical antibiotic; topical atropine 1%; and 5-fluorouracil (optional).

2. Evaluate the patient on postoperative day 1 and daily to weekly thereafter, based on examination results and presence of complications.

Titrate the frequency of topical corticosteroid administration based on the degree of conjunctival hyperemia, level of IOP, and appearance of the filtering bleb.

3. Continue a tapering course of topical corticosteroids for several weeks after surgery.

4. IOP may also be titrated by suture lysis of the scleral flap sutures or by the use of releasable suturing techniques.

5. Postoperative application regimens for the use of 5-fluorouracil vary according to the healing response. In general, administer 5 mg in 0.1 cc by subconjunctival injection, with the number of injections adjusted according to the degree of conjunctival inflammation.

6. Releasable sutures can be selectively removed by elevating the suture anterior to the flap with a 27-gauge needle, pulling the free end of the clear corneal suture, and gently pulling the suture downward with a forceps. Gentle pressure on the edge of the flap with a moistened cotton-tipped swab may cause elevation of the bleb.

COMPLICATIONS

- Intraoperative complications: choroidal hemorrhage, choroidal effusion, vitreous loss, lens injury, or hyphema
- Early postoperative complications: flat anterior chamber, hypotony, increased IOP, choroidal effusion, choroidal hemorrhage, cataract, uveitis, or nonhealing corneal epithelial defect (if subconjunctival, 5-fluorouracil is used)
- Late postoperative complications: hypotonus maculopathy, conjunctival bleb leak, bleb infection, endophthalmitis, cataract, or nonhealing corneal epithelial defect (if subconjunctival, 5-fluorouracil, or mitomycin C is used)

Chapter 30

Trabeculotomy

Pradeep Y. Ramulu, MD, PhD

Surgical incision through the trabecular meshwork is the treatment of choice for the treatment of primary congenital glaucoma, in which abnormal development of the anterior chamber angle impairs aqueous outflow and causes an intraocular pressure (IOP) elevation that responds poorly to medications. This surgical approach may also be used for other types of childhood glaucoma, including Axenfeld-Rieger syndrome, Sturge-Weber disease (encephalo-trigeminal angiomatosis), aniridia, neurofibromatosis, and juvenile open-angle glaucoma. Incision through the trabecular meshwork may be accomplished via an external approach (trabeculotomy), or an internal approach (goniotomy). Both procedures have similar efficacy, although trabeculotomy becomes the procedure of choice in eyes with corneal clouding.

PREOPERATIVE STEPS

1. If surgery cannot be scheduled promptly (within a week), acetazolamide solution may be administered every 8 hours at a total daily dose of 10 to 20 mg/kg.
2. Arrange for axial length measurements to be taken in operating room for children under the age of 2. Axial lengths are used to diagnose infantile glaucoma as well as to monitor its progression.
3. Consult with the pediatric anesthesiology and/or pediatric service regarding the need for admission in newborn infants under 60 weeks of gestational age.

INSTRUMENTATION AND SUPPLIES

- Lid speculum
- 0.12 forceps
- Conjunctival (non-toothed) forceps
- Westcott and Vannas scissors
- No. 75 blade or equivalent
- Crescent blade
- Cautery unit
- Harms trabeculotomes, leftward and rightward
- 10-0 nylon suture
- 8-0 polyglactin (Vicryl) suture
- Needle holders
- Tono-Pen
- For suture trabeculotomy only: 5-0 polypropylene (Prolene) suture and handheld thermal cautery

SURGICAL PROCEDURES

Harms Trabeculotomy

1. Measure the IOP with the Tono-Pen after intramuscular ketamine administration or sevoflurane mask. IOP is more accurately measured following ketamine anesthesia, but the use of sevoflurane will save time in cases where surgery is likely necessary.
2. Await the induction of general anesthesia.
3. Examine the eyes under anesthesia, including echographic measurement of axial length, determination of corneal diameter, and anterior segment examination.
4. Prep and drape.
5. Place the lid speculum.
6. Place an 8-0 polyglactin corneal traction suture and rotate the eye toward the area of the intended trabeculotomy (optional).
7. Perform a 4 o'clock limbal conjunctival peritomy with conjunctival forceps and Wescott scissors. Primary trabeculotomies should be done in the superonasal quadrant if possible, while repeat trabeculotomies may be done temporally.
8. Cauterize over areas of bleeding and over the area of the intended scleral flap.

9. Form a triangular or rectangular two-thirds-thickness scleral flap using a No. 75 blade and 0.12 forceps to stabilize the eye. Take care not to enter the suprachoroidal space, particularly in buphthalmic eyes where the sclera may be thin. The flap should extend at least 2.5 mm posterior to the limbus to allow for variations in the locations of Schlemm's canal.

10. Cauterize bleeding vessels within the bed of the scleral flap using fine-tip cautery.

11. Under high magnification, use a No. 75 blade to gradually perform a radial cut-down over the suspected location of Schlemm's canal (usually 1.5 to 2.5 mm posterior to the limbus).

12. Identify Schlemm's canal by the circumferentially oriented scleral fibers as well as aqueous humor egress.

13. Cannulate Schlemm's canal with the rightward Harms trabeculotome.

14. With the arm of the rightward trabeculotome inside Schlemm's canal and parallel to the plane of the iris, rotate the trabeculotome into the anterior chamber (Figure 30.1). Minimal force should be required. Bleeding and shallowing of the anterior chamber are commonplace at this stage.

15. Repeat Step 14 with the leftward Harms trabeculotome.

16. Close the radial cutdown with a 10-0 nylon suture. Rotate the knot into the sclera.

17. Tightly close the scleral flap with 3 to 5 10-0 nylon sutures. Rotate the knots into the flap.

18. Dissect into the posterior sub-Tenon's space with blunt Wescott scissors, and use a blunt cannula to inject 2 mL of 0.75% bupivacaine into this space for postoperative anesthesia.

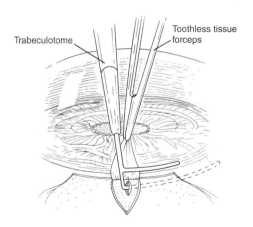

Trabeculotome

Toothless tissue forceps

Figure 30.1. Inferior prong of the trabeculotome is passed into Schlemm's canal, using the superior prong to establish orientation within the canal. The trabeculotome should pass easily. Once in position, it is rotated into the anterior chamber. Care should be taken to not tilt the trabeculotome anteriorly or posteriorly. (Reproduced, with permission, from Weinreb RN, Mills RP, eds. *Glaucoma Surgery: Principles and Techniques.* 2nd ed. Ophthalmology Monograph 4. San Francisco: American Academy of Ophthalmology; 1998:200.)

19. Close conjunctiva at both ends of the peritomy with 8-0 polyglactin suture. If a corneal traction suture was used, a portion of this suture can be employed.
20. Inject subconjunctival corticosteroid and antibiotic.
21. Place a drop of 1% atropine sulfate in the eye.
22. Place a cotton patch with a Fox shield over the eye.

Suture Trabeculotomy

For suture trabeculotomy, replace Steps 13 to 15 above with the following steps:

- Prepare the 5-0 polypropylene suture for threading Schlemm's canal. Using a hand-held thermal cautery, slightly melt the end of a 5-0 polypropylene suture to create a bulb-like terminus. Also, mark the suture at the 6-cm mark; 360° cannulation of Schlemm's canal does not require more than this length of suture.
- Thread the prepared polypropylene suture through the previously identified Schlemm's canal. In some cases, threading will have to be discontinued after resistance is encountered from catching the suture in a collector channel or because of a discontinuous canal of Schlemm. It is sometimes possible to redirect the suture by pressing over Schlemm's canal externally if the end bulb is visualized. In other cases, the suture will continue to thread past 6 cm, likely because of entry of the suture into the suprachoroidal space, in which case the suture should be withdrawn.
- Pull the suture through Schlemm's canal into the anterior chamber for 360° and remove.
- Proceed to Step 16 above.

POSTOPERATIVE CARE

1. Start prednisolone acetate 1% 4 times daily and taper over 1 month.
2. Start atropine sulfate 1% daily. Continue for 2 weeks and then discontinue.
3. Start a topical fluoroquinolone drop 4 times daily for 2 weeks and then discontinue.
4. Examine the patient the next postoperative day, and then in 4 to 6 weeks, as part of an examination under anesthesia if necessary.

COMPLICATIONS

- Hyphema (usually transient and of no long-term consequence)
- Detachment of Descemet's membrane
- Cyclodialysis cleft
- Endophthalmitis
- Iridodialysis
- Cataract
- Elevated IOP

Part IV

Strabismus Surgery

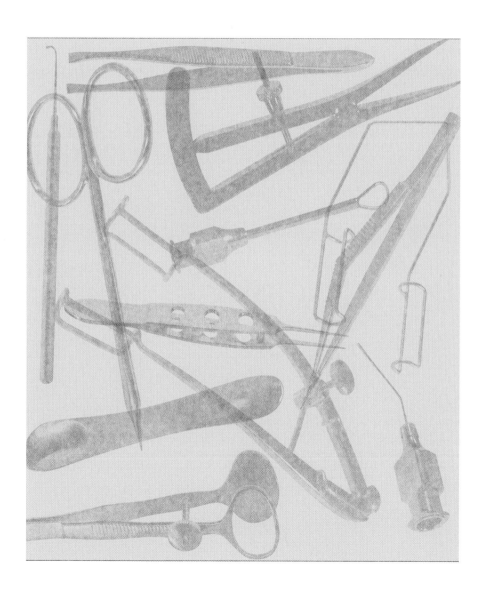

Chapter 31

Recession of Extraocular Rectus Muscle

Rudolph S. Wagner, MD
Suqin Guo, MD

Recession is the most commonly performed muscle-weakening procedure in strabismus surgery. It can be used in all forms of strabismus, unilaterally, bilaterally, or combined with muscle resection.

INSTRUMENTATION AND SUPPLIES

- Forceps: Castroviejo suture forceps 0.12 mm, 0.3 mm, or 0.5 mm; Stern-Castroviejo locking forceps 0.5 mm (for fornix-based approach)
- Westcott scissors with blunt tips
- Barraquer eye speculum with solid or wire blades
- Curved-jaw needle holder
- Caliper
- Muscle hooks (Jameson, Culler, Stevens, or Green)
- 4-0 silk suture
- 5-0 or 6-0 absorbable (Vicryl) suture, double-armed, with spatula needles
- 6-0 plain gut suture

SURGICAL PROCEDURE

1. This procedure is usually performed under general anesthesia.
2. Prep and drape.

3. Place a 4-0 silk traction suture through the conjunctiva (at the 6 and 12 o'clock limbus for surgery on the horizontal recti and at the 3 and 9 o'clock limbus for vertical rectus surgery).

4. Create a limbal peritomy or cul-de-sac (fornix) incision with Westcott scissors and 0.12 forceps (Figure 31.1).

5. Reflect conjunctival-Tenon's layer and dissect the intermuscular membrane to expose bare sclera posterior to each side of the muscle insertion. The muscle capsule should be left intact on the muscle tendon.

6. Insert a large Jameson muscle hook or Green hook under the muscle tendon, posterior to its insertion.

7. Place a double-armed, 5-0 or 6-0 absorbable suture about 1 mm posterior to the muscle insertion in the middle of the muscle; pass each arm of the suture within the muscle, exiting at each border of the muscle. Then reinsert the needles 2 mm from the muscle margin and lock on each side of the muscle (Figures 31.2A, 31.2B).

8. Disinsert the muscle from its original insertion with blunt-tipped Westcott scissors, whose tips are placed in between the muscle insertion and the suture line (Figure 31.3). Inspect the anterior and posterior of the muscle after disinsertion to ensure the muscle is contained in the suture.

9. Mark the planned amount of recession onto the sclera, posterior to the muscle stump, with a caliper (Figure 31.4).

10. Pass the spatula needles partial thickness into the sclera at the premarked points in the "crossed-sword" fashion (Figure 31.5). The muscle sutures are tied (Figure 31.6). Intrascleral needle passes should be parallel to the original muscle insertion, and entrance points should be measured about 10 mm in width to avoid sag in the middle of the muscle.

11. Close conjunctiva with a 6-0 plain gut suture.

Figure 31.1. A limbal incision is made through conjunctival and Tenon's capsule by using Westcott scissors and 0.12 forceps.

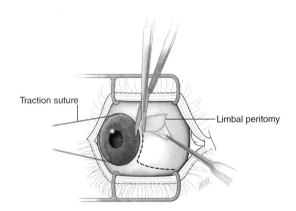

Traction suture   Limbal peritomy

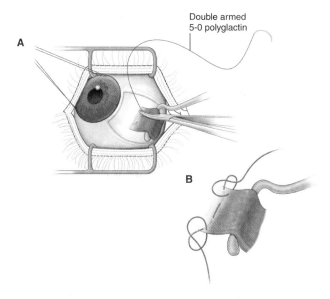

Double armed
5-0 polyglactin

A

B

Figure 31.2. Placing the suture. (A) A double-armed 5-0 or 6-0 absorbable suture is placed 1 mm posterior to the muscle insertion in the middle of the width of the muscle. (B) The double-armed suture is passed within the muscle and exited at the muscle border, but 2 mm from the edge of the muscle and locked onto itself on both borders.

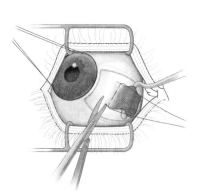

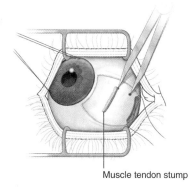

Muscle tendon stump

Figure 31.3. Blunt-tipped Westcott scissors are placed in between the muscle insertion and suture line to disinsert the muscle.

Figure 31.4. The planned amount of recession is marked onto the sclera.

COMPLICATIONS

- Hemorrhage
- Infection
- Scleral perforation
- Under- or overcorrection
- Diplopia
- Lost muscle

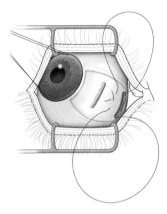
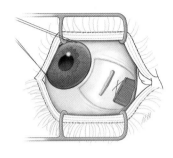

Figure 31.5. The spatula needles are passed into the partial-thickness sclera at the premarked points.

Figure 31.6. The muscle sutures are tied.

- Anterior segment ischemic syndrome
- Change in eyelid position
- Malignant hyperthermia
- Bradycardia caused by oculocardiac reflex

Hemorrhage is usually insignificant.

Infection (uncommon) includes suture abscesses, preseptal or orbital cellulitis, and endophthalmitis. The latter may be related to accidental scleral perforation. Scleral perforation is usually caused by a needle track. Incidence can be minimized by using spatula needles and wearing surgical loupes.

Under- or overcorrections are the most common complication of strabismus surgery. Undercorrection is more common than overcorrection. Poor fusion, amblyopia, and contracture of scar tissue can be underlying causes.

Diplopia can be treated with prisms, Botox injection, or additional surgery.

Lost muscle can be managed at the time of surgery by pulling the muscle sleeve of the retracted muscle in Tenon's capsule in a "hand over hand" fashion, bringing the muscle into view. Occasionally, reoperation may be required for exploration and retrieval of the lost muscle. Use of a headlamp can minimize the surgical manipulation and trauma.

Anterior segment ischemic syndrome can be caused by simultaneous surgery on 3 rectus muscles (or on 2 rectus muscles in patients with poor blood flow), as the blood supply of the anterior segment comes from the anterior ciliary arteries running in the rectus muscles. The syndrome is characterized by corneal edema, iris neovascularization, iris atrophy, and hypotony. The incidence of anterior segment ischemic syndrome may be reduced by performing surgery simultaneously on fewer than 3 muscles or sparing the anterior ciliary vessels during rectus muscle recession/resection.

Change in eyelid position can occur with surgery on vertical rectus muscles (muscle recession: pushing eyelid posteriorly and exposing bare sclera; muscle resection: pulling eyelid anteriorly and narrowing eyelid fissure). This is reduced by careful dissection of intermuscular membrane and connective tissue between the eyelids and associated vertical rectus muscles.

Malignant hyperthermia can be triggered by anesthetic agents including halothane, enflurane, and succinylcholine. Early signs include tachycardia, arrhythmia, unstable blood pressure, masseter spasm, and elevated CO_2 level. Later signs include temperature rise, respiratory and metabolic acidosis, and renal and heart failure. The treatment is to discontinue anesthetic agents, hyperventilate with oxygen, administer dantrolene, cool the patient, and monitor vital signs.

Bradycardia during extraocular muscle surgery is caused by traction on extraocular muscles intraoperatively. It is treated with intravenous atropine or release of the extraocular muscle.

Chapter 32

Resection of Extraocular Rectus Muscle

Rudolph S. Wagner, MD
Suqin Guo, MD

Muscle resection is used to strengthen or increase the effect of an extraocular muscle. It can be used unilaterally, bilaterally, or combined with muscle recession. The resection technique is commonly used on all rectus muscle. Muscle resection should be avoided in restrictive strabismus, such as Duane syndrome, dysthyroidism, or orbital trauma.

INSTRUMENTATION AND SUPPLIES

- Forceps: Castroviejo suture forceps 0.12 mm, 0.3 mm, or 0.5 mm; Stern-Castroviejo locking forceps 0.5 mm (for fornix-based approach)
- Westcott scissors with blunt tips
- Barraquer eye speculum with solid or wire blades
- Curved-jaw needle holder
- Caliper
- Muscle hooks (Jameson, Culler, Stevens, or Green)
- 4-0 silk suture
- 5-0 or 6-0 absorbable (Vicryl) suture, double-armed, with spatula needles
- 6-0 plain gut suture
- Hartman or Prince muscle clamp

SURGICAL PROCEDURE

1. This procedure is usually done under general anesthesia.
2. Prep and drape.
3. Place a 4-0 silk traction suture through the conjunctiva (at the 6 and 12 o'clock limbus for surgery on the horizontal recti and at 3 and 9 o'clock for vertical rectus surgery).
4. Create a limbal peritomy incision with Westcott scissors and 0.12 forceps. Alternatively, a fornix incision may be used.
5. Reflect the conjunctival-Tenon's layer and dissect the intermuscular membrane to expose bare sclera posterior to each side of the muscle insertion. The muscle capsule should be left intact on the muscle tendon.
6. Insert a large Jameson muscle hook at the muscle insertion.
7. Insert a second Jameson hook posteriorly under the muscle, acting as a retractor.
8. Use a caliper to mark the location of the planned resection, and place a double-armed 5-0 or 6-0 absorbable suture at the center of the full-thickness muscle belly (Figure 32 .1).
9. Pass each arm of the suture within the muscle and exit at the muscle border. Then place a locking bite of full muscle thickness on each side of the muscle border (Figure 32.2).
10. Place a Hartman or Prince clamp anterior to the suture line. Excise the muscle anterior to the clamp (Figure 32.3).
11. Remove the remaining muscle from its insertion with a blunt Westcott scissors, keeping a 1 mm stump of tendon (Figure 32.4).
12. Place sutures at the original muscle insertion with a partial-thickness scleral pass. Then tie the sutures (Figure 32.5).
13. Close the conjunctiva with a 6-0 plain suture.

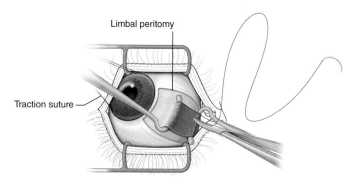

Limbal peritomy

Traction suture

Figure 32.1. After marking the site of planned resection onto the muscle, the surgeon places a double-armed 5-0 or 6-0 absorbable suture at the center of the muscle belly.

Figure 32.2. Each arm of the suture is passed into the muscle and exited at the muscle border. A locking bite of full-thickness muscle is made on each side of the muscle border.

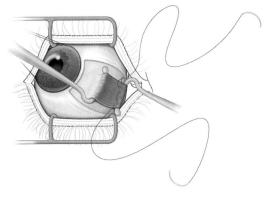

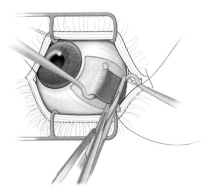

Figure 32.3. The muscle is excised anterior to the clamp and suture line.

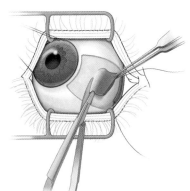

Figure 32.4. The remaining muscle segment is excised using Westcott scissors.

Figure 32.5. The spatula needles are passed under the muscle insertion. The muscle is moved anterior towards the stump and the sutures are tied.

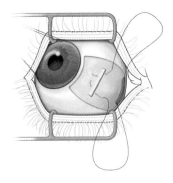

COMPLICATIONS

Refer to complications noted in Chapter 31.

Chapter 33

Adjustable Sutures for Extraocular Rectus Muscles

Rudolph S. Wagner, MD
Suqin Guo, MD

Adjustable sutures are used to improve the outcome of desired postoperative alignment with fewer operations. Their use is indicated in acquired strabismus, preoperative diplopia, reoperation, or restrictive strabismus occurring with Duane syndrome, dysthyroidism, or orbital trauma.

INSTRUMENTATION AND SUPPLIES

- Instrumentation and supplies are the same as those noted in Chapters 31 and 32.

SURGICAL PROCEDURE

1. The adjustable suture procedure is often performed on the recessed muscle. It can also be done on the resected muscle. Pass each arm of the double-armed 5-0 or 6-0 absorbable suture through the muscle stump after it is disinserted from the globe. The suture ends should emerge close together at the exit points.
2. Tie a separate sliding knot (6-0 absorbable suture) around the ends of the 5-0 absorbable sutures, sliding up and down a few times (Figure 33.1).
3. Pull the muscle forward to the insertion, and place the sliding knot at the desired distance (mm) from the muscle stump (Figure 33.2).

Figure 33.1. A sliding knot is tied around muscle sutures, sliding anteriorly and posteriorly a few times.

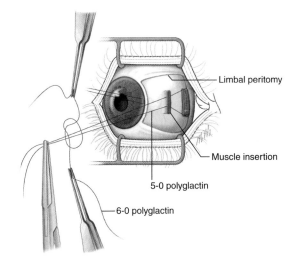

Limbal peritomy

Muscle insertion

5-0 polyglactin

6-0 polyglactin

Figure 33.2. The muscle is pulled towards the insertion, and the sliding knot is placed at the planned position (mm), measured from the muscle insertion.

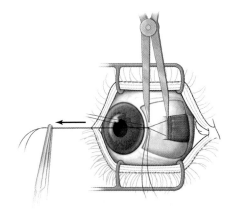

4. Reset the sliding knot back to the muscle stump, and place the muscle to the desired and recessed location (Figure 33.3).
5. Close the conjunctival over the stump with a 6-0 plain gut suture (Figure 33.4).

Postoperative Alignment Adjustment

1. The postoperative alignment is performed in the recovery room after the patient is fully awake and alert from the general anesthetic. The alignment can also be adjusted 1 to 2 days after surgery.
2. If a muscle is over-recessed (overcorrected) and needs to be advanced:
   • Pull the muscle sutures toward the cornea.
   • Move the sliding suture posteriorly to the sclera (Figure 33.5).

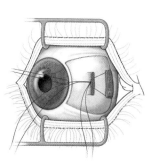

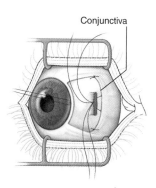

Figure 33.3. The sliding knot is moved back to the muscle stump and muscle is then placed in the planned recessed position.

Figure 33.4. The conjunctiva is closed using 6-0 plain suture.

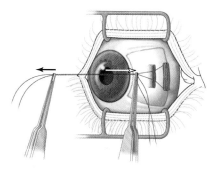

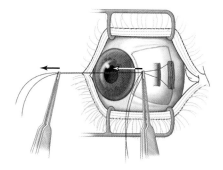

Figure 33.5. If the muscle is over-recessed, the muscle sutures are pulled towards the cornea and the sliding knot is moved posteriorly, adjusting to reach the desired alignment.

Figure 33.6. If the muscle is under-recessed, the sliding knot is pulled anteriorly towards the cornea to the desired position and placed back to the muscle stump.

- Check the alignment, tie the muscle suture, and remove all excess sutures if the alignment is as desired.
3. If a muscle is under-recessed (undercorrected) and needs to be further recessed:
   - Pull the muscle sutures toward the cornea.
   - Move the sliding suture anteriorly to the cornea (Figure 33.6).
   - Check the alignment, tie the muscle suture, and remove all excess sutures if the alignment is as desired.

COMPLICATIONS

Refer to complications noted in Chapter 31.

Chapter 34

Anteriorization of the Inferior Oblique Muscle

Rudolph S. Wagner, MD
Suqin Guo, MD

Anteriorization is a frequently performed inferior oblique muscle-weakening procedure. It may change the inferior oblique muscle from an elevator to a depressor. It can be used to treat either primary or secondary inferior oblique overaction and to correct "V" patterns. The procedure can be graded by placing the inferior oblique tendon just lateral to the inferior rectus muscle insertion, or more posteriorly for less weakening, or more anteriorly for greater effect. The procedure is usually done bilaterally and is useful in cases of inferior oblique overaction combined with dissociated vertical deviation.

INSTRUMENTATION AND SUPPLIES

- Forceps: Castroviejo suture forceps, 0.3 mm or 0.5 mm
- Westcott scissors with blunt tips
- Barraquer eye speculum—solid or wire blades
- Curved jaw Castroviejo needle holder
- Caliper
- Muscle hooks: Jameson or Green muscle hooks; small rectus muscle hooks (Culler, von Graefe, or Stevens)
- 5-0 or 6-0 absorbable suture
- 6-0 plain gut suture

SURGICAL PROCEDURE

1. This procedure is usually performed under general anesthesia.
2. Prep and drape.
3. Grasp the conjunctiva at the limbus with a 0.5 forceps in the inferior temporal quadrant, and elevate and adduct the eye.
4. Create an inferior cul-de-sac (fornix) incision with Westcott scissors and 0.3 (or 0.5) forceps parallel to the blade of the speculum about 8 mm from the limbus (Figure 34.1), then incise the intermuscular membrane inferotemporally as it is grasped with 0.3 forceps by the assistant (Figure 34.2).
5. Bare sclera is then visualized (Figure 34.3).
6. Hook the lateral rectus muscle with a Stevens hook and replace it with a Green hook. Next, pass a 4-0 silk traction suture beneath the lateral

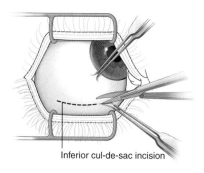

Inferior cul-de-sac incision

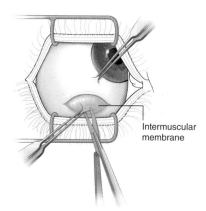

Intermuscular membrane

Figure 34.1. Creating an inferotemporal cul-de-sac or fornix incision.

Figure 34.2. Incising the intermuscular membrane.

Figure 34.3. Locating bare sclera.

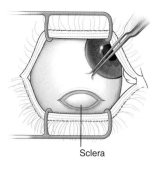

Sclera

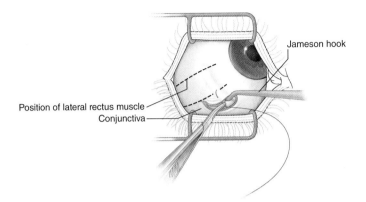

Jameson hook

Position of lateral rectus muscle
Conjunctiva

Figure 34.4. Hooking the lateral rectus muscle.

rectus muscle insertion, with the needle of the suture penetrating the conjunctiva at the superior border of the muscle (Figure 34.4).

7. Expose the inferotemporal quadrant by placing a large muscle hook through the inferior edge of the fornix incision (below the lateral rectus muscle), engaging Tenon's capsule and placing traction on it inferiorly and anteriorly. Place another muscle hook at the superior edge of the fornix incision to facilitate exposure of the inferotemporal quadrant by spreading the incision (Figure 34.5).

8. Pass a Stevens hook adjacent to the globe in the inferotemporal quadrant to engage the inferior oblique muscle. Rotate the hook 90° and elevate it, bringing the inferior oblique muscle into view (Figure 34.6).

9. Open Tenon's capsule, exposing the margins of the inferior oblique muscle (Figure 34.7).

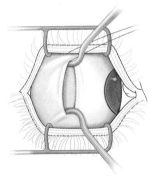

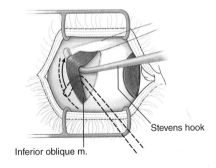

Stevens hook

Inferior oblique m.

Figure 34.5. Exposing the inferotemporal quadrant.

Figure 34.6. Hooking the inferior oblique muscle.

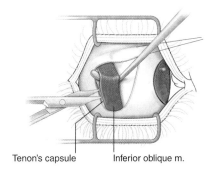

Tenon's capsule   Inferior oblique m.

Figure 34.7. Incising Tenon's capsule.

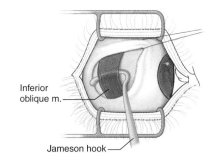

Inferior
oblique m.

Jameson hook

Figure 34.8. Isolating the inferior oblique muscle.

10. Place a Jameson hook below the muscle to create a larger opening
     (Figure 34.8).
11. Locate the insertion of the inferior oblique muscle by sliding a Jame-
     son hook toward the globe. Grasp the muscle insertion with a small
     straight clamp and disinsert the muscle with blunt Westcott scissors
     (Figure 34.9).
12. Secure the tendon with a double-armed 5-0 absorbable suture, locked
     at both sides as in rectus muscle surgery (Figure 34.10).
13. Hook the inferior rectus muscle and isolate its lateral margin
     (Figure 34.11).
14. Reattach the inferior oblique muscle to the sclera at the lateral mar-
     gin of the inferior rectus insertion with partial-thickness scleral bites
     (Figure 34.12).
15. Remove the silk traction suture and close conjunctiva with 6-0 plain
     gut suture.

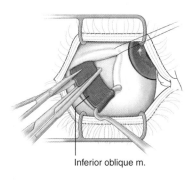

Inferior oblique m.

Figure 34.9. Disinsertion of the inferior oblique
tendon.

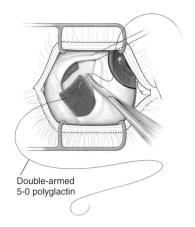

Double-armed
5-0 polyglactin

Figure 34.10. Securing the tendon with sutures.

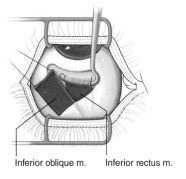

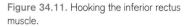

Figure 34.11. Hooking the inferior rectus muscle.

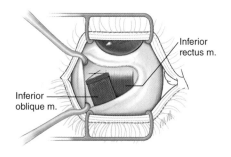

Figure 34.12. Transposing the inferior oblique muscle.

COMPLICATIONS

- Persistent or recurrent inferior oblique overaction
- Restrictive strabismus
- Laceration of the inferior temporal vortex vein
- Anti-elevation syndrome
- Complications listed for rectus muscle surgery (Chapter 31)

Persistence or recurrence of inferior oblique overaction may result from incomplete weakening; such persistence often occurs when residual posterior fibers are left intact and attached to the globe in their anatomic position.

Fat adherence resulting in restrictive strabismus occurs when Tenon's capsule is violated following blind, aggressive hooking of the inferior oblique muscle.

Laceration of the inferior temporal vortex vein can occur, resulting in excessive bleeding at the surgical site.

Excessive anterior and lateral placement of the inferior oblique muscle may result in an anti-elevation syndrome with restricted elevation in abduction.

Chapter 35

Full Tuck of the Superior Oblique Tendon

Rudolph S. Wagner, MD
Suqin Guo, MD

"Tucking" the superior oblique tendon is commonly performed to correct the extorsion, hyperdeviation, and downgaze convergence resulting from superior oblique muscle palsy or paresis.

INSTRUMENTATION AND SUPPLIES

- Forceps: Castroviejo suture forceps, 0.3 mm and 0.5 mm
- Westcott scissors with blunt tips
- Barraquer eye speculum—solid or wire blades
- Needle holder (curved and without lock)
- Caliper
- Muscle hooks: Jameson or Green muscle hooks; small rectus muscle hooks (Culler, von Graefe, or Stevens)
- 6-0 absorbable (Vicryl) suture
- 5-0 nonabsorbable (Mersilene) suture
- 6-0 plain gut suture
- Superior oblique tendon tucker (Green)

SURGICAL PROCEDURE

1. This procedure is usually performed under general anesthesia.
2. Prep and drape.

3. Create a superonasal cul-de-sac (fornix) incision by grasping the conjunctiva at the superior limbus, rotating the eye inferotemporally, and incising the superonasal conjunctiva with a Westcott scissors.
4. Secure the superior rectus muscle with a Jameson hook. Catch the superior oblique tendon with a Stevens hook about 8 mm posterior and parallel to the nasal superior rectus muscle insertion (Figure 35.1).
5. Pass a 6-0 absorbable suture below the tendon, forming a loop (Figure 35.2).
6. Pass a needle below the superior rectus muscle from its temporal aspect, grasp the free ends of the suture loop, and pull them temporally (Figure 35.3).
7. Identify the superior oblique tendon insertion (Figure 35.4).
8. Apply the tendon tucker to the superior oblique. The more lax the tendon feels, the greater the blades of the tucker are spread (total tuck range 8 to 20 mm), Figure 35.5.

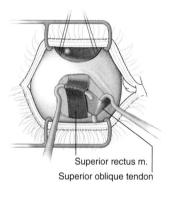

Superior rectus m.
Superior oblique tendon

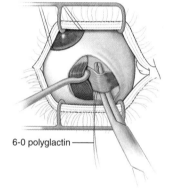

6-0 polyglactin

Figure 35.1. Hooking the superior oblique tendon medially.

Figure 35.2. Looping the superior oblique tendon with a suture.

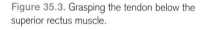

Figure 35.3. Grasping the tendon below the superior rectus muscle.

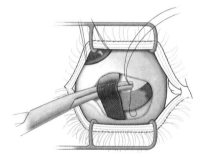

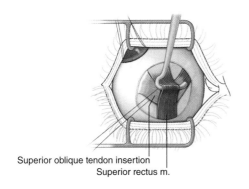

Figure 35.4. Displacing the tendon laterally.

Superior oblique tendon insertion
Superior rectus m.

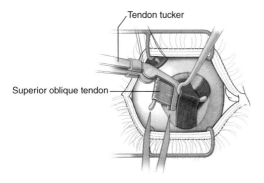

Figure 35.5. Applying the tendon tucker.

Tendon tucker

Superior oblique tendon

9. Pass a 5-0 nonabsorbable (Mersilene) suture through both sides of the tendon and tie it beneath the tucker, creating a folded tendon (Figure 35.6).

10. After removing the tucker, attach the loop of the folded tendon to the sclera temporally at the level of the original superior oblique tendon insertion (Figure 35.7).

11. Close the cul-de-sac incision with a single 6-0 plain gut suture.

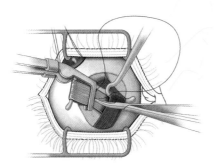

Figure 35.6. Closing the folded tendon with sutures.

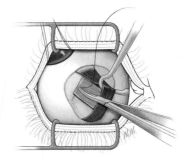

Figure 35.7. Attaching the apex of the "tucked" tendon to the sclera.

COMPLICATIONS

- Limited elevation in adduction
- Suture slippage
- Complications listed for rectus muscle surgery (Chapter 31)

Excessive tucking or advancement of the tendon loop can result in limited elevation in adduction (iatrogenic Brown syndrome).

Suture slippage can negate the effect of the procedure.

Part V

Vitreoretinal Surgery

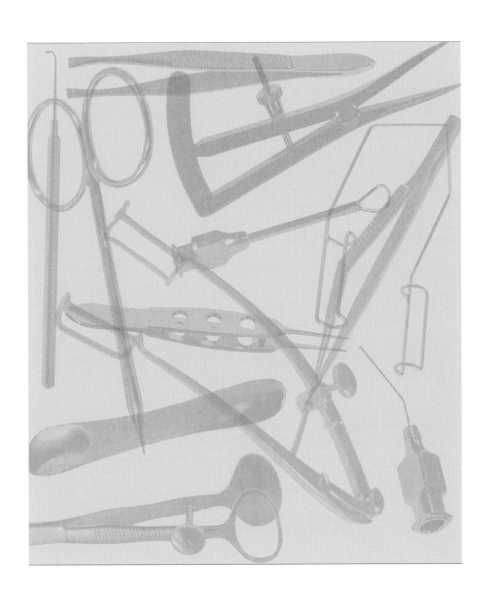

Chapter 36

Laser Photocoagulation for Macular Edema

Neelakshi Bhagat, MD, MPH, FACS
Marco A. Zarbin, MD, PhD, FACS

Laser photocoagulation is indicated for the treatment of clinically significant macular edema (CSME) associated with diabetes as well as macular edema in branch retinal vein occlusion. The decision to treat CSME with laser depends on the presence of retinal thickening on clinical examination and not solely on the presence of leakage on a fluorescein angiogram. Optical coherence tomography (OCT) can identify patients with subclinical thickening that may not be identified with biomicroscopy; however, focal laser treatment based on OCT findings alone is not recommended at this time. Consider treatment for macular edema in branch retinal vein occlusion (BRVO) if the BRVO is at least 3 months old with visual acuity 20/40 or worse and not spontaneously improving in absence of blood in the fovea or macular capillary nonperfusion.

PREOPERATIVE STEPS

1. Examine the macula with a stereoscopic contact lens.
2. Review a fluorescein angiogram less than 3 weeks old to localize precisely the leaking areas and areas of nonperfusion and to guide the laser treatment.

INSTRUMENTATION AND SUPPLIES

- Argon green (514 to 527 nm) or dye yellow laser (577 nm)
- Macular contact lens

SURGICAL PROCEDURE

1. Topical anesthesia is used.
2. Place the macular lens (magnification approximately 1.0) to identify the leakage area and landmarks.
3. For diabetic CSME:
   - Laser wavelength used: argon green or dye yellow. Check laser parameters. Spot size: 50 to 100 μm. Duration: 0.05 to 0.1 seconds. Power: as necessary to create mildly white burns (usually start with 80 mW power).
   - Identify the lesions to be treated.
     - Focal treatment: direct treatment to discrete points of leaking microaneurysms on fluorescein angiogram.
     - Grid treatment: in cases of diffuse leakage from the retinal capillary bed, place treatment in a grid pattern (50 to 200 μm spot size, burns placed 1 to 2 burn widths apart).
   - During the initial treatment, only treat lesions 500 μm or more away from the center of the macula and not at the edge of the foveal avascular zone (FAZ).
   - For follow-up treatments: if CSME persists and if vision is 20/40 or worse, consider treating the leaking lesions located 300 to 500 μm from the center of the macula.
     - Focal direct treatment (Figures 36.1A, 36.1B): apply laser spots only to the leaking lesions in thickened retina, with 50 to 100 μm spot size, 0.05 to 0.1 second duration, and enough power to create mild whitening of retinal pigment epithelium (RPE) under the treated lesion (usually start at 80 mW and titrate up).

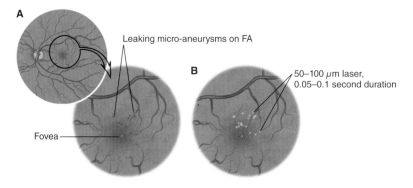

Figure 36.1. Fundus illustration, focal laser for clinically significant diabetic macular edema, noting treatment areas (A) and focal laser-treated areas with parameters (B).

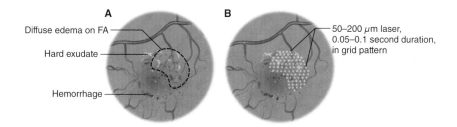

Figure 36.2. Grid laser photocoagulation for diffuse clinically significant diabetic macular edema, noting treatment area (A) and laser parameters (B).

- – Grid laser treatment (Figures 36.2A, 36.2B): apply laser spots in a grid pattern to areas of retinal thickening using 50 to 200 μm (usually 100 μm) spot size, 1 to 2 burn widths apart with 0.05 to 0.1 second (usually 0.1 second unless treating between 300 to 500 μm of FAZ center, in which case use 0.05 second and 50-μm spot size) duration. Use enough power to create mild whitening of RPE with conservative sparse treatment in the papillomacular bundle (consider using 50-μm spots in papillomacular bundle and when treating between 300 to 500 μm of FAZ center).
  - To produce resolution of retinal thickening 3 to 4 treatments (every 3 to 4 months) may be required. Obtain another fluorescein angiogram to identify treatable lesions and to assess the location of FAZ. Apply additional laser treatment to leaking lesions or in grid pattern as described above.
4. For macular edema with BRVO (Figures 36.3A, 36.B):
  - Laser wavelength used: green or yellow. Check laser parameters. Spot size: 100 μm; duration: 0.1 seconds. Power: start at approximately 80 mW and titrate up to produce mild whitening of the RPE.

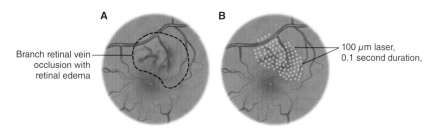

Figure 36.3. Laser photocoagulation for macular edema in an eye with branch retinal vein occlusion, noting treatment area (A) and laser parameters (B).

- Treatment may be extended up to the edge of FAZ and peripherally to the major vascular arcade (ie, 2 disc diameters from the edge of FAZ).
- Avoid direct treatment of shunt vessels and treatment of intraretinal hemorrhage.

POSTOPERATIVE CARE

1. No medications are necessary.
2. Follow up at 3 months.
3. Re-treat any treatable lesions if CSME persists.

COMPLICATIONS

- Scotomata
- Visual loss
- Inadvertent foveal burn
- Subretinal fibrosis
- Rupture of Bruch's membrane
- Choroidal neovascularization
- Choroidovitreal neovascularization
- Subretinal hemorrhage

Chapter 37

Panretinal Photocoagulation

Neelakshi Bhagat, MD, MPH, FACS
Marco A. Zarbin, MD, PhD, FACS

The goal of panretinal photocoagulation (PRP) is to induce regression of existing retinal neovascularization and prevent development of new retinal neovascularization on the disc and elsewhere in the retina, thus forestalling the development of vitreous hemorrhage or traction retinal detachment. Indications for PRP include:

- High-risk proliferative diabetic retinopathy (PDR): neovascularization on optic disc (NVD) if it covers greater than one-third of the disc area; any NVD with vitreous hemorrhage; or moderate-to-severe neovascularization elsewhere (NVE) (≥1/2 disc diameter in size) with vitreous hemorrhage (Figure 37.1A)

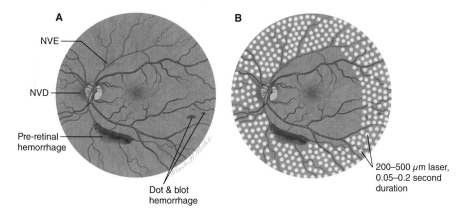

Figure 37.1. Panretinal photocoagulation. (A) Signs of proliferative diabetic retinopathy. (B) Extent of laser treatment.

207

- Patients with type II diabetes with PDR and any neovascularization, even in the absence of "high risk" characteristics
- Patients with severe nonproliferative diabetic retinopathy (NPDR) who cannot be followed regularly (for patients with bilateral severe NPDR consider treating at least 1 eye with PRP)
- Patients with nondiabetic causes of proliferative retinopathy (eg, sickle cell retinopathy, retinal venous occlusive disease, or ocular inflammatory disease such as pars planitis with NVE)

PREOPERATIVE STEPS

1. Complete a retinal examination to evaluate presence of neovascularization.

INSTRUMENTATION AND SUPPLIES

- Laser: argon green (514 to 527 nm), krypton red (647 nm), tunable dye (577 to 630 nm), or diode laser (790 to 830 nm); krypton red and diode wavelengths useful for eyes with nuclear sclerotic cataracts or vitreous hemorrhage
- Peripheral fundus lenses: Goldmann 3-mirror lens (magnification is 1:1; burn size = spot size), Rodenstock (magnification 1:2; burn size = 2 × spot size), or wide field lens (field of view: 115° to 160°; burn size = 1.9 to 2.3 x spot size [eg, Volk SuperQuad or QuadrAspheric])

SURGICAL PROCEDURE

1. Topical anesthesia is preferred unless the patient is intolerant of laser due to pain, in which case subconjunctival or retrobulbar anesthesia can be used.
2. Place the contact lens on the eye.
3. Check laser parameters. Spot size: 200 to 500 μm (500 μm for 3-mirror lens; 200 to 300 μm if using Rodenstock lens or other wide field lenses). Duration: 0.05 to 0.2 seconds (shorter duration is associated with less discomfort). Power: start at 130 mW and titrate up to produce a gray-white (not intense white) burn. Space spots 0.5 to 1 burn width from each other.

4. Consider the extent of laser treatment (indirectly reflected in the number of laser applications), Figure 37.1B:
   - PRP for PDR or retinal neovascularization associated with CRVO: apply treatment (approximately 1500 spots) over 2 sessions, extending treatment from just outside the temporal arcades to just anterior to the equator. Nasally, treatment is not brought closer than 500 μm to the optic nerve. Temporally, treatment is not brought closer than 2.5 disc diameters to the fovea.
   - Rubeosis iridis (eg, with PDR or CRVO): the laser spots should extend out to the ora serrata.
   - Sectoral photocoagulation for retinal neovascularization with BRVO: laser in the quadrant involved by the vein occlusion.

Clinical Tips

- PDR: start with the inferior periphery and then treat the superior periphery.
- Treat no closer than one-half to 1 disc diameter to the optic nerve head nasally and 2.5 disc diameters from the edge of the foveal avascular zone temporally.
- Avoid the long posterior ciliary nerves and arteries (horizontally). Treat all known areas of retinal nonperfusion. One can use intravenous fluorescein angiography to identify nonperfusion.
- Do not treat directly over retinal vessels.
- If the patient is uncomfortable, decrease the laser power and/or duration.

POSTOPERATIVE CARE

1. Topical or oral medications typically are not prescribed; however, if extensive treatment is applied (eg, rubeosis iridis with CRVO), then use prednisolone acetate 1% 4 times a day and atropine 1% twice a day as prophylaxis against development of secondary angle closure due to choroidal detachment.
2. Follow up in approximately 1 to 3 weeks.
3. Clinical response to treatment usually requires about 3 weeks. Regression is evident as a loss of the capillary brush border of the NV and development of fibrosis of the neovascularization. Separate treatment

sessions by 1 to 3 weeks. (Presence of rubeosis requires aggressive treatment, usually every week until full PRP is completed.)

COMPLICATIONS

- Inadvertent foveal burn
- Macular edema
- Constriction of peripheral visual field
- Choroidal effusion with or without associated angle-closure glaucoma
- Reduced dark adaptation
- Retinal tear formation
- Break in Bruch's membrane
- Choroidal neovascularization
- Choroidovitreal neovascularization
- Anterior segment ischemia in predisposed individuals (eg, sickle cell disease), particularly if treatment is extensive and if long posterior ciliary arteries are occluded
- Iridocyclitis if treatment is "heavy" or extensive
- Cataract
- Iris burns

Chapter 38

Demarcation Laser Photocoagulation for Retinal Tears

Neelakshi Bhagat, MD, MPH, FACS
Marco A. Zarbin, MD, PhD, FACS

Demarcation laser photocoagulation for retina tears can be used in the treatment of a retinal break, a retinal break with subclinical retinal detachment, or a retinal dialysis (with or without symptoms).

PREOPERATIVE STEPS

1. Perform a meticulous retinal examination to diagnose and locate all retinal breaks, using indirect ophthalmoscopy with scleral depression as well as a 3-mirror contact lens exam if needed (Figure 38.1A).

INSTRUMENTATION AND SUPPLIES

- Laser: argon green (514 to 527 nm), krypton red (647 nm), tunable dye (577 to 630 nm), or diode laser (790 to 830 nm)
- 20-, 28-, or 30-D lens
- Wide-angle viewing fundus contact lens (eg, Rodenstock or Goldmann 3-mirror lens)

SURGICAL PROCEDURES

Contact Lens Delivery System

1. Wavelength: argon green; however, if moderate or severe nuclear sclerotic cataract or vitreous hemorrhage is present, use krypton or diode laser, which may penetrate better and give better uptake at the level of retinal pigment epithelium-choroid.
2. Topical anesthesia is used.
3. Surround the retinal break with 3 to 5 rows of confluent laser applications using a spot size of 200 to 500 μm (200 μm with Rodenstock or wide-angle lenses and 500 μm with a 3-mirror lens), duration 0.05 to 0.2 seconds, and power to achieve a moderately white burn (Figure 38.1B).
4. If there is difficulty getting laser uptake, confirm there is no subretinal fluid present.
5. If the tear is too peripheral and the anterior edge cannot be reached using the Rodenstock lens, try the 3-mirror lens or consider switching to indirect laser delivery. If there is media opacity that precludes adequate uptake of the laser, transscleral cryopexy may be needed.

Indirect Laser Photocoagulation

1. Examine and locate the peripheral retinal tear(s).
2. Use a scleral depressor to position the edge of the tear at the tip of depression.

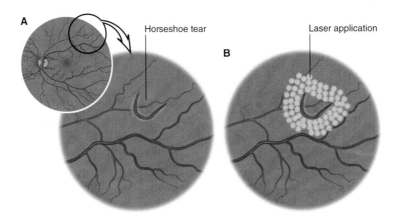

Figure 38.1. Laser demarcation of a retinal tear, showing a horseshoe-shaped tear (A) and pattern of laser application (B).

3. Use a 20-, 28-, or 30-D lens to deliver 3 to 5 rows of confluent laser around the edges of the tear.

4. Typical parameters: argon green or krypton red (in the presence of cataract or vitreous hemorrhage); duration 0.15 to 0.2 seconds; power titrate from 200 mW upwards to get a moderate white laser spot.

5. This delivery system is more painful than the contact lens method and may need to be given at a slower pace. Retrobulbar anesthesia may be needed in rare patients. Usually, topical or subconjunctival anesthesia suffices.

6. For retinal breaks located anterior to the equator, be sure to extend treatment to the ora serrata in the meridian of the tear. Also, extend treatment for one-half to 1 clock hour lateral to the anterior margins of the tear.

POSTOPERATIVE CARE

1. Usually no topical medications are given.

2. Restrict activity (vitreous fluid currents associated with eye movement may promote development of retinal detachment).

3. After the procedure, firm adhesion between neurosensory retina and retinal pigment epithelium takes 7 to 12 days to achieve. Consider double patching to reduce subretinal fluid, if any, before and after the procedure. (The treatment area may be much reduced with less morbidity.)

4. Follow up 1 week after treatment.

5. Patients should follow up emergently if new symptoms of photopsia, floaters, or decreased peripheral or central vision are noted.

COMPLICATIONS

- Failure to surround retinal break adequately, which can lead to retinal detachment
- Inadvertent treatment of the fovea
- Retinal perforation
- Choroidal rupture
- Vitreous hemorrhage
- Anterior segment ischemia if peripheral laser treatment is extensive (particularly if long posterior ciliary arteries are closed by treatment)

Chapter 39

Thermal Laser Photocoagulation for Extrafoveal Choroidal Neovascularization

Neelakshi Bhagat, MD, MPH, FACS
Marco A. Zarbin, MD, PhD, FACS

Thermal laser photocoagulation is indicated for well-defined (classic) extrafoveal choroidal neovascular membranes (the foveal edge of choroidal neovascularization [CNV] is 200 to 2500 μm from the center of the foveal avascular zone [FAZ]).

PREOPERATIVE STEPS

1. Examine the macula with a stereoscopic contact lens (Figure 39.1A).
2. Acquire a fluorescein angiogram and color fundus photographs ≤72 hours old to localize the CNV precisely and to guide the application of laser burns during treatment.

INSTRUMENTATION AND SUPPLIES

- Krypton red or argon green laser
- Macular contact lens

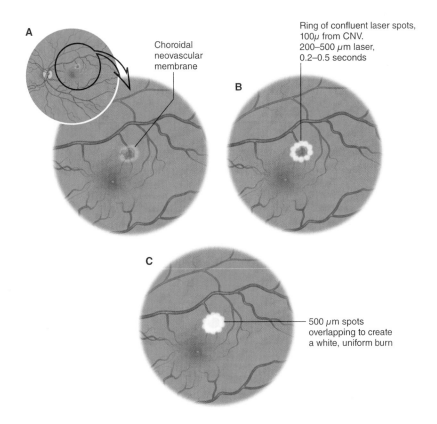

Figure 39.1. Thermal laser photocoagulation of an extrafoveal choroidal neovascular membrane (CNV). (A) CNV. (B) Ring of laser spots outlining CNV. (C) Overlapping laser spots covering CNV.

SURGICAL PROCEDURE

1. Review the fluorescein angiogram (≤72 hours old) before the treatment.
2. Anesthesia: topical anesthesia is preferred unless the patient has difficulty maintaining steady fixation, in which case retrobulbar anesthesia is recommended.
3. Place the macular contact lens (magnification approximately 1.0) to identify the leakage area and landmarks.
4. Check laser parameters. Spot size: 200 to 500 μm. Duration: 0.2 to 0.5 seconds. Power: as necessary to create uniform, intense, white burns.
5. Identify a 100 μm border around the edge of CNV (or hemorrhage) and create an outline with a 200 μm laser spot (ie, cover 100 μm beyond the leaking edge of the CNV) if the foveal edge of the CNV is ≥300 μm from the foveal center (Figure 39.1B). Fill in the area

outlined using 500 μm spots in an overlapping fashion to create uniform, intense, white burns (Figure 39.1C). At the foveal edge, if CNV is less than 300 μm from the center of the FAZ, simply cover the CNV.

POSTOPERATIVE CARE

1. No medications are necessary.
2. Consider follow up at 3 and 6 weeks; 3, 6, 9, and 12 months; and every 6 months thereafter.
3. Obtain a fluorescein angiogram at each visit and re-treat if persistence or recurrence is present. (Persistence: leakage of fluorescein at edge of CNV within 6 weeks of initial treatment; recurrence: leakage of fluorescein at the edge of the treatment scar more than 6 weeks after treatment.)

COMPLICATIONS

- Inadvertent foveal burn (in the setting of extra- or juxtafoveal CNV)
- Visual loss
- Central scotoma
- Rupture of Bruch's membrane
- Retinal or choroidal hemorrhage
- Retinal pigment epithelium
- Choroidovitreal neovascularization

Chapter 40

Photodynamic Therapy of Choroidal New Vessels

Jennifer I. Lim, MD

Photodynamic therapy (PDT) of choroidal new vessels (CNV) is indicated for the treatment of subfoveal predominantly classic CNV lesions in patients with age-related macular degeneration, subfoveal CNV lesions in patients with high myopia or ocular histoplasmosis, or juxtafoveal CNV lesions in which the treating physician believes laser photocoagulation would result in foveal damage.

PREOPERATIVE STEPS

1. Dilate the pupil.
2. Obtain a fluorescein angiogram (FA).
3. Calculate the greatest linear dimension (GLD) of the CNV lesion based upon the FA (correct for magnification factor as needed).
4. Calculate the laser treatment spot size (GLD + 1000 μm = spot size).
5. Weigh the patient and measure the patient's height.
6. Calculate the body surface area (BSA) in meters squared for the patient as the verteporfin dose is dependent on the BSA.
7. Prepare the patient's arm for the intravenous (IV) injection of verteporfin. It is prudent to use a large vein such as the antecubital vein instead of the small hand veins.

INSTRUMENTATION AND SUPPLIES

- IV catheter and IV fluids (D_5W)
- IV pump and filter
- PDT laser machine (689 nm)
- Syringe (30 cc) for IV pump and drug
- Verteporfin dye and sterile water for mixing the solution
- 5-cc syringe filled with 5% dextrose for flushing verteporfin dye at the end of infusion
- Topical anesthetic eye drops (proparacaine)
- Macular contact lens (magnification approximately 1.0 to 1.5; eg, Mainster wide field lens)

SURGICAL PROCEDURE

1. Reconstitute the verteporfin (green powder in vial) with 7 mL sterile water to yield 7.5 mg/mL.
2. Calculate the verteporfin dose needed (based upon the patient's BSA). Draw up the required verteporfin dose from the reconstituted vial.
3. Dilute the verteporfin drug using 5% dextrose to create a total infusion volume of 30 mL.
4. Set the laser to the calculated treatment spot size (GLD + 1000 μm), Figure 40.1.

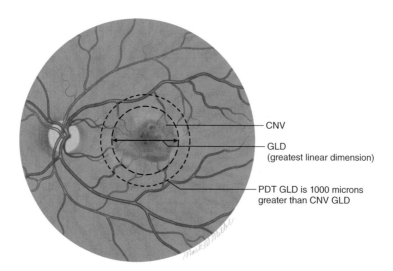

Figure 40.1. Calculating the area of treatment.

5. Infuse the drug intravenously using an IV pump (3 mL/minute rate) set for 10 minutes duration. Start the timer (900 seconds) on the laser.
6. Monitor the infusion site for any site of extravasation. If extravasation is noted, stop infusion. If more than half of the drug has been injected, proceed with the treatment. If less than half has been infused, start another IV and continue infusion. Apply cold packs to the affected area.
7. Push sterile D_5W through the IV line until it is cleared of drug at the end of 10 minutes.
8. Position the patient's head on the laser machine chin rest.
9. Apply the contact lens.
10. Turn on the slit lamp on the diode laser ($50J/cm^2$ light dose with intensity at 600 mW/cm^2).
11. Check the laser settings on the diode laser.
12. Switch the diode laser to the on position (15 minutes after the start of the infusion). (The timer should go off.)
13. Treat the lesion 5 minutes after the end of the verteporfin infusion.
14. Depress the pedal to deliver the laser.
15. Using the aiming beam, ensure that the treatment area overlies/encircles the CNV lesion.
16. Treat for 83 seconds.
17. Remove the lens from the corneal surface and rinse.

POSTOPERATIVE CARE

1. Advise the patient to avoid exposure of skin and eyes to direct sunlight or bright indoor light for 5 days.
2. Advise the patient to wear sunglasses, broad brimmed hat, long sleeve pants and shirt, and scarf to prevent skin exposure to sunlight immediately after treatment. Inform the patient that sunblock will not protect the patient from infrared sunlight, which can activate the dye and cause a burn.
3. Consider repeat treatment in 3 months if leakage or CNV growth is present on the FA.

COMPLICATIONS

- Acute severe visual acuity decrease
- Extravasation of verteporfin dye
- Infusion-related back pain
- Skin burns

Acute severe visual acuity decrease is equivalent to a decrease of 20 or more letters within 7 days of the treatment. Obtain FA to check for choroidal hypoperfusion. There is no proven therapy for this complication of treatment. Use of lower fluence (eg, 25 mJ) might help reduce likelihood of the complication, but this potential benefit has not been studied in clinical trials. Vision may spontaneously improve but not fully recover over 6 weeks.

Infusion-related back pain usually subsides in a few minutes. If severe, then evaluate the patient for any signs of other systemic illness. Otherwise, apply PDT treatment.

Skin burns are related to postoperative sunlight activation of dye. Refer the patient to a dermatologist for care of the burn.

Chapter 41

Retinal Cryopexy

Neelakshi Bhagat, MD, MPH, FACS
Marco A. Zarbin, MD, PhD, FACS

Retinal cryopexy, also known as retinal cryotherapy, is indicated in the treatment of peripheral retinal tears (especially in the presence of media opacities), the prophylaxis of selected retinal areas of abnormal vitreoretinal adhesion (eg, lattice degeneration) in selected cases, and the treatment of selected peripheral retinal tumors and vascular malformations (eg, Coats disease, retinal capillary hemangioma, or vasoproliferative tumor).

PREOPERATIVE STEPS

1. Perform a meticulous retinal examination.
2. Dilate the pupil (eg, cyclopentolate 1% + phenylephrine 2.5%).

INSTRUMENTATION AND SUPPLIES

- Indirect ophthalmoscope with 20- and 28-D lenses
- Cryosurgical unit with a transscleral retinal cryoprobe
- Lid speculum
- Lidocaine 1% or 2%
- Tuberculin syringe
- 30-gauge needle

SURGICAL PROCEDURES

Treatment of Retinal Breaks

1. Localize all retinal breaks using an indirect ophthalmoscope, a scleral depressor, and an indirect condensing lens.
2. Test the cryoprobe to check if a temperature of −60°C to −80°C can be achieved, and verify that the tip of the probe freezes and forms an iceball. (Generally, the nitrogen tank gas pressure must be 600 to 700 torr to achieve this degree of probe cooling.)
3. Anesthesia: subconjunctival lidocaine 1% or 2% to the cryo site or, rarely, retrobulbar anesthesia. (Even for treatment in all 4 quadrants, subconjunctival anesthesia usually suffices.)
4. Apply the cryoprobe directly on the conjunctiva over the retinal break so that the tip is perpendicular to globe.
5. Use the indirect ophthalmoscope to visualize the fundus (Figure 41.1A); indent the sclera with the cryoprobe tip so that the edge of the retinal tear is positioned on the indented tip.
6. Activate the cryotherapy unit by depressing the foot pedal.
7. Terminate the cryo-application as soon as retinal pigment epithelium–retina whitening is observed through the ophthalmoscope. Wait for the whitening to dissipate, and move on to a contiguous area at the edge of the break (Figure 41.1B).
8. If whitening is not observed after a few seconds of depressing the foot pedal, stop and confirm the position of the probe tip. Also, check to

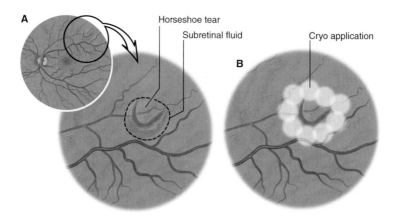

Figure 41.1. Cryopexy of a retinal tear. (A) Visualizing the retinal tear. (B) Retinal whitening due to cryo application.

see if the machine is working (eg, check the gas pressure, make sure the probe is inserted properly into the cryo unit, and make sure the cryo unit is activated).

9. Overlap the cryo marks slightly. Surround the breaks with a single freeze-thaw (1 to 2 mm of treatment). If the break is anterior to the equator, extend treatment to the ora serrata in the meridian of the break.

Cryopexy for Predisposing Lesions and Retinal Vascular Lesions

1. Lattice degeneration with atrophic holes: use the same procedure as in "Treatment of Retinal Breaks" in this chapter unless large areas are to be treated, in which case consider using laser treatment instead. Also, retrobulbar anesthesia may be needed.

2. Peripheral vascular tumors and vascular malformations (eg, retinal capillary hemangioma and Coats disease), Figure 41.2A: treat the entire lesion, tumor, or malformation with contiguous cryopexy lesions (Figure 41.2B). If significant leakage is still noted 6 weeks after the initial treatment, re-treat with cryopexy.

POSTOPERATIVE CARE

1. Prescribe Pred Forte 1% 4 times a day for 5 days and Cyclogyl 2% twice a day for 3 days.

2. Prescribe analgesic (eg, Percocet 5/325 for 2 days).

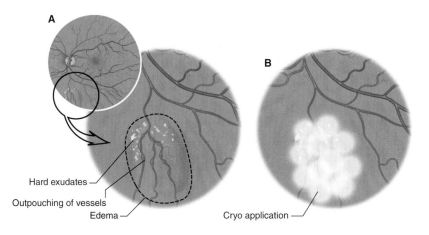

Figure 41.2. Cryopexy of a vascular tumor. (A) Fundus illustration of vascular tumor with retinal edema. (B) Area and extent of cryo application.

3. For horseshoe tears, restrict activity for 2 weeks.

4. Follow up at 1 and 3 weeks after treatment and thereafter as required.

COMPLICATIONS

- Incomplete treatment of the retinal break
- Vitreous hemorrhage
- Conjunctival hemorrhage, chemosis, or laceration
- Ablatio fugax

If treatment of the retinal break is incomplete, typically the antero-lateral margins of the break are not treated adequately in such a case.

Ablatio fugax (exudative retinal detachment) can occur after treatment of retinal capillary hemangiomata.

Chapter 42

Posterior Sub-Tenon's Injections

Christina Flaxel, MD

Posterior sub-Tenon's injections are used in several settings:

- To administer drugs, generally a corticosteroid, to the posterior segment of the eye (Figure 42.1). Triamcinolone acetonide is the most commonly administered drug; however, other corticosteroids may be used, such as betamethasone, dexamethasone, or methylprednisolone.
- To treat inflammatory conditions that do not respond to topical corticosteroid administration. These conditions include intermediate uveitis (eg, pars planitis), posterior uveitis, and cystoid macular edema after cataract surgery.
- To treat isolated ocular inflammation if systemic anti-inflammatory medications are inadequate or not tolerated (eg, unilateral cystoid macular edema in a patient with sarcoidosis who is on the maximum tolerated dose of systemic anti-inflammatory therapy).

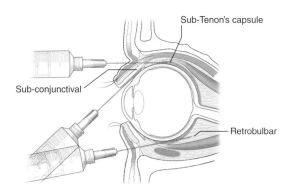

Sub-Tenon's capsule

Sub-conjunctival

Retrobulbar

Figure 42.1. Illustration showing the subconjunctival, sub-Tenon's, and retrobulbar spaces.

PREOPERATIVE STEPS

1. The surgeon should understand the epibulbar anatomy to avoid injury to extraocular muscles and their insertions as well as to avoid damage to the globe (eg, perforation) or optic nerve (if a 1.5-inch needle is used).

INSTRUMENTATION AND SUPPLIES

- 27-gauge 1/2-inch or 25-gauge 5/8-inch needle
- 1-cc tuberculin syringe or 3-cc syringe
- Cotton-tipped applicators
- Lid speculum (optional, depending on technique)
- Corticosteroid
- Anesthesia (see "Surgical Procedure")

SURGICAL PROCEDURE

1. Shake well and draw triamcinolone or other corticosteroid into the syringe using a large-bore needle (eg, 18 gauge). Push the plunger until the syringe has the desired volume of medication; 0.5 to 1 mL may be injected. For triamcinolone, the standard dosage is 20 to 40 mg per injection.
2. Anesthesia:
   - Topical drops, such as proparacaine 0.5%, or
   - Topical anesthetic drops followed by a cotton-tipped applicator soaked in topical anesthesia, placed under the eyelid at the site of the planned injection for 1 to 5 minutes, or
   - Topical Xylocaine gel applied in the inferior fornix.
3. Place a drop of povidone-iodine into the fornix (optional).
4. A lid speculum may be used for a superior sub-Tenon's injection; it is optional for an orbital floor injection.
5. For superior sub-Tenon's corticosteroid injection:
   - Using the 27-gauge 1/2-inch or 25-gauge 5/8-inch needle, bevel down, enter the sub-Tenon's space close to the fornix (within several millimeters).
   - Advance the needle, following the curvature of the globe, using frequent, small, lateral movements to ensure that the needle does not enter the globe (Figure 42.2). The needle should freely move in

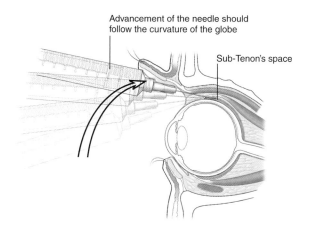

Advancement of the needle should follow the curvature of the globe

Sub-Tenon's space

Figure 42.2. Advancement of the needle using frequent, small, lateral movements.

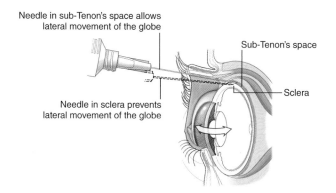

Needle in sub-Tenon's space allows lateral movement of the globe

Sub-Tenon's space

Sclera

Needle in sclera prevents lateral movement of the globe

Figure 42.3. The needle's movement indicating its location in sclera or the sub-Tenon's space.

the sub-Tenon's space. If the sclera is penetrated, the needle will not move freely, and the globe will rotate with the lateral motion of the needle (Figure 42.3).

- If scleral engagement occurs, pull back slightly and then advance slowly again.

6. For orbital floor, retroseptal corticosteroid injection:
   - Using the 27-gauge 1/2-inch or 25-gauge 5/8-inch needle, either through the eyelid or through the conjunctiva (preferred) with the bevel of the needle up, entering in the outer one-third of the lower lid or fornix, advance the needle below the globe to its full length.
   - Ask the patient to look right and left to make sure the globe has not been penetrated or caught with the needle. If there is suspicion that the globe is engaged, pull back again and advance slowly.
   - Palpate the globe through the lids to monitor the IOP. A rock-hard globe may indicate intraocular injection and central retinal artery occlusion.

7. Pull back the plunger to ensure the injection is not in an intravascular space.
8. Inject the corticosteroid so that the depot is close to the globe.
9. Withdraw the needle and, if necessary, apply pressure at the injection site with a cotton-tipped applicator to achieve hemostasis.
10. Remove the lid speculum.

POSTOPERATIVE CARE

1. Usually no topical medications are given. One may also patch and give oral Tylenol for comfort if needed.
2. The patient may apply an icepack for 1 to 2 hours after the injection, as there may be mild lower lid edema with the inferior orbital floor injection.

COMPLICATIONS

- Ptosis of upper lid (with superior injection)
- Scarring with restriction of eye movement
- Subconjunctival hemorrhage
- Globe perforation with inadvertent injection of medication intraocularly
- Chronically high IOP
- Cataract

Globe perforation with inadvertent injection of medication intraocularly is the most serious of the complications listed. Generally, no treatment is necessary unless the retina is perforated or the globe ruptures, but it is wise to do a dilated retinal examination or obtain a retina specialist's opinion. The patient will need close monitoring to follow IOPs and may need pars plana vitrectomy with removal of intravitreal corticosteroid for chronically elevated IOP unresponsive to the maximum tolerated dose of medical therapy.

Cataract associated with a sub-Tenon's injection is usually corticosteroid-induced following repeated injection. Occasionally, it is associated with lens damage during injection.

Chapter 43

Intravitreal Injections

Neelakshi Bhagat, MD, MPH, FACS
Marco A. Zarbin, MD, PhD, FACS

Intravitreal injections are commonly used to administer intravitreal antibiotics for endophthalmitis, intravitreal anti-VEGF medications for choroidal neovascularization, and intravitreal corticosteroid for macular edema due to retinal vascular disease.

PREOPERATIVE STEPS

1. Complete a retinal evaluation and a scleral-depressed, peripheral retinal examination.
2. Obtain ultrasonography of the posterior segment to identify retinal detachment or choroidal detachment if there is no view of the fundus (eg, in endophthalmitis).

INSTRUMENTATION AND SUPPLIES

- Indirect ophthalmoscope and 20-D lens
- Lid speculum (preferably wire-type)
- Povidone-iodine swabs
- Tuberculin syringes with 30-gauge needles
- Intravitreal medications, each in a separate tuberculin syringe with a 30-gauge needle

- Sterile eye drapes (elective)
- Topical antibiotics and topical anesthetic

SURGICAL PROCEDURE

1. Place topical anesthetic drops. In lieu of or in addition to topical drops, one can place sterile lidocaine 2% gel. (Generally, it is easiest to administer the gel after the lid speculum is in place—Step 2.) Alternatively, one can use (1) a pledget soaked in anesthetic against the site of injection for 2 minutes or (2) a subconjunctival injection of lidocaine 2% without epinephrine (also easiest to administer after Step 2).
2. Place the lid speculum.
3. Prep the eyelids and the conjunctiva with povidone-iodine (Betadine) swabs. If lidocaine gel is administered, one can use the swab to displace the gel from the conjunctival surface. One can then repeat administration of topical povidone-iodine. Wait for the Betadine to dry before proceeding (usually serveral minutes).
4. Use a sterile caliper or the blunt end of a sterile tuberculin syringe (approximately 4 mm) to mark the location of the injection site (3 mm from limbus in a pseudophakic/aphakic eye or 4 mm from the limbus in a phakic eye), Figures 43.1A, 43.1B.
5. Prepare the volume to be given (usually 0.05 to 0.1 mL).

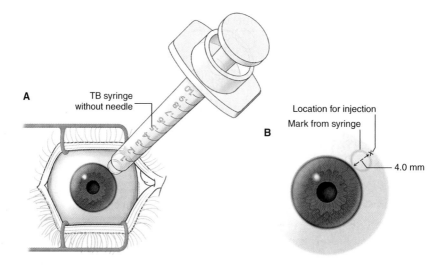

Figure 43.1. Using the blunt end of tuberculin syringe (A) to mark the location of the injection site (B).

6. Use a 30-gauge needle for the injection at a marked location on the pars plana. The needle tip should enter perpendicular to the sclera (Figure 43.2).
   • If a vitreous biopsy is to be done (eg, for endophthalmitis), it is performed before the intravitreal injection is given.
   • After 3 or 4 mm is marked from the limbus, a 26-gauge needle (3/8-inch) on tuberculin syringe is used to aspirate vitreous fluid. The amount aspirated usually depends on the volume to be injected. If the vitreous is not syneretic, one may not aspirate any fluid ("dry tap").
   • Alternatively, use a bedside portable vitrector (eg, Intrector, Insight Instruments, Stuart, Florida) instead of a needle for vitreous biopsy. The tip of the vitrector has a 23-gauge, sharp blade to traverse the conjunctiva and sclera in a smooth manner; the vitrectomy probe is connected to a short length of tubing that is attached a tuberculin syringe. Use the sharp tip to enter the eye at the marked site (Figure 43.3). Activate the

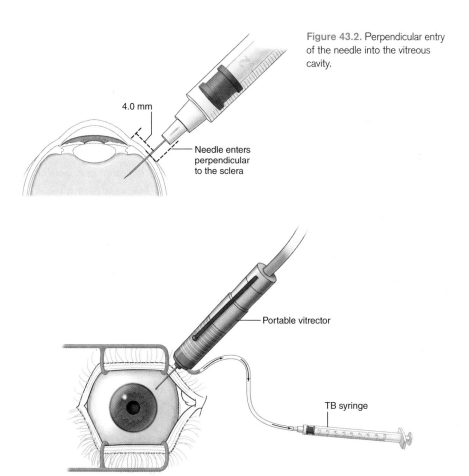

4.0 mm

Needle enters perpendicular to the sclera

Figure 43.2. Perpendicular entry of the needle into the vitreous cavity.

Portable vitrector

TB syringe

Figure 43.3. Vitreous biopsy using a 23-gauge portable vitrector.

vitrector using the switch on the handpiece and aspirate the cut vitreous into the tuberculin syringe; next, remove the vitrector from the eye. Use a sterile cotton-tipped swab against the entrance site and rub the conjunctiva over it gently to prevent any fluid outflow from the vitreous cavity and extrusion of vitreous from the wound.

7. Remove the speculum.

8. Place a drop of antibiotic solution.

9. Examine the fundus with indirect ophthalmoscopy to confirm the perfusion of the central retinal artery and to assess any complications (vitreous hemorrhage, retinal tear, or detachment).

10. Check the IOP 15 to 30 minutes after the injection. Treat with glaucoma medications if the IOP remains 25 to 35 mm Hg, or consider performing paracentesis if the IOP remains >35 mm Hg 1 hour after the injection.

POSTOPERATIVE CARE

1. Prescribe topical antibiotic (the frequency ranges from 4 times a day to every hour while awake, depending on the surgeon's choice) for 3 days unless one is treating endophthalmitis, in which case long-term topical and systemic antibiotics may be used.

2. Recommend an analgesic such as ibuprofen or extra-strength acetaminophen (usually a non-narcotic analgesic is sufficient).

3. For intravitreal injections to treat conditions other than endophthalmitis (eg, Kenalog for macular edema, anti-VEGF medication for AMD), one can follow up in 3 to 7 days; however, for patients with endophthalmitis, the follow-up examination usually is the next day.

COMPLICATIONS

- Endophthalmitis
- Vitreous hemorrhage
- Central artery occlusion
- Retinal tear
- Retinal detachment
- Choroidal hemorrhage
- Subconjunctival hemorrhage and chemosis
- Sterile endophthalmitis in the case of triamcinolone (Kenalog) injection
- Cataract

Chapter 44

Anterior Vitrectomy

Neelakshi Bhagat, MD, MPH, FACS
Marco A. Zarbin, MD, PhD, FACS

Anterior vitrectomy is indicated for the management of vitreous loss during cataract surgery. The goal is to excise enough vitreous to avoid vitreous prolapse anterior to the plane of the iris diaphragm.

INSTRUMENTATION AND SUPPLIES

- Vitrectomy suction/cutting instrumentation
- 23-gauge butterfly infusion needle
- Fiber-optic light source
- Cyclodialysis spatula
- Acetylcholine chloride (Miochol-E)
- Cellulose sponge

SURGICAL PROCEDURE

1. Once capsular rupture is encountered at the time of cataract surgery and once the decision has been made that an anterior vitrectomy is indicated, take all instruments out of the eye to set up anterior vitrectomy. One should consider lowering the infusion pressure (bottle height) and infusing viscoelastic material into the anterior chamber to prevent hydraulic forces from enlarging a lens capsular tear, if present.

2. Decide to use the cataract incision (limbal approach) or the pars plana approach to perform vitrectomy. (Pars plana vitrectomy is described in Chapter 47.) The limbal approach is described below.

3. Insert the vitrectomy probe through the cataract incision into the center of pupillary space, keeping the probe in the anterior one-third of the vitreous cavity.

4. Make sure the cutting port is in view at all times.

5. There are 2 options for infusion, a sleeve or a second instrument.
   - Sleeve: enlarge the limbal incision, if necessary, since the sleeve delivers infusion fluid and vitreous removal through a single incision. Since the infusion is next to the cutting port, it can push the vitreous away from the probe tip and opposes the entrance of the vitreous into the probe, a relatively inefficient way of performing vitrectomy (Figure 44.1).
   - Second instrument: use a 23-gauge butterfly infusion needle through the paracentesis site for a 2-port vitrectomy. Here, the infusion flow is far from the probe and does not interfere with vitreous incarceration into the probe (Figure 44.2).

6. For illumination, use a fiber-optic probe or coaxial illumination of the operating microscope. Place the fiber-optic probe at the limbus for visualization by scleral scatter (Figure 44.3). It offers better visualization of anterior chamber vitreous strands than coaxial illumination of the operating microscope. The fiber-optic probe also can be placed inside the eye through a second port (paracentesis port), which needs to be approximately 1.4 mm wide for a 20-gauge probe.

7. Take extra care to avoid vitreous prolapse into the anterior chamber when the instrument is removed. Some helpful maneuvers include lowering of the IOP and infusion of air into the anterior chamber.

Figure 44.1. Anterior vitrectomy using an infusion sleeve.

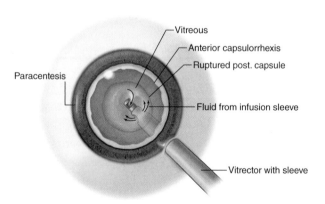

Vitreous

Anterior capsulorrhexis

Ruptured post. capsule

Paracentesis

Fluid from infusion sleeve

Vitrector with sleeve

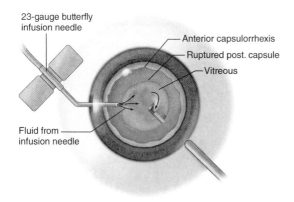

23-gauge butterfly
infusion needle

Anterior capsulorrhexis

Ruptured post. capsule

Vitreous

Fluid from
infusion needle

Figure 44.2. A 2-port anterior vitrectomy.

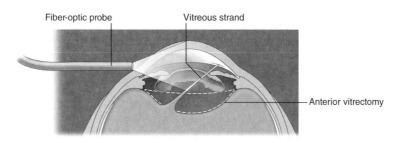

Fiber-optic probe   Vitreous strand

Anterior vitrectomy

Figure 44.3. Scleral scatter illumination of the anterior segment structures.

8. Place the intraocular lens in the bag, the sulcus, or the anterior chamber angle depending on the integrity of the lens capsule.
9. Inject acetylcholine chloride (Miochol-E) to constrict the pupil. A peaked pupil indicates presence of a vitreous strand in the anterior chamber. Use a cyclodialysis spatula to sweep the strand from the wound or perform vitrectomy to cut it.
10. Place the cataract wound sutures, if needed, and test the wound for any leaks or incarcerated vitreous using a cellulose sponge (eg, Weck-Cel).

POSTOPERATIVE CONSIDERATIONS

1. Follow up on the first postoperative day.
2. Use topical antibiotics (eg, Vigamox 4 times a day) for 1 week and corticosteroid drops (eg, prednisolone acetate 1%) as the degree of inflammation warrants.
3. Follow-up examination is the same as for cataract surgery (Chapter 1).

COMPLICATIONS

- Transient increase in the IOP
- Hyphema
- Vitreous strands remaining incarcerated in the wound
- Cystoid macular edema
- Corneal edema
- Retinal tear or detachment
- Endophthalmitis
- Choroidal hemorrhage
- Vitreous hemorrhage
- Epithelial downgrowth

Chapter 45

Pneumatic Retinopexy

Neelakshi Bhagat, MD, MPH, FACS
Marco A. Zarbin, MD, PhD, FACS

In pneumatic retinopexy, a gas bubble is injected into the vitreous cavity to tamponade the retinal breaks until the retina is reattached. Indications include rhegmatogenous retinal detachment with no proliferative vitreoretinopathy; retinal break(s) located in the superior 240° periphery (ie, between 8 and 4 o'clock positions clockwise), no larger than 1 clock hour; and all retinal tears within 90° of each other.

Contraindications include the patient's inability to properly position the head after surgery; a history of advanced glaucoma, sickle cell disease, or other eye diseases in which a significant increase in IOP is contraindicated; the presence of extensive lattice degeneration outside of the area to be treated; and pseudophakia (a relative contraindication).

PREOPERATIVE STEPS

1. Dilate the pupil (tropicamide 1%, phenylephrine 2.5%).
2. Perform a meticulous retinal examination to localize all retinal breaks and the extent of the retinal detachment.

INSTRUMENTATION AND SUPPLIES

- Sterile lid speculum
- Povidone-iodine swabs

- Lidocaine 2% without epinephrine or 2% lidocaine gel
- Topical antibiotic drops
- Tuberculin syringes
- 5/8-inch, 30-gauge needles
- Castroviejo calipers
- Cryopexy unit
- Indirect ophthalmoscope with 20-, 28-, or 30-D lens
- Intraocular gas: either sulfur hexafluoride (SF_6) or perfluoropropane (C_3F_8) with Millipore filter

SURGICAL PROCEDURE

1. With the patient reclining, place the lid speculum.
2. Anesthesia: topical 2% lidocaine gel, subconjunctival lidocaine 2% in the quadrant to be treated, or retrobulbar anesthesia.
3. Using an indirect ophthalmoscope, identify the retinal tears and perform transscleral cryopexy (see Chapter 41).
4. Sterilize the eyelids, eyelashes, and ocular surface using a swab of 10% Betadine; let the iodine dry on the skin and ocular surface.
5. Draw up pure intraocular gas through the Millipore filter into a tuberculin syringe.
6. Mark the site of the gas injection, 3 mm (aphakia/pseudophakia) or 4 mm (phakic eye) posterior to the limbus superotemporally.
7. Direct the needle tip to the center of the globe (Figure 45.1A).
8. Inject 0.3 cc C_3F_8 or 0.5 cc SF_6 at the marked site, using a tuberculin syringe attached to a 30-gauge needle. Inject rapidly and smoothly to avoid formation of multiple small bubbles (Figure 45.1B).
9. Tamponade the injection site with a sterile cotton-tipped applicator to prevent egress of gas.
10. Position the patient's head so that the bubble is away from the location of the retinal break. Have the patient first positioned face down; 6 hours later, the patient should rotate the head so that the bubble is against the tear. If the break is small and the bubble is large, there is little chance for the gas to enter the subretinal space, and one can position the bubble against the break 10 to 15 minutes after the intravitreal gas injection. Instruct the patient, before he or she is sent home, how to position the head in order to place the bubble against the tear once it has expanded.

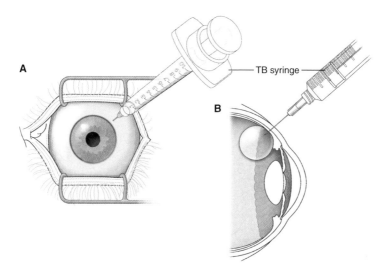

Figure 45.1. Inject the gas rapidly and smoothly to avoid formation of multiple small bubbles.

11. Visualize the central retinal artery with indirect ophthalmoscopy to verify its patency and to assess any complications (eg, subretinal gas or vitreous hemorrhage).

12. If small clusters of bubbles ("fish eggs") are noted, gently tap the globe in the quadrant of bubbles several times to coalesce them into a single large bubble (Figure 45.2).

13. If subretinal gas is present, consider vitrectomy. If the tear is large and the bubble is relatively small, one can sometimes force the bubble out of the subretinal space by proper rotation of the patient's head in a manner that brings the bubble to the meridian of the retinal break.

14. Check the IOP in 10 minutes. If central retinal artery remains closed for ≥5 minutes or if the IOP is ≥40 mm Hg, perform anterior chamber paracentesis sterilely to lower the IOP.

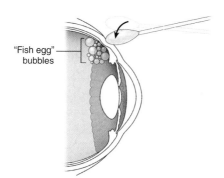

"Fish egg" bubbles

Figure 45.2. Tap the globe to coalesce all the gas bubbles into a single large bubble.

Figure 45.3. A 28-D lens may facilitate viewing through the gas bubble.

Face is tilted to the right

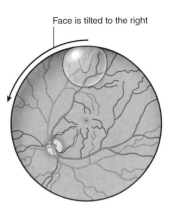

15. Instill 1 to 2 drops of topical antibiotic into the eye.
16. Prescribe Tylenol for pain (unless contraindicated).
17. If a cryopexy unit is not available or if the detachment is bullous so that one cannot apply optimal cryopexy treatment to the retinal pigment epithelium at the margins of the break (due to parallax), one can use indirect laser photocoagulation. In this case, the following steps apply:
    • No cryopexy is performed; only gas is injected. (Follow the same steps above, with the exception of Step 3.)
    • Perform laser demarcation once the retina is attached via bubble tamponade (usually postoperative day 1 to 3). Rotate the head so that the gas bubble is directed to the quadrant away from the tear and apply 3 to 5 rows of laser photocoagulation away from the margin of the tear, taking care to treat for 1 clock hour on either side of the edges of the tear all the way up to the ora serrata. A 28-D lens may facilitate viewing through the gas bubble (Figure 45.3).

POSTOPERATIVE CARE

1. Instruct the patient to call the surgeon for pain unrelieved by Tylenol, as this symptom may be due to elevated IOP or endophthalmitis.
2. Follow up on the first postoperative day.
3. Examine the fundus, especially to rule out any inferior retinal tears. Normally all or most subretinal fluid will have resorbed within several days, depending on the extent and duration of the detachment.
4. If the retina is attached, follow up at 1, 3, and 6 weeks after surgery. The patient may still need to position the head 50% of the time so that the bubble is against the tear during the first 2 weeks after treatment.

(Experimental studies indicate that cryoretinopexy requires 2 weeks to achieve maximum scar strength, and laser treatment requires somewhat less time.)

COMPLICATIONS

- Endophthalmitis
- Lack of retinal attachment due to persistent vitreous traction on the retinal tear
- Secondary retinal break formation (particularly in cases with inferior lattice degeneration)
- Subretinal gas
- Extension of retinal break
- Vitreous hemorrhage
- Cataract

Chapter 46

Repair of Retinal Detachment With a Scleral Buckle

Neelakshi Bhagat, MD, MPH, FACS
Marco A. Zarbin, MD, PhD, FACS

The scleral buckle procedure is indicated to repair rhegmatogenous retinal detachment. (Proliferative vitreoretinopathy, if present, should be less than grade L-2 [full-thickness fixed retinal folds in 2 quadrants], and retinal break[s] are located anterior to the equator.) The technique can used as prophylaxis against retinal detachment in selected fellow eyes of patients with giant retinal tears. It also can be used in selected cases of stage 4a retinal detachment (subtotal, extrafoveal) associated with retinopathy of prematurity, although lens-sparing vitrectomy is generally the preferred approach in this condition.

INSTRUMENTATION AND SUPPLIES

- Lid speculum
- Toothed tissue forceps (0.12, 0.3, and 0.5 mm)
- Westcott scissors
- Curved Stevens scissors
- Sutures (5-0 nylon or 4-0 white silk and 6-0 black silk on spatula needle, 8-0 polyglactin [Vicryl] or 6-0 gut)
- Muscle hooks (including fenestrated hook)
- Needle holder
- Schepens retractor
- Indirect ophthalmoscope and indirect lenses (eg, 20 or 28 D)
- Straight scleral depressor

- Gass localizer
- Marking pen
- Cryosurgical unit with transscleral cryoprobe
- Silicone buckling elements
- Schiøtz tonometer
- Tuberculin syringe with 5/8-inch, 30-gauge needle
- Air, SF_6, C_3F_8 gas (in selected cases)
- Bacitracin antibiotic solution to soak the buckling element

SURGICAL PROCEDURE

1. Anesthesia: local anesthesia with sedation or general anesthesia.
2. Prep and drape the eye in a sterile manner.
3. Place the lid speculum.
4. Perform a 360° conjunctival peritomy at the limbus with Westcott scissors and tissue forceps (Figure 46.1).
5. Perform blunt dissection in Tenon's space between the rectus muscles with Westcott scissors (Figure 46.2).
6. Isolate rectus muscles using the muscle hook.
7. Sling each rectus muscle with a 2-0 silk suture using a fenestrated muscle hook (Figure 46.3, Figure 46.4). The muscle hook should be passed in a temporal-to-nasal direction while slinging superior rectus muscle to avoid slinging the superior oblique tendon. Tie a knot at the distal end of each suture.
8. Inspect the sclera for any thinning in all 4 quadrants.

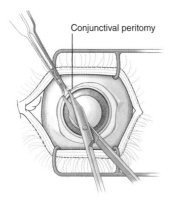

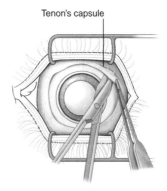

Figure 46.1. A 360° conjunctival peritomy at the limbus.

Figure 46.2. Blunt dissection of Tenon's capsule between the recti muscles.

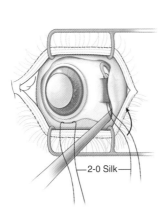

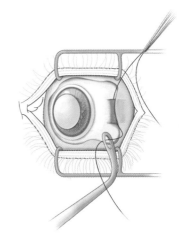

Figure 46.3. Isolate the rectus muscle.

Figure 46.4. Sling the rectus muscle with a 2-0 silk suture.

9. Examine the retina completely with scleral depression and indirect ophthalmoscopy.

10. Localize and mark the location of all retina holes and tears along with the anterior, posterior, medial, and lateral extent. Also, mark the location of the ora serrata in each quadrant (eg, using Gass localizer and marking pen) if the ora is not located at the level of the muscle insertions.

11. Perform cryopexy (see Chapter 41 in addition to the following steps):
    - Position the cryotherapy probe under the tears and create whitening of all the edges of the tears (Figures 46.5, 46.6) taking care not to treat the bare retinal pigment epithelium (RPE) exposed to the

Figure 46.5. Placement of the transscleral cryoprobe probe under the retinal tear.

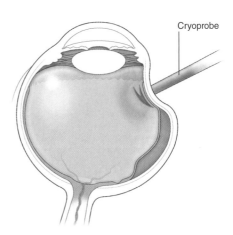

Cryoprobe

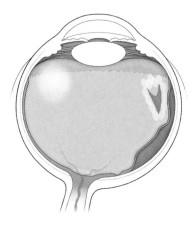

Figure 46.6. Whitening of the edges of the tear.

vitreous cavity. Terminate the freeze as soon as whitening of the retina-RPE is evident. The eye can be rotated using the 2-0 silk sutures.

- If retina is bullously detached, one may not be able to create any whitening of the neurosensory retina. Whitening of the underlying RPE is sufficient.
- Wait for the cryoprobe to thaw before moving the probe to adjacent area around the break. Cryo spots must overlap each other slightly to completely seal the break with 1 to 2 mm of treatment surrounding the edges of the break.
- Treatment should extend to the posterior margin of the vitreous base in the meridian of the tear.

12. Select the style (sponges, or silicone bands and tires) and the size of the buckling element to be used. (A silicone band is a thin strip of silicone used to encircle the eye in order to support the vitreous base. A tire is a wide silicone element used in a segmental or an encircling fashion [usually with a band] to relieve focal [with a segmental element] or posterior vitreoretinal traction that extends more than 4 mm posterior to the ora serrata). Decide if a segmental or an encircling buckling element is needed.
   - Factors favoring placement of a segmental element:
     - A single break
     - Multiple retinal breaks anterior to the equator in different quadrants
     - A history of Sickle cell disease or sickle trait
     - A history of glaucomatous optic atrophy

- Factors favoring placement of an encircling element:
  - Multiple retinal breaks anterior to the equator in the same or different quadrants
  - The presence of peripheral lattice degeneration or retinal thinning
  - The presence of proliferative vitreoretinopathy (eg, star-fold formation)
  - All breaks not definitively localized
  - Aphakic/pseudophakic detachment
  - Re-operation

13. Soak buckling elements in bacitracin solution before use (unless the patient is allergic, in which case substitute alternate antibiotic).
    - Pre-place mattress sutures to be used in securing the buckle (5-0 nylon or 4-0 white silk).
    - Suture passes should be placed parallel to the buckling element and should be approximately 4 mm long through partial-thickness sclera. Visualize the needle tip as it is placed through the sclera, to avoid perforating globe (Figure 46.7).
    - For circumferential buckles, the anterior suture pass should be at the ora serrata, and the posterior pass should be at least 3 mm posterior to the posterior margin of the most posterior retinal break (see Figure 46.7). The width of the buckle selected depends on the location of the pathology to be supported by the buckle. Encircling 240 or 42 bands are usually used to support the vitreous base. Larger elements (eg, 287 explant) are used to support those posteriorly located pathology.

14. Place the scleral buckle under the rectus muscles, and temporarily tie the buckle into position using the pre-placed mattress sutures.

Figure 46.7. Suture is passed through partial-thickness sclera.

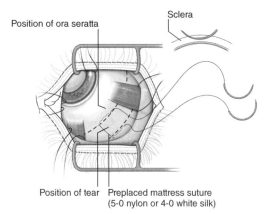

Position of ora seratta

Sclera

Position of tear   Preplaced mattress suture
(5-0 nylon or 4-0 white silk)

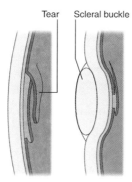

Tear   Scleral buckle   Figure 46.8. Placement of the scleral buckle to support the retinal tear.

15. Verify the proper positioning of the buckle over the retinal breaks by indirect ophthalmoscopy (Figure 46.8).

16. If drainage of subretinal fluid is anticipated, choose a location that will be supported by the buckle, if possible. Untie sutures to loosen the buckle and drain subretinal fluid if indicated.

- Drainage may be indicated in cases of high retinal detachment, evident vitreoretinal traction that would prevent retina–choroid apposition, a giant retinal tear, the presence of a macular hole, longstanding retinal detachment (ie, viscous subretinal fluid), in the setting of significant glaucomatous optic atrophy or sickle cell disease/trait, or if no retinal breaks are identified.

- Choose an area under bullous detachment, away from the retinal tear, to avoid retinal perforation/incarceration.

- Avoid vortex veins (preferable to drain near horizontal rectus muscles).

- Drainage from a nasal quadrant reduces the chance for submacular hemorrhage if bleeding occurs during drainage.

- Create a radial incision in the sclera down to the suprachoroidal space (dark blue tissue visible), approximately 3 mm long with a sharp blade (eg, No. 69 Beaver blade), Figure 46.9A.

- Examine exposed choroid for any large vessels, which should be avoided when performing drainage.

- Pre-place double-armed 5-0 nylon or 6-0 silk mattress suture around the sclerotomy, particularly if the drainage site is not to be supported by the buckle.

- Perform drainage using a 30-gauge needle or the tip of a 2.5-mm diathermy pin by carefully introducing the needle approximately 1 mm through choroid into subretinal space tangentially to avoid retinal damage until a trickle of fluid is noted to egress (Figure 46.9B).

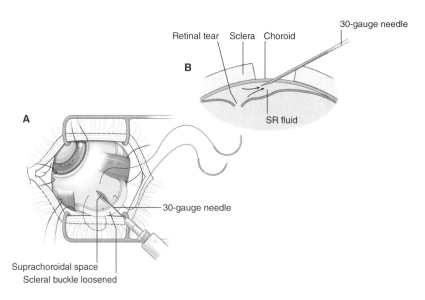

Figure 46.9. Creating a radial incision (A), then draining the subretinal fluid (B).

- Release all traction on the eye and gently press the globe with a cotton-tipped applicator to help express subretinal fluid.
- Tie off the pre-placed mattress suture around the drainage sclerotomy.

17. Secure the element by tying the sutures temporarily.

18. Examine the retina by indirect ophthalmoscopy to verify the buckle location over the breaks and inspect the drainage site for retinal incarceration. If incarceration is present, treat the site with cryopexy and support the site on a buckle.

19. If a break has fish-mouthed or if there is a break inadequately supported by a buckle, consider either revising the buckle location or adding a radial element or injecting intravitreal gas (both are very effective in managing fish-mouthing).

20. Confirm the patency of the central retinal artery.

21. Join the ends of the encircling element with a Watzke sleeve (or tantalum clip, depending on the width of the element) and trim the buckling elements with silicone cutting scissors as necessary.

22. Check the IOP with the Schiøtz tonometer. Perform an anterior chamber tap if the IOP is high. Alternatively, consider vitreous aspiration (eg, using a long 27-gauge needle or vitrectomy probe) if anterior chamber paracentesis is not successful (particularly if repeated) in lowering the IOP.

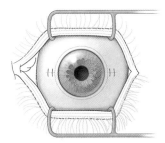

Figure 46.10. Closure of the conjunctival peritomy.

23. Remove the 2-0 silk sutures and close the peritomy. Secure Tenon's capsule directly to episclera with 8-0 polyglactin suture, ensuring coverage of silicone sponge elements to prevent postoperative extrusion. Close the conjunctiva with absorbable suture (8-0 polyglactin or 6-0 gut), Figure 46.10.

24. Inject subconjunctival cefazolin (100 mg)—if the patient is allergic to penicillin, consider vancomycin 50 mg—and Decadron (4 to 8 mg) or Kenalog (40 mg).

25. Remove the lid speculum, apply topical atropine 1% drops and antibiotic ointment, and patch.

26. Administer intravenous acetazolamide (Diamox, 250 to 500 mg), if unacceptably high postoperative IOP is probable (unless the patient is allergic to sulfa or has another contraindication; acetazolamide should be used with caution in renal dialysis patients since it is eliminated via the kidney).

POSTOPERATIVE CARE

1. Keep the patch on until examining the patient on the first postoperative day.

2. Limit strenuous activity. Head positioning may be indicated if a gas bubble has been used. In the absence of intravitreal gas, having the patient recline on his or her back encourages settling of the retina, as the specific gravity of the retina is greater than that of the vitreous.

3. Follow up on the first postoperative day; postoperative weeks 1, 3, 6, and 12; postoperative month 6; and then annually. Start topical antibiotics 4 times a day, prednisolone acetate 1% drops 4 times a day, and atropine 1% up to 4 times a day.

4. Start Percocet (7/500), 1 tablet orally every 6 hours for eye pain (unless contraindicated).

COMPLICATIONS

- Central retinal artery occlusion
- Increased IOP
- Subretinal hemorrhage
- Serous or hemorrhagic choroidal detachment
- Retinal or vitreous incarceration in drainage sites
- Vitreous hemorrhage (and, in some cases, secondary hyphema)
- Anterior segment ischemia
- Infection or extrusion of buckling element
- Erosion of the buckle into the vitreous cavity (particularly with the use of silicone sponge material)
- Endophthalmitis
- Strabismus
- Proliferative vitreoretinopathy

Chapter 47

Pars Plana Vitrectomy With Specialized Techniques

Neelakshi Bhagat, MD, MPH, FACS
Marco A. Zarbin, MD, PhD, FACS

Indications for pars plana vitrectomy include the following:

- Removal of media opacities (eg, nonresolving vitreous hemorrhage)
- Repair of a tractional or traction-rhegmatogenous retinal detachment (eg, proliferative vitreoretinopathy, proliferative diabetic retinopathy)
- Repair of a rhegmatogenous retinal detachment
- Removal of an epiretinal membrane
- Repair of a macular hole
- Submacular surgery to remove subfoveal blood or subfoveal choroidal neovascularization in selected patients
- Removal of intraocular foreign bodies
- Vitreous biopsy
- Removal of a cataractous lens with zonular dehiscence using the pars plana approach
- Repositioning of a subluxated intraocular lens (IOL) implant

PREOPERATIVE STEPS

1. Conduct a thorough preoperative retinal examination or an ultrasound examination of retina and vitreous if media opacity precludes it.
2. Dilate the pupil.

INSTRUMENTATION AND SUPPLIES

- Lid speculum
- Fine-toothed tissue forceps (eg, 0.12 mm or 0.3 mm)
- Westcott scissors
- Cautery with attachments both for external and intraocular use
- Castroviejo calipers
- 20-gauge microvitreoretinal (MVR) blade
- 25- or 23-gauge inserter-cannula system
- Needle holders
- Infusion cannula (2.5, 4.0, or 6.0 mm depending on the presence of choroidal detachment/cyclitic membrane)
- Sutures (7-0 and 8-0 polyglactin [Vicryl])
- Vitrectomy suction/cutting instrumentation
- Fiber-optic endoilluminator
- Corneal lens ring
- Contact lenses. Traditional lens system (TLS): 30° and 60° prism, wide angle, macular, and biconcave lenses. Wide-angle lens system (WAS): wide-angle lens (eg, Ocular 155-D lens or Volk Mini Quad/Quad XL), equator lens (eg, Ocular 91-D lens or Volk Central Retinal lens), or macular lens (eg, Ocular 66-D lens or Volk Super Macula lens). Biome noncontact system: macular and wide-angle lenses.
- Scleral plugs
- Cotton-tipped applicators
- Indirect ophthalmoscope with 20- and 30-D lenses
- Intraocular forceps, scissors, and pick
- Charles fluted needle
- Intraocular pick (eg, Michels, Awh), scissors (eg, horizontal, vertical), forceps, diamond-dusted cannula (eg, Tano)
- Laser (endo or indirect)
- Cryo unit (transscleral cryotherapy) plus appropriate probes
- Perfluorocarbon liquid
- Gas (SF_6, C_3F_8) and silicone oil, depending on the case
- Inverting system for the wide-angle vitrectomy lenses (eg, Volk ROLS)

SURGICAL PROCEDURE

1. Anesthesia: general or retrobulbar +/- a lid block.
2. Prep and drape the patient in a sterile manner.
3. Place the lid speculum.

4. Perform focal conjunctival peritomies (Figures 47.1A, 47.1B) using Westcott scissors and toothed forceps.
5. Perform the sclerotomy and infusion.
   - 20-gauge:
     - Make 3 sclerotomies 3 to 4 mm from the limbus as measured with calipers, parallel to the limbus at 2 and 10 o' clock positions and inferotemporally (5 o'clock in the left eye and 7 o'clock in the right eye).
     - Pre-place the infusion line at the inferotemporal sclerotomy site using 7-0 polyglactin sutures through partial-thickness sclera (Figure 47.2A). Create the sclerotomy with the MVR blade perpendicular to the sclera, aiming toward the center of the globe. Visualize the MVR tip through the pupil.
     - Place the infusion cannula through the sclerotomy and secure it with pre-placed suture (Figure 47.2B). Confirm the location of the cannula tip in the vitreous cavity by using the endoillumina-tor probe to look directly through the pupil. Do not start the infusion if the cannula cannot be visualized.
     - Perform superior sclerotomies at the 2 and 10 o'clock positions using an MVR blade (Figure 47.2B). Apply scleral plugs.

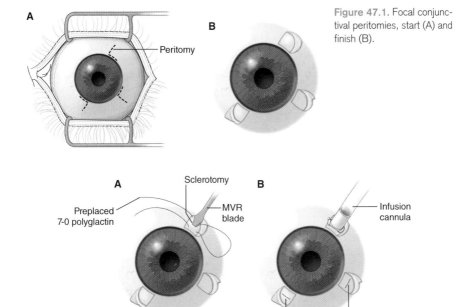

Figure 47.1. Focal conjunc-tival peritomies, start (A) and finish (B).

Figure 47.2. 20-gauge vitrectomy. (A) Sclerotomy with the MVR blade perpendicular to the sclera. (B) Placement of infusion cannula.

- 23-gauge and 25-gauge: focal peritomies are not made since a transconjunctival entrance is performed.
  - Mark the site of entry with a caliper. Displace the conjunctiva over it with a 0.12 forceps or a cotton-tipped applicator. Take the sharp inserter-cannula system (eg, Alcon, Bausch and Lomb, or DORC), which is either a sharp trocar or a stiletto blade preloaded with a cannula.
  - Make a beveled incision in the inferotemporal quadrant for the infusion line (Figure 47.3). The stiletto blade or the sharp trocar is inserted at a 30° angle through the conjunctiva and the sclera for 1 mm and then angled directly towards the optic nerve. (For the 25-gauge vitrectomy, some surgeons still prefer to make a nonbeveled transconjunctival entry perpendicular to the sclera with the inserter-cannula system.) Hold the cannula with a forceps and remove the inserter (trocar or stiletto blade).
  - Connect the infusion line to the cannula. Confirm the location of the cannula tip in the vitreous cavity.
  - Perform the other two entries at 2 and 10 o'clock positions similarly.
6. Suture the lens ring 3 mm from the limbus with 7-0 polyglactin suture at 3 (or 6) and 9 (or 12) o' clock positions (see Figure 47.4). Place viscous coupling medium on the cornea (eg, Goniosol).
7. Place the contact lens on the cornea.
   - For surgeons using the traditional Machemer lens system (TLS), usually begin with the wide-angle lens (−50 D). For macular dissection (eg, stripping of the internal limiting membrane, dissection of the epiretinal membrane), use the macula lens. For peripheral vitreous dissection, use the prism (30°, 60°) lens.

Figure 47.3. Small-gauge vitrectomy showing beveled incision in the sclera for the infusion line.

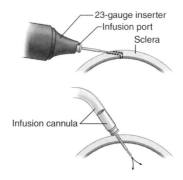

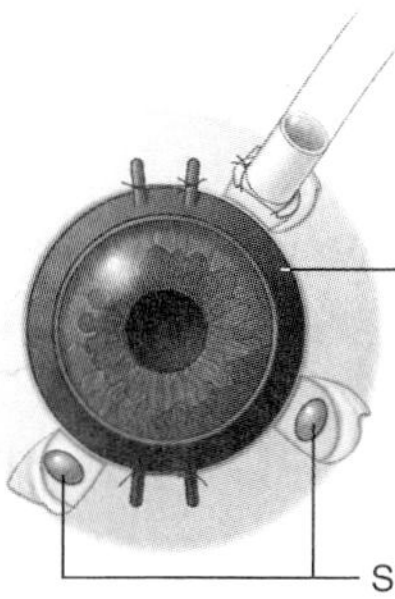

Figure 47.4. Placement of the lens ring.

Lens ring

Scleral plugs

- For surgeons using the wide-angle lens system (with contact lenses or Biome), the inverter should be connected in the microscope. Usually begin with the wide-angle lens (155 D). For macular dissection, use the macula lens (66 D). For equatorial dissection, use the equator lens (91 D).

8. Insert the fiber-optic endoilluminator and vitrectomy probe after removing the scleral plugs (Figure 47.5).

9. Turn off the room light and microscope light.

10. Set vitrectomy instrument parameters:
    - 20-gauge vitrectomy
      - Cutting rate: approximately 600 cpm for regular cutting probe (RCP), or 1200 to 2000 cpm for high-rate cutting probes (HCP). Core vitrectomy 600 cpm (HCP: Innovit [HCP-I] 1200 cpm; guillotine (HCP-G) 2000 cpm). Vitreous base: 800 cps (HCP-I: 1800 cpm; HCP-G: 2500 cpm). Extraction of dense membranes:

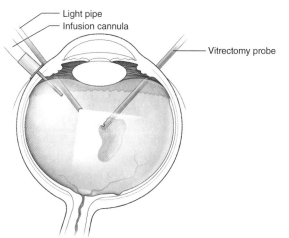

Light pipe
Infusion cannula

Vitrectomy probe

Figure 47.5. Endoilluminator highlighting the vitreous and tip of the vitrector.

low cutting rate of 200 to 400 cpm (HCP 600 to 800 cpm) and high suction. If close to detached retina: HCP 800 cpm (HCP-I: 1800 cpm; HCP-G: 2500 cpm) and low suction.

  – Suction: 80 to 180 mm Hg and adjust as necessary (HCP: 150 to 200 mm Hg). Core vitrectomy: 180 mm Hg (HCP: 200 mm Hg). Vitreous base: 25 to 50 mm Hg (HCP: 80 to 100 mm Hg). Extraction of dense membranes or induction of posterior vitreous detachment: high suction 200 to 250 mm Hg. If close to detached retina, decrease the suction to 25 to 50 mm Hg (HCP: 80 to 100 mm Hg). With high suction, one may need to increase infusion pressure to prevent globe collapse.

- 23-gauge vitrectomy:
  – Uses 2500 cpm, high-speed, 23-gauge pneumatic vitreous cutter. The infusion is usually kept at 30 mm Hg. Core vitrectomy: 1500 cpm and a vacuum of 400 mm Hg. Vitreous base: 2500 cpm and a vacuum of 150 mm Hg. Induction of posterior vitreous detachment: increase suction to 500 mm Hg.
- 25-gauge vitrectomy:
  – Uses 1500 cpm, high-speed, 25-gauge pneumatic vitreous cutter. The infusion is usually kept at 40 mm Hg. Core vitrectomy: 1100 cpm and a vacuum of 600 mm Hg. Vitreous base: 1500 cpm and a vacuum of 250 mm Hg. Induction of posterior vitreous detachment: increase suction to 600 mm Hg.

11. Perform vitrectomy; remove the central (core) vitreous.
12. Remove the lens if cataract hinders an adequate view of the posterior segment (see Chapter 48).
13. Identify the posterior hyaloid face.
    - Induce a posterior vitreous detachment (PVD) if the hyaloid face is still attached to the macula and optic nerve. Use the vitrector in aspiration mode with high suction (200 to 250 mm Hg for 20 gauge; 600 mm Hg for small-gauge vitrectomy) over the optic nerve.
    - If unsuccessful, incise the posterior hyaloid face near the optic nerve head with a bent-tipped, 20-gauge needle or barbed MVR blade and extend the vitreous detachment to the equator (Figure 47.6).
14. Perform a 360° scleral-depressed peripheral vitrectomy, and shave the vitreous base without touching the posterior surface of the lens. Use prism lenses (TLS) or the wide-angle 166 D (WAS) lens to visualize peripheral vitreous. When using the TLS system, the assistant can improve visualization of the periphery (even when using prism lenses) by providing scleral indentation.

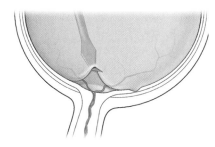

Figure 47.6. Induction of posterior vitreous detachment using a barbed MVR blade.

15. Perform the next step as indicated for the particular vitreoretinal pathology, including membrane peel, air-fluid exchange, use of perfluoro-octane (eg, Perfluoron) to flatten the posterior retina and express subretinal fluid through the retinal hole (Figure 47.7), and endophotocoagulation.

16. If using the WAS system, check the peripheral retina for any tears or breaks, especially at the sclerotomy sites. Use a light pipe through one of the sclerotomy ports and place a scleral plug in the other remaining superior port. Depress the sclera with the other hand and look for any peripheral tears under the microscope. If using the TLS lens system, use the indirect ophthalmoscope and scleral indentation to check the retinal periphery once the instruments are removed from the eye.

17. Treat retinal breaks.
   • If the retinal breaks are small and no vitreoretinal traction is present and there is no or minimal subretinal fluid, perform fluid-air exchange. Change balance salt solution infusion to air and drain over the retinal tear using the Charles fluted needle (Figure 47.8) or using active suction (the silicone-tip cannula attached to vitrectomy machine to achieve maximum suction of 100 to 150 mm Hg). Perform

Figure 47.7. Use of Perfluoron.

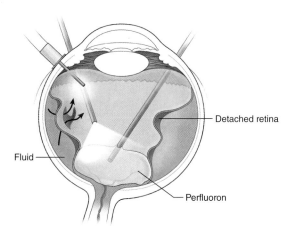

Detached retina

Fluid

Perfluoron

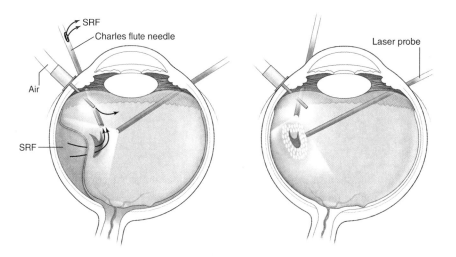

Figure 47.8. Fluid-air exchange.

Figure 47.9. Endolaser photocoagulation around the retinal tear.

an endolaser (Figure 47.9) or indirect laser procedure around the flattened retinal tear.

- If large retinal breaks are present and there is vitreoretinal traction on the break, consider placing a scleral buckle (usually a No. 240 or No. 42 band) to support the vitreous base (Figure 47.10); see Chapter 46.
- If significant peripheral retinal detachment is present, consider using Perfluoron to flatten the retina up to the tear; perform fluid-air exchange, and then demarcation endolaser or indirect laser around the tear (see Figures 47.7, 47.8, and 47.9).

18. Remove the instruments from the eye.

19. If vitreous prolapses through sclerotomy sites, cut it flush with sclera using Westcott scissors. Alternatively, one can use the vitrectomy probe at a high cutting rate and low suction to excise vitreous from the sclerotomy area.

20. Close each sclerotomy site with 7-0 polyglactin suture in a figure-eight shape (Figures 47.11A, 47.11B, 47.11C, and 47.11D).

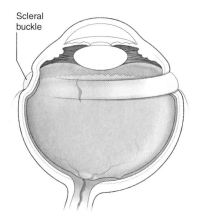

Figure 47.10. Scleral buckle supporting the retinal tear.

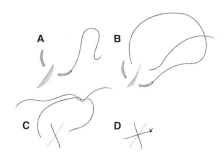

Figure 47.11. Closure of the sclerotomy site (A to D).

VARIOUS TECHNIQUES USED IN POSTERIOR SEGMENT SURGERY

Relieve Vitreoretinal Traction (Membrane Peel)

1. Use a Michels or Awh pick, a bent MVR blade, a bent 22-gauge or 25-gauge needle, or a diamond-dusted cannula (eg, Tano) to identify and develop a cleavage plane between the retina and epiretinal membranes.
2. Grasp the free edge of epiretinal tissue with intraocular forceps and peel meticulously and gently from the retinal surface (ie, epiretinal membrane peeling).
3. Alternatively, remove the preretinal membrane from the surface of the retina using intraocular scissors in an en-bloc fashion (ie, delamination, Figures 47.12A, 47.12B) or segment the membrane into tiny islands (Figures 47.13A, 47.13B) of adherent epiretinal tissue that are left in place but all the surrounding traction is relieved (eg, vitrectomy for proliferative diabetic retinopathy).

Air-Gas Exchange

1. Infuse a nonexpansile concentration of SF_6 (20%) or C_3F_8 (12% to 15%). SF_6 dissipates in about 2 weeks, and C_3F_8 dissipates in 6 weeks.
2. Use SF_6 or C_3F_8 for tamponade, depending on the duration of the tamponade needed.

Figure 47.12. Removal of the preretinal membrane from the surface of the retina using intraocular scissors (A) in an en-bloc fashion (B).

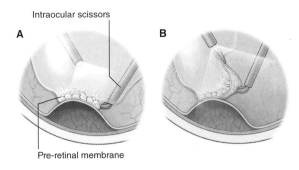

Figure 47.13. Removal of preretinal membrane (A) by segmenting the membrane into tiny islands of adherent epiretinal tissue that are left in place (B).

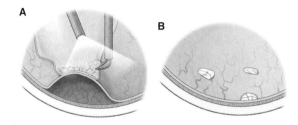

3. With the sclerotomies sewn shut, insert the tuberculin syringe (without a plunger) attached to a 5/8-inch, 30-gauge needle 3 mm (aphakia/pseudophakia) or 4 mm (phakic eye) posterior to the limbus and introduce a 20- or 60-cc syringe attached to a short 30-gauge needle containing a nonexpansile concentration of gas 3 or 4 mm posterior to the limbus (Figure 47.14).

4. Have the assistant gently depress the syringe to release the gas.

Silicone Oil Infusion

1. Introduce the silicone oil into an air-filled eye using a machine-pressurized mechanism (eg, viscous fluid controller system in Alcon's Accurus); the oil is forced into the vitreous cavity. Infusion is stopped when the silicone meniscus reaches the posterior lens capsule or the posterior surface of the iris diaphragm.

2. In aphakic eyes, an inferior iridectomy (Ando) should be created at the 6 o'clock position to prevent the development of secondary angle-closure glaucoma.

3. Check the IOP using a Schiøtz tonometer.

4. Close the sclerotomy with 7-0 polyglactin suture and the conjunctiva with 8-0 polyglactin (or 6-0 gut) suture.

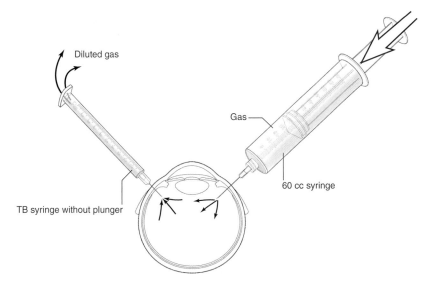

Figure 47.14. Air-gas exchange.

5. Inject subconjunctival cefazolin (100 mg)—if the patient is allergic to penicillin, consider vancomycin (50 mg)—and Decadron (4 to 8 mg) or Kenalog (40 mg).
6. Administer acetazolamide (250 to 500 mg in adults) intravenously if postoperative IOP elevation is anticipated, and the patient does not have a contraindication (eg, sulfa allergy) or relative contraindication (eg, renal failure).
7. Remove the lid speculum, apply topical antibiotic ointment and atropine 1% drops, and apply a patch.

SPECIAL APPLICATIONS OF VITRECTOMY

Endophthalmitis

Vitreous biopsy is best performed through a pars plana 1-, 2-, or 3-port vitrectomy (1-port vitrectomy is described in Chapter 44):

1. Perform core vitrectomy; excision of cortical or peripheral vitreous can be hazardous (inflamed retina is friable and more likely to tear).
2. Use an infusion light pipe with 2-port pars plana vitrectomy if the view precludes confirmation of cannula tip placement in the vitreous cavity.

3. If an infusing light pipe is not available, use a 23-gauge butterfly needle to achieve infusion via limbal entry into the anterior chamber until the view improves, thus permitting visualization of the tip of the infusion cannula in the vitreous cavity.

4. Obtain an undiluted vitreous biopsy sample. Attach a 3-cc tuberculin syringe to the vitrectomy aspiration line. Gently withdraw plunger of syringe with probe activated to remove vitreous material.

5. After obtaining approximately 0.3 to 1.0 cc (depending on when globe collapse occurs) of undiluted vitreous, stop vitrectomy, and turn on the infusion.

6. Submit the specimen for smear and culture immediately.

7. Attempt to continue to remove core vitreous until the retina is visible, or, if visualization is inadequate, a bright red reflex is obtained.

8. Close the sclerotomies with 7-0 polyglactin suture.

9. Inject the following intravitreal antibiotics: vancomycin 1 mg/0.1 mL and ceftazidime 2.25 mg/0.1 cc. (If the patient is allergic to penicillin, consider substituting tobramycin 400 μg/0.1 cc in that case.) Consider using amphotericin B (5 μg/0.1 mL) or fluconazole (25 mg/0.1 mL) in cases of fungal endophthalmitis or intravitreal voriconazole (100 μg/0.1 mL).

Repositioning and Suturing of Posteriorly Dislocated Intraocular Lens (IOL)

1. Perform 3-port vitrectomy.
2. Excise vitreous adherent to the IOL.
3. Grasp the IOL with intraocular forceps and deliver it into anterior chamber.
4. The surgeon may infuse perfluorocarbon to float the IOL into the retroiridal space.
5. Use 2 intraocular forceps to manipulate IOL haptics into the ciliary sulcus (posterior chamber IOL [PCIOL], assuming adequate capsular support) or anterior chamber angle (anterior chamber IOL [ACIOL]), Figure 47.15.
6. If the PCIOL is dislocated and inadequate capsular support exists for sulcus fixation, consider replacing the PCIOL with an ACIOL via limbal incision rather than suturing the PCIOL in position.
7. PCIOLs with inadequate capsular support can be stabilized by suturing the haptics to the iris, which is associated with a fixed pupil.
8. Technique for transscleral PCIOL suturing:

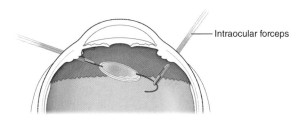

Figure 47.15. Repositioning of a posteriorly displaced IOL.

Intraocular forceps

- Create half-thickness triangular scleral flaps centered on the 3 and 9 o'clock meridians (Figure 47.16).
- Insert a long 27-gauge bent needle 1 mm from the limbus at the 9 o'clock position and exit at the 3:15 o'clock position, 1 mm from the limbus (at the ciliary sulcus). Place the swaged end of a 16-mm straight needle, 10-0 polypropylene suture into the barrel of the 27-gauge needle (Figure 47.17).
- Draw the 27-gauge needle into the vitreous cavity (Figure 47.18).
- Redirect the needle so that it exits the globe 1 mm from the limbus at the 2:45 o'clock position, under the scleral flap creating a small loop of suture in the vitreous cavity (Figure 47.19).
- Create a scleral tunnel incision superiorly or make a beveled limbal incision from the 10 to 2 o'clock positions with a No. 69 Beaver blade.
- Externalize the 10-0 Prolene polypropylene loop through the tunnel incision using a Sinskey hook (Figure 47.20).

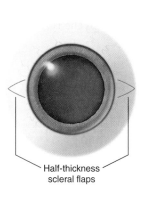

Half-thickness scleral flaps

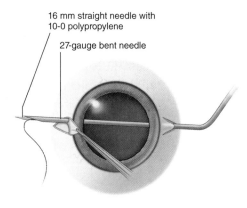

16 mm straight needle with 10-0 polypropylene

27-gauge bent needle

Figure 47.16. Technique of transscleral PCIOL suturing (shown in Figures 47.16 to 47.23). Triangular partial-thickness scleral flaps 180° apart.

Figure 47.17. Placement of a long 27-gauge bent needle under the flaps, and insertion of 10-0 straight polypropylene suture inside the 27-gauge needle.

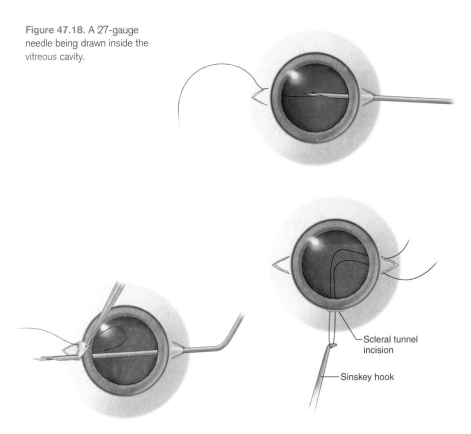

Figure 47.18. A 27-gauge needle being drawn inside the vitreous cavity.

Figure 47.19. Creation of a 10-0 polypropylene loop in the vitreous cavity.

Figure 47.20. Externalization of 10-0 polypropylene loop.

- Repeat the same maneuver (second through fifth bullet, above) using a bent 27-gauge needle at the 3 o'clock position.
- Each loop is passed through the eyelet of the lens and is looped around the haptic without a knot (Figure 47.21).
- Pull the ends and tie 10-0 Prolene polypropylene suture in bed of scleral flaps (Figure 47.22).
- Close scleral flaps with a single 10-0 nylon suture, burying the knot (Figure 47.23).

Macular Pucker

1. Perform 3-port vitrectomy.
2. Place the high-magnification macular contact lens on the cornea.
3. Create the cleavage plane between the epiretinal membrane (ERM) and the retina, using a blunt pick if possible (Figure 47.24).

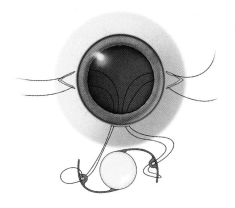

Figure 47.21. Looping 10-0 polypropylene around the IOL haptic.

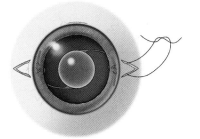

Figure 47.22. The 10-0 polypropylene suture knots buried under the scleral flaps.

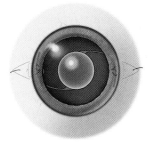

Figure 47.23. Closure of the scleral flaps.

Epiretinal membrane

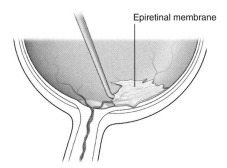

Figure 47.24. Macular pucker. Removal of the epiretinal membrane.

4. If one cannot develop the edge with a blunt pick, use a bent MVR blade to create cleavage plane: indent the MVR blade against the lid speculum or other hard surface to create a fine bend in the tip; next, use a diamond-dusted cannula (eg, Tano) to scrape epiretinal tissue off the retinal surface.

5. After creating the edge, peel the ERM using intraocular forceps.
6. If the retina is detached, the cleavage plane can also be extended using viscodissection.
7. Close the eye as above.

Macular Hole

1. Perform 3-port vitrectomy with excision of the posterior hyaloid face away from the optic nerve head and the macula.
2. Perform dissection of the internal limiting membrane (ILM). This is important for closure of stage III or IV macular holes of duration greater than 6 months.
   • Gently scrape the retinal surface around the macular hole with a diamond-dusted cannula (eg, Tano), Figure 47.25. Begin about 1.5 disc diameters away from margin of hole and scrape centripetally.
   • Alternatively, incise the ILM with the MVR blade about 1.5 disc diameters from the edge of the hole (Figure 47.26A). Use end-grasping forceps (eg, Tano) to grasp and elevate the free edge of the ILM.
3. When the ILM is elevated, grasp the edge with intraocular forceps and peel in a circumferential fashion (ie, capsulorrhexis) away from the edge of the macular hole (Figure 47.26B).
4. Perform air-fluid exchange as described above.

Endophotocoagulation

1. Perform 3-port vitrectomy as described above.
2. After membrane peeling and retinal reattachment, introduce the endophotocoagulation probe into the superior sclerotomy.

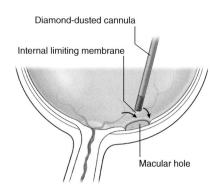

Figure 47.25. Dissection of the internal limiting membrane with a diamond-dusted cannula.

Diamond-dusted cannula

Internal limiting membrane

Macular hole

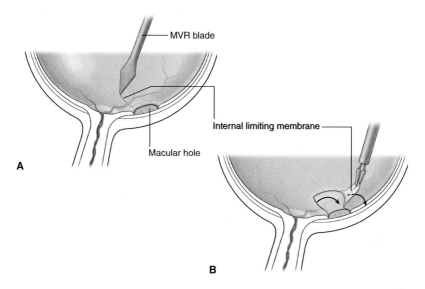

MVR blade

Internal limiting membrane

Macular hole

A

B

Figure 47.26. (A) Dissection of the ILM using an MVR blade. (B) ILM peel in a circumferential fashion around the macular hole.

3. Instruct the circulating nurse to provide protective goggles (appropriate to laser wavelength being used) to all operating room personnel not shielded by the filter on the operating microscope.

4. Instruct the circulating nurse to turn laser on "Treat" with settings at 0.2 to 0.3 seconds duration, and power setting of 150 to 300 mW power (depending on the degree of pigmentation of the fundus).

5. Apply laser treatment as follows:
   - Retinal break: surround the retinal break with 3 rows of confluent white burns, each about 300 to 500 μm in diameter (see Figure 47.9). If the break is anterior to the equator, consider extending treatment out to the ora serrata in the meridian of the break.
   - Panretinal photocoagulation (PRP): apply moderate burn intensity, spacing burns 1 to 2 burn widths apart (see Figure 37.1B). Do not bring treatment closer than 500 μm to the optic nerve head nasally or 2.5 disc diameters to the fovea temporally.

6. Wide-angle viewing system: using the wide-angle lens or the equator lens permits a wide field of view for laser application, even with the endophotocoagulation probe.

7. A biconcave contact lens in the fluid- or air-filled eye also permits a wide field of view for PRP application.

8. The indirect laser ophthalmoscope can also be used to deliver laser burns in periphery with a 20- or 28-D lens.

POSTOPERATIVE CARE

1. Keep an eye patch in place until examining the patient on the first postoperative day unless there is a need to administer medications earlier (eg, anti-glaucoma drops in appropriately selected patients).
2. Advise patient to limit strenuous activity. Face-down positioning may be required in the gas-filled phakic eye.
3. Prescribe topical antibiotics 4 times a day for 1 week; prednisolone acetate 1% 4 times a day for 3 to 6 weeks, tapered as inflammation permits; and atropine 1% twice a day for cycloplegia.
4. Control the IOP with topical medications, including beta-blockers (eg, timolol), alpha agonists (eg, apraclonidine twice a day), and carbonic anhydrase inhibitors (including topical Trusopt 2% 3 times a day) as needed and as tolerated. Add systemic carbonic anhydrase inhibitors (eg, methazolamide [eg, 25 mg orally 3 times a day] or acetazolamide [eg, 250 mg orally 4 times a day]) as needed and as tolerated.
5. Examine at 1, 3, and 6 weeks postoperatively and then as necessary.

COMPLICATIONS

- Cataract formation
- Transient elevation in the IOP
- Central retinal artery occlusion
- Anterior chamber shallowing and secondary angle-closure glaucoma
- Persistent corneal epithelial defect (especially in diabetic patients)
- Vitreous hemorrhage
- Choroidal hemorrhage
- Iatrogenic retinal breaks and detachment (including proliferative vitreoretinopathy)
- Cystoid macular edema
- Epiretinal membrane
- Rubeosis iridis and neovascular glaucoma (particularly in diabetic patients)
- Endophthalmitis

Chapter 48

Pars Plana Lensectomy

Neelakshi Bhagat, MD MPH, FACS
Marco A. Zarbin, MD, PhD, FACS

Pars plana lensectomy is indicated in the management of cataract during pars plana vitrectomy, subluxed or fully dislocated cataractous lens, or retained lens material following cataract surgery. At this time, only the 20-gauge vitrectomy unit can be used for pars plana lensectomy; the fragmatome is not available in 23 or 25 gauge.

PREOPERATIVE STEPS

1. Perform a thorough preoperative retinal examination or an ultrasound examination of retina, vitreous, and epiciliary space (using ultrasound biomicroscopy) if cataract precludes it.
2. Dilate the pupil (tropicamide 1%, Cyclogyl 1%, phenylephrine 2.5%).

INSTRUMENTATION AND SUPPLIES

- Lid speculum
- Tissue forceps (0.12 mm and 0.3 mm)
- Westcott scissors
- Castroviejo calipers
- 20-gauge microvitreoretinal (MVR) blade
- Needle holders

- 4- or 6-mm infusion cannula depending on associated pathology (6-mm cannula if cyclitic membrane is present)
- Sutures (7-0 and 8-0 polyglactin [Vicryl])
- 23-gauge butterfly needle
- Vitrectomy machine and vitrectomy suction/cutting instrument, fiber-optic endoilluminator, and ultrasonic phacofragmentation unit with 20-gauge tip
- Corneal ring with contact lenses. Traditional lens system (TLS): 30° and 60° prism, wide-angle, macular, and biconcave lenses. Wide-angle lens system (WAS): wide-angle lens (Ocular 155-D lens or Volk Mini Quad/Quad XL lens), equator lens (Ocular 91-D lens or Volk Central Retinal lens); macular lens (Ocular 66-D lens or Volk Super Macula lens); or, Biome noncontact system (macular and wide-angle lenses).
- Scleral plugs
- Indirect ophthalmoscope with 20- and 28-D lenses
- Charles fluted needle
- Retinal cryopexy unit or indirect laser ophthalmoscope
- Liquid perfluorocarbon (eg, perfluoro-octane)

SURGICAL PROCEDURE

1. General or retrobulbar anesthesia is used.
2. Prep and drape the patient in a sterile manner.
3. Place the lid speculum.
4. Perform focal conjunctival peritomies using Westcott scissors and toothed forceps (see Figures 47.1A, 47.1B).
5. Pre-place the infusion line at the inferotemporal sclerotomy site using 7-0 polyglactin (or 4-0 white silk) sutures through partial-thickness sclera (see Figure 47.2).
6. Create a sclerotomy for the infusion line with the MVR blade (see Figure 47.2). Insert the blade perpendicular to the sclera, aiming toward the center of globe, and visualize the blade tip through the pupil.
7. Place the infusion cannula through the sclerotomy and secure it with pre-placed sutures (see Figure 47.2). View and confirm the presence of the cannula tip in the vitreous cavity by directly looking through the pupil, using the endoilluminator probe. Do not start the infusion if the cannula cannot be visualized.
8. Fashion superior sclerotomies at the 2 and 10 o'clock positions using the MVR blade, and apply scleral plugs.

9. Use a 23-gauge butterfly needle through a limbal incision for irrigation until enough lens material is removed to allow direct visualization, if the infusion cannula tip cannot be confirmed in the vitreous due to cataract (Figures 48.1A, 48.1B).
10. Through a superior sclerotomy (usually on the side of the surgeon's dominant hand), incise the lens capsule at the equator with the MVR blade.
11. Insert the ultrasonic phacofragmentation probe through the sclerotomy and into the lens through the incised capsule.
12. Remove the lens nucleus with the ultrasound probe (see Figure 48.1B). Suggested settings: suction, 150 to 200 mm Hg and vary as needed; ultrasound, 15% to 50% power and pulse mode (8/sec) to fragment the nucleus.
13. Remove the ultrasonic probe.
14. Insert the vitrectomy probe to remove remaining peripheral lens cortex. Suggested settings: regular cutting probe (RCP) approximately 300 to 500 cps; high-rate cutting probe (HCP): Innovit (I) 1000 cps; guillotine (G) 1500 cps; suction: approximately 150 to 180 mm Hg.
15. Attempt to aspirate cortex using only suction mode if it aspirates easily.
16. Peripheral cortex can be visualized using scleral indentation with the nondominant hand.

A

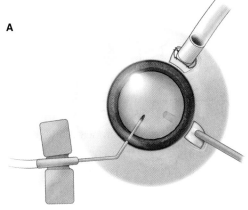

B

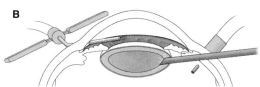

Figure 48.1. Pars plana lensectomy. (A) A 23-gauge butterfly needle for irrigation in the anterior chamber, since the infusion cannula tip cannot be confirmed in the vitreous due to cataract. (B) Fragmatome through the sclerotomy for lensectomy.

17. Attempt to leave the posterior capsule intact. The surgeon can preserve or remove anterior capsule, depending on surgeon preference (sulcus fixation permits leaving anterior capsule intact; fixation in the bag requires a central anterior capsulotomy).
18. Complete the posterior vitrectomy (as described in Chapter 47).
19. If lens fragments fall posteriorly, perfluorocarbon liquid can be used to float the lens into the mid-vitreous cavity to avoid retinal damage during phacoemulsification.
20. Aspirate out perfluorocarbon liquid at the end of the case.
21. If not done previously, perform core vitrectomy and then excise posterior hyaloid (as described in Chapter 47) out to the equator.
22. Place the intraocular lens if indicated.
23. Examine the peripheral retina with indirect ophthalmoscopy and scleral depression.
24. Close sclerotomies with 7-0 polyglactin suture in a figure-eight shape (see Figure 47.11).
25. Close conjunctiva with 8-0 polyglactin suture.
26. Inject subconjunctival cefazolin (100 mg)—if the patient is allergic to penicillin, consider vancomycin (50 mg)—and Decadron (4 to 8 mg) or Kenalog (40 mg).
27. Remove the lid speculum.
28. Apply atropine 1% drops, patch, and place a Fox shield.
29. Administer systemic antiglaucoma agents (eg, acetazolamide) if indicated.

POSTOPERATIVE CARE

1. Examine on the first postoperative day.
2. Prescribe topical antibiotics (eg, moxifloxacin [Vigamox]) 4 times a day for 1 week; corticosteroid drops (eg, prednisolone acetate 1%) tapered over 3 to 6 weeks, as inflammation warrants; and atropine 1% up to 4 times a day for cycloplegia.
3. Control the IOP with medications and drops as necessary.
4. Follow up postoperative week 1, 3, and 6 and then as necessary.

COMPLICATIONS

- Retinal tear or detachment
- Vitreous hemorrhage
- Hemorrhagic/serous choroidal detachment
- Endophthalmitis
- Corneal decompensation
- Scleral burn with pathological enlargement of the sclerotomy site

Chapter 49

Vitreous Implants

Lawrence P. Chong, MD

Vitreous implants are used to insert a drug delivery device through the pars plana of the eye. These include the Vitrasert (Bausch & Lomb) or the Retisert (Bausch & Lomb), both FDA-approved. The Vitrasert implant is for zone 1 or zone 1-threatening CMV retinitis. The implant delivers ganciclovir into the vitreous cavity and delivers drug for up to 6 to 8 months. The Retisert is for the treatment of chronic noninfectious posterior uveitis. It delivers fluocinolone acetonide (0.3 to 0.4 ug/day) into the vitreous cavity and delivers drug for up to 30 months.

PREOPERATIVE STEPS

1. Conduct a thorough preoperative retinal examination or an ultrasound examination of retina and vitreous if cataract precludes it.
2. Dilate the pupil.
3. Confirm a platelet count greater than 10,000.
4. Exclude patients with viral (especially herpetic) diseases of the conjunctiva and the cornea (for Retisert).

INSTRUMENTATION AND SUPPLIES

- Calipers
- Fine-toothed forceps

- Wescott tenotomy scissors
- Wet-field diathermy cautery: eraser tip and forceps tip
- 20-gauge microvitreoretinal (MVR) blade
- Vannas capsulotomy scissors
- Mechanical vitreous cutter and vitrectomy unit
- 8-0 nylon suture with spatula needle
- Indirect ophthalmoscope and handheld 20-D lens
- Subconjunctival injections

SURGICAL PROCEDURE

The operative procedure is similar for both implants. The only difference is the size of the implant and consequently the size of the scleral opening.

1. Anesthesia: retrobulbar injection.
2. Prep and drape the patient in a sterile manner.
3. Place the lid speculum.
4. The implant should be placed in 1 of the 2 inferior quadrants. Make a limbal-based conjunctival peritomy long enough to allow exposure of the pars plana 3.5 mm posterior to the limbus when the conjunctiva is retracted. Usually this peritomy spans the complete insertions of the recti muscles bordering that quadrant (Figure 49.1).
5. Control episcleral bleeding with diathermy.
6. Pass a double-armed 8-0 nylon suture through the eyelet of the implant. Make a single knot and set aside the implant (Figure 49.2).
7. Using the MVR blade, make an incision 3.5 mm parallel to the limbus and extend it to a length of 3 mm for the Retisert implant and 5 mm for the Vitrasert implant (Figure 49.3).
8. Carefully examine the uvea and incise it with Vannas scissors (Figure 49.4).

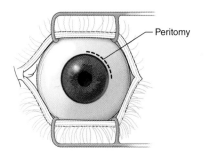

Figure 49.1. Conjunctival peritomy.

Peritomy

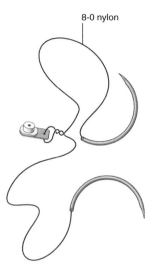

Figure 49.2. Prepare the implant by passing a double-armed 8-0 nylon suture through the eyelet of the implant and tying a single knot.

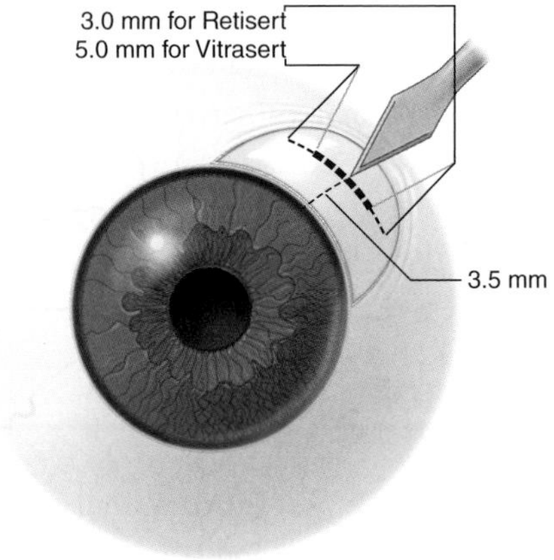

Figure 49.3. Scleral incision for inserting the implant.

9. Remove prolapsing vitreous with mechanical vitrectomy at the surface of the sclerotomy (Figure 49.5).
10. Place the implant through the sclerotomy with the body of the implant facing away from the crystalline lens (Figure 49.6).
11. Pass the needles of the double-armed suture through the edge of the wound, from the surface of the sclera and exiting from the inside of the wound. The finished knot will remain buried within the wound (Figure 49.7).

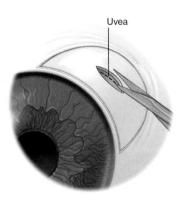

Figure 49.4. Incise the uvea with Vannas scissors.

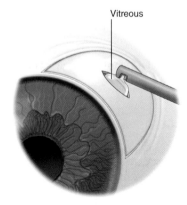

Figure 49.5. Cut the prolapsed vitreous with the vitrector.

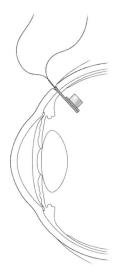

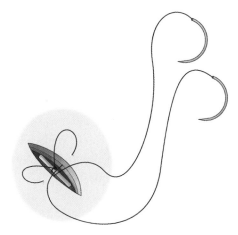

Figure 49.6. Placement of the implant.

Figure 49.7. Suture the implant to the sclerotomy edges burying the knot in the wound.

12. Close the length of the sclerotomy with a running 8-0 nylon suture in such a way that the knot remains buried within the wound. Alternatively, the wound can be closed with interrupted nylon sutures over the long tails of the suture securing the implant to the scleral wound. The wound is tested. The eye can be reinsufflated with balanced salt solution if the IOP is low.

13. Verify that the implant's position is completely through the uvea by indirect ophthalmoscopy.

14. Close the conjunctiva by apposing the edges of the conjunctiva at the nasal or temporal limbus and diathermizing with the forceps. Alternatively, the conjunctiva can be closed by suture.

15. Subconjunctival injections are administered.

16. The implant is replaced every 6 to 8 months (Vitrasert) or 30 months (Retisert) for recurrent disease or relapse.

17. Retisert implants may be difficult to remove and replace through some incisions. Often, another implant is placed in another location along the pars plana. If a Retisert implant must be removed or replaced in an eye that has undergone a vitrectomy, it is imperative to have a pars plana infusion canula to maintain eye pressure during the procedure.

POSTOPERATIVE PROCEDURE

1. Keep a patch in place until the patient is examined on the first postoperative day.
2. Limit strenuous activity.
3. Prescribe topical antibiotics 4 times a day for 1 week; prednisolone acetate 1% 4 times a day for 3 to 6 weeks, tapered as inflammation permits; and atropine 1% twice a day for cycloplegia.
4. Examine at 1, 3, and 6 weeks postoperatively and then as necessary.
5. These devices can be replaced when the delivery system is empty with recurrent infection (for the Vitrasert implant) or inflammation (for the Retisert implant).

COMPLICATIONS

- Endophthalmitis
- Vitreous hemorrhage
- Choroidal hemorrhage
- Iatrogenic retinal breaks and detachment
- Increased IOP (with the Retisert implant, up to 60% of patients need IOP-lowering medications within 9 months)
- Cystoid macular edema
- Epiretinal membrane
- Cataract formation
- Implant extrusion

Chapter 50

Drainage of Choroidal Detachments

Neelakshi Bhagat, MD, MPH, FACS
Marco A. Zarbin, MD, PhD, FACS

Drainage of a choroidal detachment is indicated for management of accumulated persistent serous or hemorrhagic suprachoroidal effusions as a result of trauma, hypotony after glaucoma surgery, or other intraocular surgeries. Drainage of an appositional choroidal detachment ("kissing choroidal detachment") is indicated to restore normal anatomy and avoid retinal injury.

PREOPERATIVE STEPS

1. Perform an ocular examination.
2. Use ultrasonography to evaluate the extent of choroidal detachment (in the presence of media opacity), to ascertain the nature of the suprachoroidal fluid (ie, blood vs serous fluid), and to assess the presence of nonlysed hemorrhagic clots.

INSTRUMENTATION AND SUPPLIES

- Lid speculum
- Toothed tissue forceps (0.12, 0.3, and 0.5 mm)
- Westcott and Stevens scissors
- Curved Stevens scissors
- Sutures (2-0 black silk on spatula needle, 8-0 polyglactin [Vicryl] or 6-0 gut)

- Muscle hooks (including fenestrated hook)
- Needle holder
- Schepens retractor
- Beaver blade, super sharp blade
- Indirect ophthalmoscope and indirect lenses (eg, 20 or 28 D)
- Straight scleral depressor
- Anterior chamber maintainer (eg, 23-gauge needle connected to an infusion line)
- Viscoelastic solution

SURGICAL PROCEDURE

1. Local anesthesia with sedation or general anesthesia is used.
2. Prep and drape the eye in a sterile manner.
3. Place the lid speculum.
4. Perform a 360° conjunctival peritomy at the limbus with Westcott scissors and tissue forceps (see Figure 46.1). If a glaucoma filtration bleb is present, avoid instrumentation of the conjunctiva in the quadrant of the bleb.
5. Bluntly dissect the Tenon's space between muscles with Stevens scissors (see Figure 46.2).
6. Isolate rectus muscles using a muscle hook.
7. Sling each isolated rectus muscle with a 2-0 silk suture using a fenestrated muscle hook (see Figures 46.3, 46.4). The muscle hook should be passed in a temporal-to-nasal direction while slinging superior rectus muscle to avoid slinging the superior oblique tendon. Tie a knot at the distal end of each suture.
8. Inspect the sclera for any thinning in all exposed quadrants.
9. Examine the retina completely with scleral depression and indirect ophthalmoscopy. Use ultrasound as a guide if needed.
10. Make a paracentesis using a super-sharp blade at the corneal limbus. Place an anterior chamber maintainer connected to balanced salt solution bottle (BSS) on the vitrectomy machine.
11. Turn the infusion on to perfuse BSS into the anterior chamber.
12. Choose an area under highly elevated choroidal detachment. One can either make either a radial or a circumferential incision.
    - Radial incision: create a radial incision in the sclera, 3 to 4 mm long, 3 to 5 mm from the limbus with a sharp blade (eg, No. 69

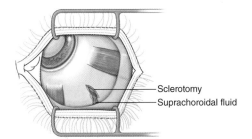

Figure 50.1. Drainage of a choroidal detachment.

Sclerotomy
Suprachoroidal fluid

Beaver blade), Figure 50.1, down to the suprachoroidal space and suprachoroidal effusion will gush out.

- Circumferential incision: make a circumferential incision 3 to 4 mm in chord length, 3 to 4 mm posterior to the limbus. If there is trapped suprachoroidal fluid (versus a clot), a more posteriorly situated sclerotomy may be needed. Sclerotomies can be circumferential or radial, depending on the anatomy of the choroidal detachment.

13. Release all traction on the eye and gently press the globe with a cotton-tipped applicator to help express suprachoroidal fluid. Some-times the traction exerted by the assistant pulling on the stay sutures may help egress of fluid.

14. Examine the retina by indirect ophthalmoscopy to evaluate the extent of residual choroidal detachment. Repeat the drainage procedure in areas of residual choroidal detachment.

15. Do not attempt to drain areas with residual suprachoroidal clot, as demonstrated by pre- or intraoperative echography.

16. Examine the retina with indirect ophthalmoscopy; if necessary, create sclerotomies in all quadrants until all the suprachoroidal fluid is drained.

17. Remove the 23-gauge infusion system. Viscoelastic injection may be needed to maintain the anterior chamber and an IOP between 15 to 20 mm Hg. Suture the limbal incision with 10-0 nylon.

18. Remove the 2-0 silk sutures and close the peritomy with absorbable suture (8-0 polyglactin or 6-0 gut), see Figure 46.10.

19. Inject subconjunctival cefazolin (100 mg)—if the patient is allergic to penicillin, consider vancomycin (50 mg)—and Decadron (4 to 8 mg) or Kenalog (40 mg).

20. Remove the lid speculum, apply topical atropine 1% drops and antibi-otic ointment, and patch.

POSTOPERATIVE CARE

1. Examine the patient on the first postoperative day.
2. Prescribe topical antibiotics (eg, Vigamox 4 times a day) for 1 week and corticosteroid drops (eg, prednisolone acetate 1%) as the degree of inflammation warrants as well as atropine 1% 4 times a day.
3. Follow-up examination is the same as for pars plana vitrectomy surgery (Chapter 47).

COMPLICATIONS

- Transient increase in the IOP
- Hypotony
- Vitreous hemorrhage
- Hyphema
- Retinal tear or detachment
- Endophthalmitis
- Recurrent suprachoroidal hemorrhage

Part VI

Ophthalmic Plastic Surgery

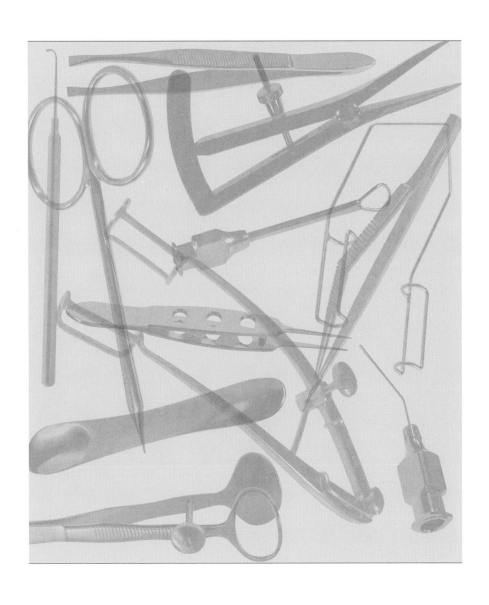

Chapter 51

Skin Grafts

Susan R. Carter, MD

This chapter covers 2 types of skin grafts the ophthalmic surgeon may be tasked to perform: full-thickness skin grafts and split-thickness skin grafts.

FULL-THICKNESS SKIN GRAFTS

Full-thickness skin grafts are placed during the reconstruction of the eyelids when the amount of the patient's own skin is deficient. Skin grafting may be required in the setting of cicatricial changes that need to be corrected, such as with a cicatricial ectropion of the upper or lower eyelid, or when tumor excision has left a defect that necessitates graft placement rather than flap formation.

Preoperative Steps

1. Estimate the amount of skin graft needed to determine the best site to harvest the graft. The closest matches to eyelid skin are eyelid skin from an unaffected lid and retroauricular skin. Other sites that are used include preauricular, supraclavicular, and inner upper-arm skin.
2. Examine the chosen donor site to ensure sufficient amount and lack of skin lesions.

Instrumentation and Supplies

- Marking pen
- Anesthetic eye drops
- 2% lidocaine with epinephrine 1:100,000
- 27-gauge, 1 1/2-inch needle with syringe
- Betadine swabs
- Bard-Parker No. 15 blade scalpel
- Castroviejo 0.5 mm forceps
- Westcott scissors
- Needle holder
- Cotton-tipped swabs
- 4-0 silk traction suture
- 4-0 monofilament suture for retroauricular closure
- 6-0 silk suture
- Eye pads
- 1 inch paper tape with Mastisol

Surgical Procedure With Eyelid Skin Graft

1. Mark the upper eyelid crease.
2. Measure and mark the redundant skin superior to the lid crease with the eyelids in a closed position.
3. Place an anesthetic drop on the eye and infiltrate the donor and graft sites with 2% lidocaine with epinephrine 1:100,000 mixed with hyaluronidase.
4. Prep and drape the patient in a sterile manner.
5. Place a 4-0 silk traction suture through the gray line of the middle of the lower eyelid, if the graft is to be placed in the lower lid. Clamp the suture to the drape superior to the eyebrow.
6. Prepare the recipient site for the skin graft with judicious use of cautery and create as flat a bed of orbicularis muscle as possible for graft placement.
7. Measure the length and width of the defect in its greatest dimensions with the surrounding skin on slight stretch to measure the maximum possible dimensions, or create a template.
8. If the eyelid skin graft needed is smaller than the ellipse of tissue drawn on the upper lid, less skin is removed if desired.
9. Incise the eyelid skin with a No. 15 blade scalpel through dermis (Figure 51.1).

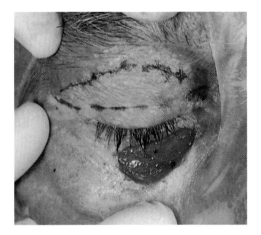

Figure 51.1. A No. 15 blade scalpel is used to incise the skin of the upper lid in preparation for a skin graft to fill a lower lid defect. (Reproduced, by permission, from Rathbun JE, *Eyelid Surgery* [Boston: Little Brown, 1990], Figure 2-13A.)

10. Excise the skin at the deep border of dermis with Wescott scissors, leaving orbicularis behind.

11. Dissect any residual subcutaneous tissue from the graft with the scissors flush to the graft until a "peau d'orange" appearance of the graft is achieved.

12. Cauterize the orbicularis muscle and proceed as with the blepharoplasty procedure (Chapter 63). Close the eyelid crease incision with a running 6-0 suture. A similar procedure can be performed on the opposite upper lid for purposes of symmetry.

13. Place the graft in the recipient site.

14. Suture the graft in place with interrupted or running 6-0 silk or plain gut sutures. If the graft is placed on a concave surface, place mattress sutures in the center of the graft to affix it to the recipient bed.

15. If the graft is placed in the lower eyelid, place Steri-Strips to fixate the 4-0 silk lower lid traction suture to the forehead skin, and place the lid on slight stretch (Figure 51.2).

16. Place a Telfa pad over the graft, followed by several eye pads, some cut to match the graft shape, to put uniform pressure over the skin graft with a full eye patch. Use Mastisol on the skin where the tape is to be placed. Alternatively, a petrolatum gauze and cotton bolster is sutured over the graft with mattress sutures.

17. Remove and change eye patch after 3 days. Leave the second patch in place for 2 to 3 more days.

18. Remove sutures at 1 week postoperatively.

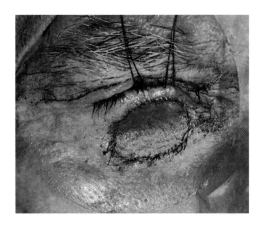

Figure 51.2. The upper lid incision is closed, the skin graft is sutured in place in the lower lid, and lower lid traction sutures are affixed to the forehead. (Reproduced, by permission, from Rathbun JE, *Eyelid Surgery* [Boston: Little Brown, 1990], Figure 2-13B.)

Surgical Procedure With Retroauricular Skin Graft

1. Anesthesia: topical drops and local infiltration with 2% lidocaine with epinephrine 1:100,000 mixed with hyaluronidase of recipient and donor graft sites.
2. Prep and drape the patient in a sterile manner.
3. Obtain the retroauricular graft from the non-hair bearing skin behind the ear. Center the graft with the midline on the line where the ear meets the skull (Figure 51.3).
4. Incise the skin with a No. 15 blade scalpel once the graft dimensions have been drawn in the retroauricular region.
5. Excise the graft with sharp and blunt dissection with minimal subcutaneous tissue (Figure 51.4).
6. Remove any subcutaneous tissue until a "peau d'orange" appearance is achieved.
7. Close the skin incision with multiple 4-0 monofilament interrupted sutures, leaving the ends long for easy removal (Figure 51.5).
8. Remove retroauricular sutures at 1 to 2 weeks postoperatively, depending on the degree of wound tension.
9. Proceed with placement of the graft as described in "Procedure With Eyelid Skin Graft" in this chapter.

Complications

- Bleeding
- Infection
- Graft failure
- Wound dehiscence

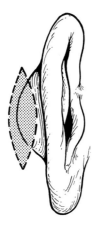

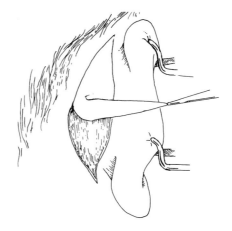

Figure 51.3. The retroauricular skin graft is centered on the junction of the ear with the skull. (Reproduced, by permission, from Tanenbaum M, McCord CD, Nunnery WR, eds, *Oculoplastic Surgery* [Philadelphia: Lippincott Williams & Wilkins, 1995], Figure 1.8B.)

Figure 51.4. The full-thickness skin graft is excised from the retroauricular region. (Reproduced, by permission, from Rathbun JE, *Eyelid Surgery* [Boston: Little Brown, 1990], Figure 2.16B.)

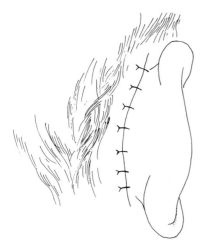

Figure 51.5. The retroauricular region is closed with suture ends left long. (Reproduced, by permission, from Rathbun JE, *Eyelid Surgery* [Boston: Little Brown, 1990], Figure 2-16C.)

Bleeding is managed with direct pressure, and rarely with surgical intervention, for both donor and recipient sites.

Infection is usually managed with oral and topical antibiotics and warm compresses. Oral antibiotics may be used prophylactically in the setting of a patch placed for multiple days to prevent this complication.

Graft failure presents as a blue purple discoloration of a portion or of the entire skin graft, which may turn black. Graft failure occurs because of inadequate blood supply to the graft from inadequate vascularity of the graft bed or inadequate contact between the graft and the graft bed, which may be due to blood beneath the graft. Management includes observation initially, as some grafts may survive, and initiation of massage and corticosteroid injections after the surgical wounds have healed. Defer additional surgical intervention for at least 6 months, if possible.

Retroauricular wound dehiscence should be managed by observation alone, as the wound will usually granulate closed.

SPLIT-THICKNESS SKIN GRAFTS

Split-thickness skin grafts are placed in the setting of large areas of skin loss or of a poorly vascularized bed, such as an exenterated orbital socket.

Preoperative Steps

1. Inspect the anterior thigh as a site for harvesting a split-thickness skin graft.

Instrumentation and Supplies

- Dermatome
- Mineral oil
- Tongue blade
- Skin graft mesher

Surgical Procedure

1. Prep and drape the anterior surface of the thigh.
2. Shave the anterior surface of the thigh if excessive hair is present.
3. Lubricate the skin with mineral oil.
4. Set the dermatome at 12/1000 to 15/1000 of an inch.
5. Hold the skin taught with 2 wooden tongue blades.
6. Excise the split-thickness skin graft using the dermatome. Multiple pinpoint sites of bleeding should be visible (Figure 51.6).
7. Expand the graft in the 1:1 1/2 times mesher (ie, the graft is expanded to 1 1/2 times its previous size), if desired, with the epidermis side up on the mesher plate (Figure 51.7).
8. Wipe away the oil on the anterior thigh.
9. Use antibiotic-impregnated gauze or transparent wound dressings on the thigh. Tight circumferential bandages should be avoided.

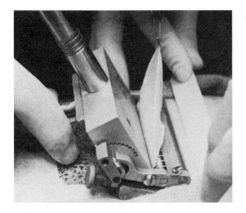

Figure 51.6. The dermatome is used to excise a split-thickness skin graft from the anterior thigh, with a tongue blade used to flatten the skin in front of the dermatome. (Reproduced, by permission, from Tanenbaum M, McCord CD, Nunery WR, eds, *Oculoplastic Surgery* [Philadelphia: Lippincott Williams & Wilkins, 1995], Figure 1.10B.)

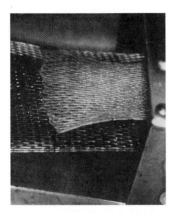

Figure 51.7. The split-thickness skin graft is fed through a mesher. (Reproduced, by permission, from Tanenbaum M, McCord CD, Nunery WR, eds, *Oculoplastic Surgery* [Philadelphia: Lippincott Williams & Wilkins, 1995], Figure 1.11C.)

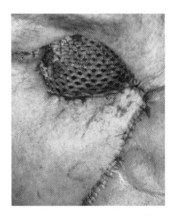

Figure 51.8. A meshed graft is sutured into an exenterated orbit. (Reproduced, by permission, from Tanenbaum M, McCord CD, Nunery WR, eds, *Oculoplastic Surgery* [Philadelphia: Lippincott Williams & Wilkins, 1995], Figure 1.11C.)

10. Suture the graft in position (Figure 51.8).
11. Prescribe prophylactic antibiotics for the first week postoperatively.

COMPLICATIONS

- Dermal resection
- Graft failure

Unintended full-thickness dermal resection at the graft site should be covered with split-thickness skin.

Graft failure may occur due to lack of vascular supply of the recipient bed. Vascularized flaps may be needed instead of split-thickness skin graft in this setting.

Chapter 52

Basic Skin Flaps in Ophthalmic Plastic Surgery

Edward J. Wladis, MD
Roberta E. Gausas, MD

Skin flaps are indicated in the reconstruction of periocular defects, particularly after trauma or the resection of skin neoplasms. The advantages of flaps are that they provide their own vasculature, usually match the surrounding skin pigmentation and texture, and generally heal with minimal cosmetic deformity. In addition, flaps are recruited to fill subcutaneous defects, as they are usually thicker than skin grafts. Each flap carries advantages and disadvantages, and knowledge of when to employ these flaps leads to improved functional and aesthetic outcomes.

INSTRUMENTATION AND SUPPLIES

- 1% lidocaine with epinephrine 1:100,000 on a 30-gauge needle
- Desmarres retractor
- Castroviejo needle driver
- 0.5 forceps (2)
- Westcott scissors
- Bovie monopolar cautery
- No. 15 blade scalpel
- 5-0 or 6-0 polyglactin (Vicryl), 6-0 polypropylene (Prolene), 6-0 fast-absorbing gut, and 6-0 silk sutures

RECTANGULAR ADVANCEMENT FLAP

Advancement flaps allow for the repair of defects without the excessive tension that often results from direct closure. Furthermore, rectangular advancement flaps may be designed without superior or inferior tension vectors, making them particularly useful in the reconstruction of periocular defects. These flaps are best employed if the flap needs to be advanced only a short distance to achieve wound closure.

Surgical Procedure

1. With a marking pen, identify a line that extends from the inferior aspect of the defect. Similarly, mark a line that extends superiorly from the superior aspect of the wound. As such, the flap delineated has a narrower apex than base. The length-to-width ratio should not exceed 3:1 (Figure 52.1A).
2. Infiltrate the flap site using 1% lidocaine with epinephrine 1:100,000.
3. Incise the skin with a No. 15 blade scalpel along the previously drawn lines.
4. Undermine the flap with Westcott scissors, mobilizing the flap. Continue undermining immediately deep to the orbicularis until the flap can easily be advanced into the wound.
5. Anchor the deep tissues of the orbicularis muscle into the recipient bed with several interrupted 5-0 or 6-0 polyglactin sutures (Figure 52.1B).
6. Close the superficial tissues with running 6-0 polypropylene or fast-absorbing gut sutures. Excision of Burow's triangles may be required at the base of the flap.

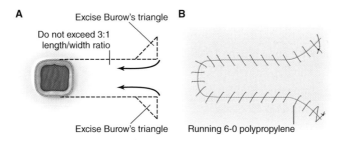

A Excise Burow's triangle B
Do not exceed 3:1
length/width ratio

Excise Burow's triangle   Running 6-0 polypropylene

Figure 52.1. Rectangular advancement flap. (A) After identifying lines that extend from the superior and inferior aspects of the wound, the intervening tissue is carefully undermined and advanced into the defect. (B) The deep tissues are anchored into the recipient bed, and the superficial skin is closed with a running suture.

Complications

- Necrosis
- Lid retraction

Excessively long flaps are at risk of necrosis. In order to ensure the health of an advancement flap, the length-to-width ratio should be less than 3:1. If a longer flap is required, maintain a thicker pedicle to allow for a robust vasculature. Avoid excessive thinning of the flap in patients with a risk of vascular compromise, such as smokers or people with diabetes.

Lid retraction may occur despite careful flap design.

BILOBED FLAP

The bilobed flap is a double transposition flap that facilitates closure of wounds in which the defect is under tension and the surrounding skin is relatively immobile. This flap allows the surgeon to transfer more tissue over a greater distance than would be possible with a single transposition flap. It is well suited for the repair of circular medial canthal and nasal dorsum defects.

Surgical Procedure

1. Determine the location of adequate skin laxity to decide the orientation of the flaps. Excise a surrounding Burow's triangle of skin to create a teardrop-shaped defect.
2. Mark a semicircle adjacent to the defect with a diameter that is slightly narrower than that of the defect. Draw an additional semicircle 90° from the defect with a diameter that is one-half of that of the defect. Connect the flap lines (Figure 52.2A).
3. Infiltrate the entire distribution of the flap and defect using 1% lidocaine with epinephrine 1:100,000.
4. Incise the flap sites with a No. 15 scalpel. Undermine the flap in a plane immediately deep to the subcutaneous fat (ie, superficial to the nasalis muscle).
5. Anchor the adjacent flap into the defect bed with several interrupted 5-0 polyglactin sutures. Rotate the distant semicircle into the larger lobe (Figure 52.2B), and anchor it into position with several interrupted 5-0 polyglactin sutures. Close the smaller flap directly with several interrupted 5-0 polyglactin sutures.

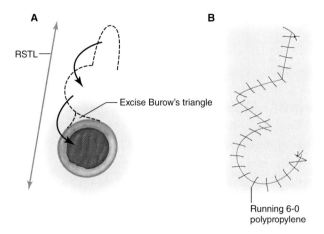

Figure 52.2. Bilobed flap. (A) Semicircular flaps are identified adjacent to the defect, and the tissue is undermined. (B) The flaps are rotated to fill the defects, and the tissues are anchored into position.

6. Close all skin wounds with superficial running 6-0 polypropylene or fast-absorbing gut sutures.

Complications

- Necrosis
- Redundant tissue

Excessively thin flaps may not recruit adequate vascular supply, and may therefore necrose.

At the time of closure, surgeons should examine the flap site to ensure that no redundant tissue ("dog ear") is present. Trim any residual tissue to avoid this complication.

RHOMBIC FLAP

The rhombic flap allows for closure of larger defects, as it mobilizes larger amounts of tissue. Incisions that are parallel to the relaxed skin tension lines (ie, those with minimal associated skin tautness) heal with less strain and "puckering," and identifying these lines facilitates optimal postoperative results. The lines of maximum extensibility are perpendicular to the relaxed skin tension lines.

Surgical Procedure

1. Draw a rhombus around the defect (ie, equilateral triangles, placed base to base).
2. Extend a line of the same length as the base of the imagined triangles horizontally, adjacent to the rhombus. At the outward tip of the horizontal line, draw lines at an angle of 60° that are parallel and equal to the sides of the rhombus (Figure 52.3A).
3. Choose the sides that are parallel to the lines of maximum extensibility (ie, perpendicular to the relaxed skin tension lines), Figure 52.3B.
4. Infiltrate the defect and the appropriately chosen lines using 1% lidocaine with epinephrine 1:100,000.
5. Incise the skin along the marked distribution with a No. 15 scalpel, and undermine with Westcott scissors.
6. Rotate the flap into the defect, and anchor it into position with several 5-0 polyglactin sutures. Close the donor site directly with several 5-0 polyglactin sutures (Figure 52.3C).
7. Close all skin wounds with running 6-0 polypropylene sutures (Figure 52.3D).

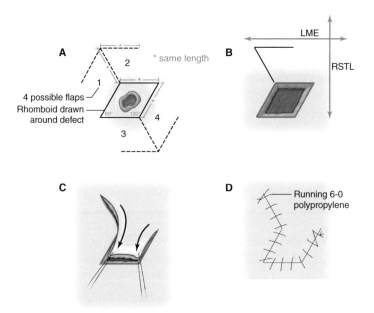

Figure 52.3. Rhombic flap. (A) After drawing a rhombus around the defect, lines of equal length are drawn adjacent to its base. Lines are then drawn at the external tips, creating a 60° angle. (B) The lines that are parallel to the lines of maximum extensibility are identified. (C) The flap is carefully undermined, rotated into position, and anchored. (D) The skin is closed.

Complications

- Puckering
- Excessive tension

The success of this flap relies on the design of the rhombus and the recognition of the surrounding relaxed skin tension lines. If these lines are violated, the closure will appear "puckered" and excessive tension may result.

To avoid excessive tension, make sure that the outlying lines are equal in length to the sides of the rhombus.

O-TO-Z-PLASTY

This flap effectively converts vertical tension to a horizontal plane. As a result, it is particularly useful in cases of lower eyelid reconstruction, as it facilitates the avoidance of a retracting force. The O-to-Z-plasty generally allows for closure of circular periocular defects with only minimal evidence of scarring.

Surgical Procedure

1. Identify a circular defect. Delineate semicircular lines, extending inferiorly from the superior aspect of the defect and superiorly from the inferior aspect. These lines should be equal in length and should extend to points along lines that are parallel to the relaxed skin tension lines (Figure 52.4A).
2. Infiltrate the entire distribution using 1% lidocaine with epinephrine 1:100,000.

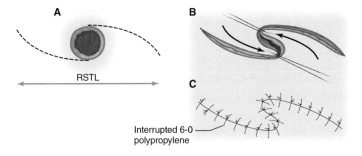

Figure 52.4. O-to-Z-plasty. (A) Semicircular lines are drawn, radiating from the superior and inferior aspects of a circular defect. (B) The flaps are undermined and reflected into the recipient bed. (C) The flaps are anchored into position, and the tissues are closed.

3. Incise the skin, and undermine in a suborbicularis plane.
4. Reflect both arms of the flap into the center of the defect (Figure 52.4B).
5. Close the flap with interrupted 6-0 polypropylene sutures (Figure 52.4C).

Complications

While this technique effectively reduces and redirects the skin tension surrounding a circular defect, attention must be paid to the size of the defect in order to prevent eyelid retraction and lagophthalmos. O-to-Z-plasties should be avoided in anterior lamellar defects exceeding 50% of the length of the eyelid. In cases where a larger defect needs to be repaired, the use of an alternative flap or a skin graft is recommended.

Z-PLASTY

The Z-plasty can be employed to reduce the appearance and retracting effects of a contracted scar. This flap facilitates the redirection of an elevated scar into the lines of relaxed tension, and enables surgeons to lengthen contracted scars. As a result, eyelid retraction and cosmetically unacceptable scars can be relieved with this technique.

Surgical Procedure

1. Measure the length of the entire scar. At each end, draw a line at a 60° angle that is equal to the length of the scar, creating a Z. Draw an ellipse around the scar site (Figure 52.5A).
2. Infiltrate the entire site using 1% lidocaine with epinephrine.
3. Excise the ellipse around the scar with a No. 15 scalpel, and incise the remainder of the Z (Figure 52.5B).
4. Undermine the flaps with Westcott scissors, allowing enough laxity to rotate these flaps into the recipient bed.
5. Rotate the flaps (Figure 52.5C).
6. Close the subcutaneous tissue with several interrupted 5-0 or 6-0 polyglactin sutures. Close the superficial tissues with running 6-0 polypropylene sutures.

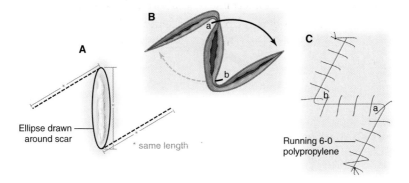

Figure 52.5. Z-plasty. (A) Lines are drawn, equaling the length of a scar at 60° angles to its superior and inferior edges and creating a Z shape. (B) The scar is excised in an elliptical pattern, and the flaps are undermined. The flaps are rotated into the recipient bed. (C) The flaps are anchored into position, and the overlying tissues are closed.

Complications

- Tissue distortion
- Necrosis

While the Z-plasty often improves the contour of the surrounding tissue, tissue distortion may develop if the Z-plasty is under excessive tension. In such cases, consider the application of a skin graft.

Observe the flap tips for signs of necrosis. Although this problem often improves with time, if significant necrosis develops, consider debridement and the placement of a skin graft.

V-TO-Y-PLASTY

The V-to-Y-plasty can be used to reduce tension lines in areas of skin contractures. Converting the shape of a defect from a V to a Y shape alleviates tissue-shortening in the direction parallel to the stem of the Y and increases the length between structures along this dimension.

Surgical Procedure

1. At the site of contracture, identify a V-shaped structure. Incise the skin of the V with a No. 15 scalpel (Figure 52.6A).

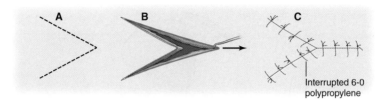

Figure 52.6. V-Y-plasty. (A) A V-shaped scar is identified. (B) With careful undermining, this V is converted to a Y. (C) All overlying tissues are then closed.

2. Undermine the tissues in a suborbicularis plane, creating adequate tissue laxity.
3. Once sufficient laxity has been created, advance the flap as a Y shape. The tip of the Y should be apposed first with a 6-0 polypropylene suture (Figure 52.6B).
4. Close the surrounding sides of the V with interrupted 6-0 polypropylene sutures (Figure 52.6C).

Complications

Avoid undue tension when advancing the tip of the V shape. Excessive skin tension creates an imbalanced wound and distracts the surrounding structures.

Y-TO-V-PLASTY

The Y-to-V-plasty is particularly useful in the reconstruction of medial canthal defects and epicanthal folds. In addition, distances between structures can be shortened with this flap, making it particularly useful in the management of telecanthus.

Surgical Procedure

1. Once a Y-shaped defect has been identified, incise the dimensions of the Y with a No. 15 scalpel (Figure 52.7A).
2. Carefully undermine all the bars of the Y in a suborbicularis plane with Westcott scissors, creating a triangle-shaped defect. Proceed with tissue dissection until the triangular flap of skin can be easily advanced to fill the resulting defect (Figure 52.7B).
3. Advance the triangular skin-and-muscle flap to the tip of the distal edge of the defect, and appose it with interrupted 6-0 polypropylene sutures (Figure 52.7C).

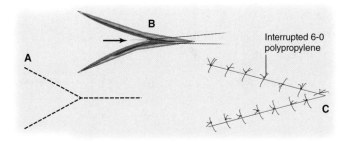

Figure 52.7. Y-V-plasty. (A) A Y-shaped scar is identified. (B) The tissues are carefully undermined to allow sufficient laxity, and advanced as a V shape. (C) All tissues are closed.

Complications

Careful tissue undermining is critical to the success of this flap. If excessive tension is placed on the flap, the surrounding tissues will be distracted medially or laterally.

GLABELLAR FLAP

This flap represents a variant of the rhombic flap. The tissue surrounding a defect in the medial canthus is often only minimally mobile, and the closure of such defects can be particularly challenging. Nonetheless, glabellar tissue can usually be mobilized, and a glabellar flap can be used to repair midsized anterior lamella defects.

Surgical Procedure

1. Starting at the lateral aspect of the defect, mark an inverted V shape superiorly, ending at the medial aspect of the contralateral eyebrow (Figure 52.8A).
2. Infiltrate the entire distribution using 1% lidocaine with epinephrine 1:100,000.
3. Incise the inverted V with a No. 15 scalpel, and undermine it with Westcott scissors immediately deep to the subcutaneous fat.
4. Reflect the flap into the recipient bed, and anchor it into position with several subcutaneous 5-0 polyglactin sutures.
5. Close the forehead site with buried subcutaneous 5-0 polyglactin sutures and superficial 6-0 polypropylene sutures.
6. Excise the excess flap tissue with Westcott scissors.

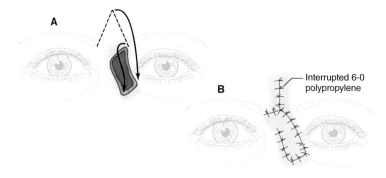

Figure 52.8. Glabellar flap. (A) An inverted V shape is drawn, pointing superiorly from the defect. The V is incised, undermined, and rotated into the defect. (B) The deep and superficial tissues are apposed.

7. Close the remainder of the flap site with subcutaneous 5-0 polyglactin sutures and superficial 6-0 polypropylene sutures (Figure 52.8B).

Complications

- Mismatched margins
- Redundant tissue

Make sure that the flap is carefully apposed in the recipient bed, and that all margins are properly matched. Failure to approximate the margins at the medial canthus may mimic the appearance of telecanthus.

After closure of the flap site, there is often redundant tissue (a "dog ear"). Generally, this problem is best managed by leaving the tissue in place for roughly 2 months. If the redundant tissue persists after wound healing and contracture have taken place, it may be trimmed at that point.

MIDLINE-FOREHEAD FLAP

The midline-forehead flap can be used to repair large medial canthal or lower eyelid defects, as it recruits vasculature from the supratrochlear, terminal, and supraorbital branches of the angular arteries. In addition, the midline-forehead flap is useful in the reconstruction of deep defects, as the deep musculature of the forehead can be rotated into the defect site.

Surgical Procedure

1. Some surgeons advocate identifying the supratrochlear or supraorbital arteries with a Doppler ultrasound, and marking these vessels for inclusion into the flap (Figure 52.9A).
2. Draw a flap with a maximum pedicle width of 1.5 cm, based at the midpoint of the nasal bridge. This flap should extend superiorly along the middle of the forehead, coming to a point at a length adequate to cover the existing defect.
3. Infiltrate the skin in the distribution of the flap using 1% lidocaine with epinephrine 1:100,000.
4. Incise the skin with a No. 15 scalpel, and undermine the flap in a plane immediately anterior to the perichondrium with Westcott scissors, leaving the pedicle intact.
5. Reflect the newly elevated flap into the defect, and anchor it into position with several interrupted 5-0 polyglactin sutures in the deep plane (Figure 52.9B).
6. Close all skin wounds with running 6-0 polypropylene or fast-absorbing gut sutures.
7. Close the forehead wound with deep 5-0 polyglactin sutures and superficial running 6-0 polypropylene or fast-absorbing gut sutures.
8. A second-stage excision of the redundant tissues at the base of the flap can be performed 6 weeks after the initial surgery.

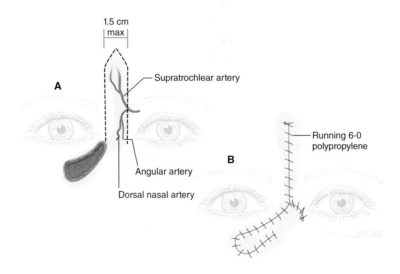

Figure 52.9. Midline-forehead flap. (A) A superiorly directed flap is identified, with the base at the midpoint of the nasal bridge. (B) This flap is incised, rotated into position, and anchored.

Complications

- Vascular compromise
- Arterial ischemia
- Hematoma

When excessively wide flaps are reflected into the recipient bed, they are at risk for vascular compromise. As such, the pedicle of the flap should not exceed 1.5 cm.

Postoperatively, if the flap appears to be cooler and paler than the surrounding tissue, arterial ischemia may be present. This may necessitate debridement of any ischemic sections.

Hematoma development beneath the flap may slow vascular ingrowth and can result in infection. Intraoperative control of bleeding will help to avoid this problem.

Chapter 53

Enucleation, Evisceration, and Exenteration

David R. Jordan, MD
Louise Mawn, MD

Enucleation, evisceration, and exenteration are the main surgical techniques by which all or parts of the orbital contents are removed.

ENUCLEATION SURGERY

Enucleation involves removal of the entire globe while preserving other orbital tissues. Enucleation may be indicated in primary intraocular malignancies (eg, melanoma or retinoblastoma) not amenable to alternative modes of therapy such as external, or proton, beam irradiation, or episcleral plaque brachytherapy.

In the severely traumatized eye with extensive prolapse of uveal tissue, enucleation within the first 10 to 14 days is considered if the risk of sympathetic ophthalmia and harm to the remaining eye is judged to be greater than the likelihood of recovering useful vision in the traumatized eye. The infrequency of sympathetic ophthalmia coupled with improved medical therapy for uveitis has made early enucleation strictly for prophylaxis a debatable practice.

Blind, painful eyes for which the ophthalmic history is well known (eg, following end-stage glaucoma, trauma, hypotony, or phthisis) are managed by enucleation or evisceration with dramatic relief from discomfort. The choice between enucleation and evisceration is controversial and varies by the surgeon's preference. Enucleation is preferred if a complete histopathologic examination of the globe is required. For debilitated patients with blind, painful eyes unable to undergo surgery and rehabilitation, a retrobulbar injection of ethanol or Thorazine may provide adequate pain relief.

If the eye is blind, unsightly, and phthisical with no possibility of a tumor, the patient may be a candidate for a scleral shell (a thin ocular prosthesis that fits over the blind eye). The shell provides a natural appearance and allows patients to keep their eye. If the eye is not phthisical, a scleral shell will make the eye appear proptotic and is not a good option; however, a painted contact lens may improve the appearance of the eye.

Preoperative Steps

1. Take a careful history and examine the eye to diagnose the problem. Review the goals of surgery: remove the eye, restore orbital volume, and provide movement to the ocular prosthesis.
2. Review the surgical procedure with patient including the temporary use of a conformer and the plan for prosthesis fitting 6 to 7 weeks after surgery. Review local versus general anesthesia, expected postoperative pain, time away from work, and follow-up visits. The potential complications of implant infection, exposure, extrusion, and migration should be discussed.
3. Decide on the orbital implant to use (porous versus nonporous). Proper selection of implant volume helps minimize superior sulcus deformity and enophthalmos. In general, a 20 to 22 mm diameter sphere allows reasonable volume return following enucleation surgery in an adult.
4. Decide on implant wrapping to use. When using a porous orbital implant (eg, hydroxyapatite/aluminum oxide/porous polyethylene), a wrap facilitates placement of the implant into the eye socket. It also allows precise fixation of the extraocular muscles to the implant surface and may provide a barrier function over the rough porous implant surface. One type of porous polyethylene implant is modified on the anterior surface for placement without a wrap.

Instrumentation and Supplies

- Magnifying loupes
- Headlight
- Bipolar cautery with bayonet forceps
- Implant (eg, polymethylmethacrylate sphere, hydroxyapatite/aluminum oxide/porous polyethylene)
- Wrap for implant (sclera, polyglactin [Vicryl] mesh, or other)
- Topical anesthetic eye drops

- 2.5% topical phenylephrine eye drops
- 2% lidocaine with epinephrine 1:100,000 for local infiltration
- Bacteriostatic saline to mix with 2% lidocaine
- 0.75% bupivacaine solution
- Topical thrombin, 4% cocaine solution
- Lid speculum
- Castroviejo 0.5-mm toothed forceps
- Westcott tenotomy scissors (curved right, blunt tips)
- Adson toothed forceps
- Castroviejo needle holder
- Stevens curved tenotomy scissors
- Small muscle hook
- Large muscle hook
- Double-pronged skin hooks (2)
- Malleable ribbon retractors
- Enucleation scissors
- Carter sphere introducer

Surgical Procedure

1. Develop a presurgery routine to ensure that the correct eye is removed. The patient should point to or touch the eye to be removed. Confirm that this eye corresponds to the consent form and to your chart notes. Place several obvious marks around the eye to be removed.
2. If there is a tumor in the eye, dilate the eye in the presurgery holding area so you can carry out direct visualization of the mass when the patient arrives in the operating room.
3. Local anesthesia with intravenous sedation or general anesthesia can be used. If local anesthesia is used, block the upper and lower eyelids with 2% lidocaine in combination with epinephrine 1:100,000, mixed half-and-half with bacteriostatic saline (approx 1.5 to 2 cc in each lid and lateral canthus). In all cases, administer a retrobulbar, intraconal injection of 2% lidocaine in combination with epinephrine 1:100,000, mixed half-and-half with 0.75% bupivacaine (5 to 7 cc), followed by pressure application to the orbit for 5 to 10 minutes.
4. Place the lid speculum.
5. Perform a 360° conjunctival limbal peritomy using Wescott scissors.
6. Dissect Tenon's tissue away from the globe in each muscle quadrant using Stevens tenotomy scissors (Figure 53.1).
7. One at a time, localize each rectus muscle and place it on a large muscle hook to ensure the entire muscle has been isolated.

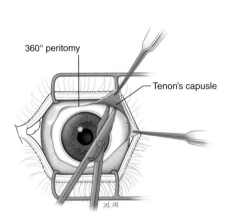

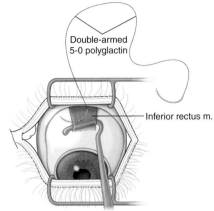

Figure 53.1. Tenon's tissue is dissected away from the globe.

Figure 53.2. A double-armed 5-0 polyglactin suture is passed, locked on either side of the muscle.

8. Gently apply cautery to the arteries at the muscle insertion.

9. Pass a double-armed 5-0 polyglactin suture locked on either side of the muscle (Figure 53.2).

10. Severe the muscle from the globe. Leave a 1 to 2 mm stump of muscle tendon attached to the globe over the medial and lateral rectus insertions so traction sutures can be applied later in the procedure.

11. Hook the inferior oblique muscle in the inferior and temporal quadrant with the tip of the muscle hook, sweeping from posterior to anterior (staying adjacent to the globe) toward the inferior rectus muscle. The muscle is held between 2 muscle hooks, clamped with a straight hemostat, cauterized in the clamped section, cut, then recauterized if the muscle stumps are bleeding. Optionally, secure the inferior oblique with a 5-0 polyglactin suture, in a similar fashion to the recti muscles, for later attachment to the implant (Figure 53.3).

12. Locate the superior oblique tendon in the superior nasal quadrant by sweeping the muscle hook from anterior to posterior (staying adjacent to the globe) toward the superior rectus muscle. Simply cut the superior oblique tendon (clamping is not required). The superior oblique is left untagged (Figure 53.4).

13. Attach a 4-0 silk suture to the lateral, +/− medial rectus insertion sites to allow traction of the globe anteriorly.

14. Place the closed enucleation scissors behind the globe and localize the optic nerve by strumming the nerve with the closed scissors. Then open the scissor tips and place the tips on either side of the optic nerve (Figure 53.5). To get as much optic nerve stump as possible, move the

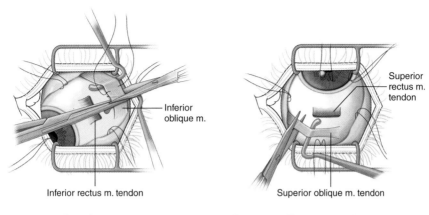

Figure 53.3. The inferior oblique tendon is cut.   **Figure 53.4.** The superior oblique tendon is cut.

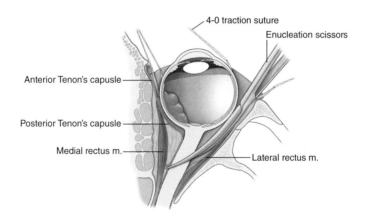

Figure 53.5. The tips of the enucleation scissors are positioned on either side of the optic nerve.

tips of the scissors directly posteriorly several millimeters. In cutting the optic nerve, maintain posteriorly directed pressure to prevent the scissors tips from sliding off the optic nerve. Once the nerve has been transected, the entire globe moves forward. Cut the remaining Tenon's tissue away from the posterior aspect of the eye, staying as close as possible to the globe (Figure 53.6).

15. Once the eye is out, apply pressure to the socket with thrombin or 4% cocaine-soaked sponges (or simply saline) for 5 minutes to achieve some hemostasis.

16. Use malleable ribbon retractors to gently retract orbital fat away from the optic nerve stump. Cauterize active bleeders in this area under direct visualization.

17. Place the implant within the socket. Prior to insertion, the implant is immersed in an antibiotic solution (eg, 500 mg of cefazolin in 500 cc

Figure 53.6. Once the optic nerve has
been transected, the entire globe moves
forward.

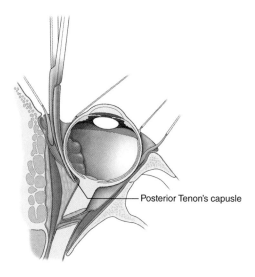

Posterior Tenon's capusle

of normal saline) within a 60-cc syringe, and the air is withdrawn.
The exact location for implant placement varies among ophthalmic
surgeons. The authors prefer to have the orbital implant remain partly
within Tenon's space and partly behind Tenon's, in the intraconal
space (Figure 53.7). Other surgeons prefer placing the implant entirely

Figure 53.7. Plac-
ing the implant in the
socket.

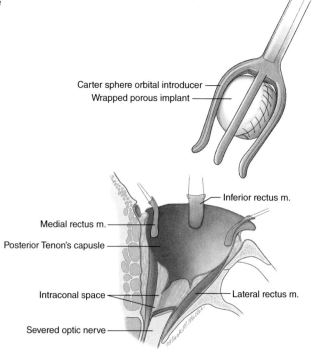

Carter sphere orbital introducer
Wrapped porous implant

Inferior rectus m.

Medial rectus m.
Posterior Tenon's capusle

Intraconal space
Lateral rectus m.

Severed optic nerve

within the intraconal space. An implant introducer (eg, Carter sphere introducer) facilitates implant placement. Avoid dragging anterior Tenon's tissue posteriorly while inserting the implant (a common problem with porous orbital implants). Once the implant is placed into the orbit, the authors routinely "seat" the implant. To perform this maneuver, apply gentle posterior pressure to the anterior implant surface using a cotton-tipped applicator while an Adson toothed forceps is used to unravel any rolled Tenon's edge for 360° around the implant. Apply additional posterior pressure to the implant with the cotton-tipped applicator while pulling anteriorly on Tenon's if a deeper implant placement is preferred (Figure 53.8).

18. Secure the rectus muscle sutures to the anterior portion of the wrapped implant, just anterior to their normal anatomic insertion sites. The authors generally attach the rectus muscles to the implant so that they are approximately 8 to 10 mm away from the antagonist rectus muscle (Figure 53.9).

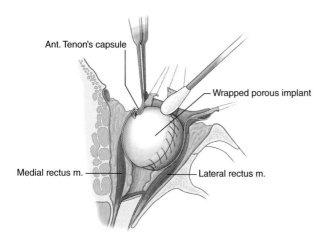

Ant. Tenon's capsule

Wrapped porous implant

Medial rectus m.

Lateral rectus m.

Figure 53.8. Applying additional posterior pressure to the implant if a deeper implant placement is preferred.

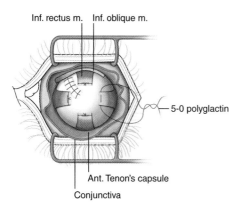

Inf. rectus m.   Inf. oblique m.

5-0 polyglactin

Ant. Tenon's capsule

Conjunctiva

Figure 53.9. The rectus muscle sutures are secured to the anterior portion of the wrapped implant.

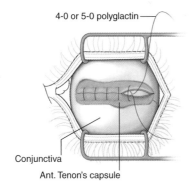

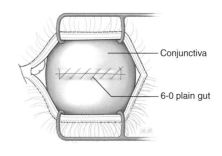

Figure 53.10. Anterior Tenon's is closed under no tension.

Figure 53.11. The conjunctiva is closed with a running 6-0 plain gut suture.

19. Meticulously close anterior Tenon's, under no tension, with a buried 4-0 or 5-0 polyglactin suture in an interrupted fashion (Figure 53.10).
20. Close conjunctiva with a running suture (6-0 plain gut suture). Rapid absorbing 6-0 plain gut suture is not recommended, as the absorption is too quick (Figure 53.11).
21. Apply antibiotic ointment to the conjunctival fornices; insert a small, medium, or large conformer depending upon the tissue space; and apply 2 eye patches. Plan on leaving the patch in place for 3 to 5 days.

Postoperative Care

1. Analgesics (such as acetaminophen with codeine) are usually prescribed.
2. Once the eye patches are removed, no special cleaning is required; the patient may shower or gently wash the face.
3. Start topical antibiotic–corticosteroid eye drops or ointment (tobramycin-dexamethasone) 4 times daily for 3 weeks. A broad-spectrum antibiotic (eg, cephalexin) is taken for 5 days.
4. The temporary conformer is left in the fornix until the patient is fitted with an "impression-fitted" prosthesis 6 to 7 weeks after surgery.
5. Follow-up examination is at 1 to 2, 4 to 6, 8 to 12, 24, and 52 weeks after surgery.

Complications

- Pain
- Nausea
- Swelling

- Infection
- Implant exposure

Pain in most patients is controlled with acetaminophen with codeine (eg, Tylenol #3), but some will require a stronger narcotic (eg, morphine).

Nausea is generally not a problem but its severity varies individually among patients. Prescribe anti-nausea medication if required.

Eyelid and conjunctival swelling may be severe when the patch is removed, and the conformer may spontaneously extrude. Advise the patient to use cool compresses 4 times daily for 30 to 60 minutes for a few days after the patch is removed. Once the swelling settles, the conformer can be replaced. If the conjunctiva is so swollen that it balloons out the palpebral aperture, it must be kept moist with lubricating ointment or antibiotic ointment every 2 hours while the patient is awake to prevent the conjunctiva from becoming dry and irritated. Persistent conjunctival dryness prolongs the swelling.

Infection is very rare in the immediate postoperative period. All patients should be on a broad-spectrum antibiotic (eg, cephalexin) during the first postoperative week. If infection occurs, topical and systemic antibiotics are required. Removal of the implant becomes necessary if the infection is refractory or extrusion appears likely. A secondary implant can be placed once the infection has resolved completely.

Implant exposure is unlikely in the first 1 to 2 weeks. If it occurs, it is most commonly due to improper wound closure, placement of an oversized implant, or infection. Providing there is no infection, additional surgery with reclosure or a patch graft (eg, sclera, temporalis fascia) is required as soon as possible whether a porous or nonporous implant is used. Do not wait for spontaneous closure when a porous implant is in place as the patient is quite vulnerable to infection in this early phase. If infection is suspected, topical and systemic antibiotics are required as discussed above.

EVISCERATION SURGERY

Evisceration involves removal of the entire intraocular contents, leaving the sclera intact. It is typically performed with keratectomy (Chapter 23). The decision to perform evisceration or enucleation has stimulated controversy over the years. Since evisceration leaves the sclera, Tenon's capsule, extraocular muscle attachments, orbital connective tissue framework, and suspensory ligaments virtually undisturbed, evisceration is thought to be associated with better postoperative appearance and motility than with enucleation (regardless of the implant used). Evisceration is simpler and quicker to perform than enucleation. Evisceration can be the first choice in all patients where the ophthalmic history of the diseased eye is well known, there is no intraocular tumor or possibility of an intraocular tumor, and the posterior pole is visible. It should not be performed if a complete histopathologic examination of the globe is required. Ultrasonography with or without computed tomography is performed before evisceration is considered in any eye in which the posterior pole cannot be visualized, even if the past history is known.

Phthisical eyes may not be ideal for evisceration, depending on the degree of contraction of the eye. If the eye is only mildly contracted, a standard evisceration can still be preformed. If the eye is severely contracted, a larger posterior sclerotomy may be required, or a complete sclerotomy where the scleral shell is bisected into 2 complete halves (from superior temporal quadrant to inferior nasal quadrant). Occasionally, the implant must be placed immediately behind the sclera (ie, posterior to posterior Tenon's) in order to insert an adequately sized implant.

Preoperative Steps

1. Obtain a careful history and perform a complete ocular examination. Review the goals of surgery: remove the intraocular contents, restore orbital volume, and provide movement to the ocular prosthesis.
2. Review the surgical procedure with the patient, including the temporary use of a conformer and the plan for prosthesis fitting 6 to 7 weeks after surgery. Review local versus general anesthesia, expected postoperative pain, time away from work, and follow-up visits required. The potential complications of implant infection and exposure should be discussed.
3. Decide on the appropriate implant (eg, polymethylmethacrylate or silicone sphere, hydroxyapatite or another porous implant, or a shaped pseudo-integrated implant (eg, universal implant made of polymethylmethacrylate).

Instrumentation and Supplies

Instrumentation and supplies needed are similar to those required for enucleation surgery with the addition of the following. An implant wrap is not required.

- Evisceration spoon
- Absolute alcohol

Surgical Procedure

1. Always ask the patient on the day of surgery to point to or touch the eye to be eviscerated. Ensure this eye corresponds to the consent form and to your chart notes. Use a marker to place several obvious marks around the eye to be eviscerated.
2. Local anesthesia with intravenous sedation or general anesthesia can be used. If local anesthesia is used, the upper and lower eyelids are blocked with 2% lidocaine in combination with epinephrine 1:100,000, mixed half-and-half with bacteriostatic saline (approximately 1.5 to 2 cc in each lid and lateral canthus). In all cases, a retrobulbar, intraconal injection of 2% lidocaine in combination with epinephrine 1:100,000, mixed half-and-half with 0.75% bupivacaine, is administered (5 to 7 cc), followed by pressure application to the orbit for 5 to 10 minutes.
3. Two types of evisceration are performed: evisceration without keratectomy and evisceration with keratectomy. The latter is far more commonly performed and will be described below.
4. Place the lid speculum.
5. Perform a 360° limbal conjunctival peritomy with Westcott scissors.
6. Undermine the conjunctiva for approximately 5 mm for 360° (Figure 53.12).
7. Enter the anterior chamber with a No. 11 scalpel blade at the 11 o'clock position, and perform a 360° keratectomy (see Figure 53.12). Remove the cornea with Westcott scissors.
8. Place an evisceration spoon into the space between choroid and sclera, and attempt to remove the intraocular contents en bloc (although it usually comes out piecemeal), Figure 53.13. Once the intraocular contents have been removed, maintain hemostasis with suction and bipolar cautery.

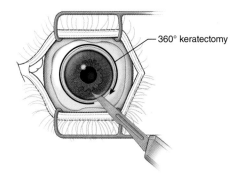

360° keratectomy

Figure 53.12. Evisceration with keratectomy. The conjunctiva is undermined.

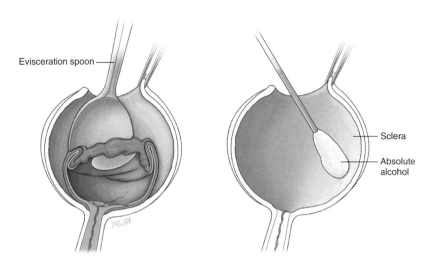

Figure 53.13. An evisceration spoon is placed prior to the removal of the intraocular contents.

Figure 53.14. The entire internal scleral surface is cleaned with cotton-tipped applicators soaked with absolute alcohol.

9. Wipe the entire internal scleral surface with cotton-tipped applicators soaked with absolute alcohol (Figure 53.14).

10. Remove a V-shaped piece of sclera 3 to 6 mm in length at 3 and 9 o'clock positions with Stevens tenotomy scissors; these can be increased in length as required up to the insertions of the medial and lateral rectus muscles and beyond the insertions to accommodate a larger implant (Figures 53.15A, 53.15B).

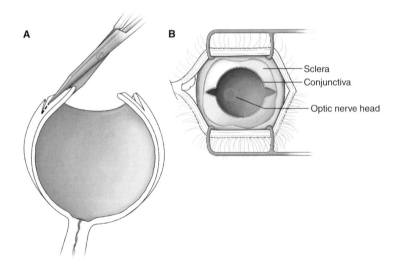

Figure 53.15. A V-shaped piece of sclera (A) is removed 3 to 6 mm in length at the 3 and 9 o'clock positions (B).

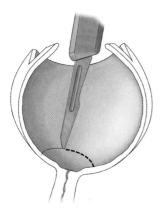

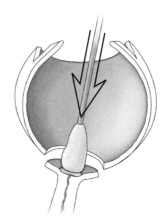

Figure 53.16. Posterior sclerotomy. A small scleral incision is made posteriorly, about 5 to 10 mm away from the optic nerve head.

Figure 53.17. The posterior sclera (with attached optic nerve) is pushed into the retrobulbar space with a cotton-tipped applicator.

11. Perform a posterior sclerotomy. Make a small scleral incision posteriorly with a No. 11 scalpel blade about 5 to 10 mm away from the optic nerve head (Figure 53.16). Incise the posterior sclera for 360° around the nerve head with Stevens scissors. Push the posterior sclera (with attached optic nerve) into the retrobulbar space with a cotton-tipped applicator (Figure 53.17).

12. Make several 10 to 15 mm radial scleral incisions with Stevens scissors in 4 to 6 positions around the posterior sclerotomy site (Figure 53.18). The radial sclerotomies open the posterior scleral shell widely, allowing placement of a larger implant (eg, 20 mm sphere) and facilitating vascularization into the posterior surface of the implant. Alternatively, a complete sclerotomy can be performed. The sclera is transacted from the superior nasal scleral edge posteriorly toward the optic nerve and from the inferior temporal scleral edge posteriorly toward the optic nerve. Sclera is then trimmed away from the optic nerve and the optic nerve is gently moved posteriorly with a cotton-tipped applicator. This technique will allow placement of even larger orbital implants (eg, 21, 22 mm spheres).

13. Place an implant into a Carter sphere introducer and inject it into the scleral cavity. If the anterior scleral opening is too small to allow entry of the implant, the V-shaped scleral incisions are opened further using Westcott scissors or a No. 11 scalpel blade to incise sclera immediately beneath the medial and lateral rectus insertion sites. An unwrapped, moistened porous implant often sticks to the scleral walls as it is being injected into the scleral shell and may not completely enter the shell. To seat the implant within the scleral shell so that the anterior scleral

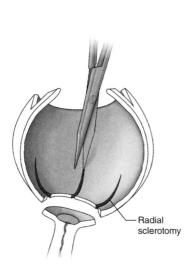

Figure 53.18. Radial sclerotomies are created to allow placement of the implant and facilitate vascularization into the posterior surface of the implant.

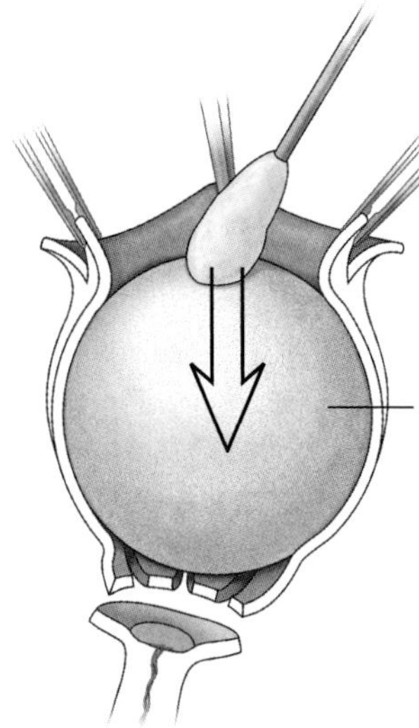

Figure 53.19. The implant is pushed posteriorly until the anterior scleral edges can be closed without tension over the implant.

edges can be closed without tension, an Adson toothed forceps is used to hold the anterior scleral lip (in several positions) while pressure is applied to the implant with a cotton-tipped applicator. The implant is pushed posteriorly until the anterior scleral edges can be closed without tension over the implant. The implant is not pushed posterior to the posterior sclerotomy. Any bits of cotton fluff are removed from the surface of the implant, and the surface is irrigated with the cefazolin solution (Figure 53.19).

14. Close the anterior scleral wound with 3 equally spaced interrupted, double-armed 5-0 polyglactin sutures so that the scleral edges are overlapped by 5 to 7 mm and are under no tension. Between each 5-0 suture, single-armed 4-0 polyglactin sutures are placed through sclera to reinforce the closure (Figure 53.20).

15. Approximate the conjunctiva and Tenon's and close without tension using a running 6-0 polyglactin suture. Rapid absorbing 6-0 plain gut suture is not recommended, as the absorption is too quick (Figure 53.21).

16. Apply antibiotic ointment, followed by a medium-sized to large plastic conformer.

17. Apply 2 eye patches and leave in place for 3 to 5 days.

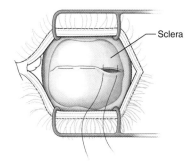

Sclera

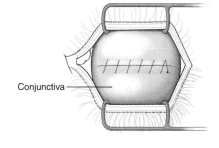

Conjunctiva

Figure 53.20. The anterior scleral wound is closed with 3 equally spaced interrupted, double-armed 5-0 polyglactin sutures so that the scleral edges are overlapped by 5 to 7 mm and are under no tension.

Figure 53.21. The conjunctiva and Tenon's capsule are approximated, and the wound is closed.

Postoperative Care

Refer to postoperative care noted in "Enucleation Surgery" in this chapter.

Complications

Refer to complications listed in "Enucleation Surgery" in this chapter.

EXENTERATION SURGERY

Exenteration involves the removal of all orbital tissues, including the eye, extraocular muscles, optic nerve, periorbita, and part or all of the eyelids. It may be performed for various reasons: ocular and eyelid neoplasms with orbital invasion; some primary orbital tumors; lacrimal gland malignancies; tumors extending into the orbit from adjacent paranasal sinuses; diffuse squamous cell carcinoma of the conjunctiva; diffuse sebaceous cell carcinoma of the eyelids and conjunctiva; and aggressive fungal infections, such as mucormycosis or aspergillosis, that extend into the orbit.

Recent studies suggest that exenteration may offer no benefit over enucleation with local excision in the management of choroidal melanomas with extrascleral extension. In the management of certain neoplasms such as rhabdomyosarcoma, radiation and chemotherapy have replaced exenteration as the primary therapeutic modality. In each case, a review of recent treatment advances for the tumor in question is recommended. In some cases of orbital

metastases or advanced orbital disease, palliative exenteration may be war-
ranted for tumor debulking or pain control. On rare occasions, exenteration
may be indicated in the treatment of nonmalignant conditions such as severe
trauma, meningioma, orbital contracture caused by sclerosing pseudotumor
and congenital deformities (eg, neurofibromatosis).

Preoperative Steps

1. Obtain a careful history and perform a complete ophthalmic examination to assess the problem. Evaluate the extent of the lesion by physical
   examination, computed tomography, and magnetic resonance imaging.
   Establish a definite pathologic diagnosis based on permanent histologic
   sections before proceeding with the exenteration. Do not base the
   decision to exenterate on a frozen section specimen.
2. The surgical procedure may be modified depending on the extent and
   location of the disease process. For tumors involving the posterior
   aspect of the orbit, the eyelid skin and orbicularis muscle may be preserved to line the exenterated socket. For invasive, poorly defined tumors involving the eyelids and conjunctiva, partial or complete excision
   of the eyelids is usually required (eg, invasive basal cell or squamous
   cell carcinoma of the eyelid and conjunctiva, diffuse sebaceous cell ad-
   enocarcinoma involving conjunctiva and lid skin). Malignancies arising
   from the nose, paranasal sinuses, or cranial cavity require collaboration
   with a neurosurgeon and an otolaryngologist for optimal management.
3. Prepare the patient for the loss of the eye and orbital soft tissue and
   the resulting cosmetic deformity. Review the goals of surgery and the
   extent of tissue removal required as well as fitting for an oculofacial
   prosthesis 2 to 3 months postoperatively. Review potential postoperative problems, such as hypesthesia of the forehead and cheek owing
   to the loss of branches of the fifth nerve. Discuss the expected level of
   pain, the recommended time away from work, and required follow-up
   visits.

Instrumentation and Supplies

- Magnifying loupes
- Headlight
- Bipolar cautery with bayonet forceps
- Colorado needle (a fine, needle-like tipped, unipolar cautery unit that
  can be used to simultaneously cut and cauterize tissues)
- 2% lidocaine with epinephrine 1:100,000 for local infiltration

- Bacteriostatic saline to mix with 2% lidocaine
- 0.75% bupivacaine solution
- 4% cocaine solution, topical thrombin
- Castroviejo 0.5 mm toothed forceps
- Westcott tenotomy scissors (curved right, blunt tips)
- Adson toothed forceps
- Castroviejo needle holder
- Stevens curved tenotomy scissors
- Periosteal elevator
- Malleable ribbon retractors
- Enucleation scissors
- Enucleation snare (eg, Storz e3670 or e3671)
- Pronged rake retractors (4)
- Bone wax

Surgical Procedure

1. Develop a presurgery routine to ensure the correct eye socket is removed. Ask the patient to point to or touch the eye socket to be exenterated immediately before the surgery. Be sure the touched side corresponds to the consent and to your chart notes. Use a marker to place several obvious marks around the eye socket to be exenterated.
2. General anesthesia is used.
3. For an eyelid-sparing exenteration, use a gentian violet marking pen to outline the incision for 360° around the upper and lower eyelids, staying 2 to 3 mm away from the eyelashes. If the eyelid skin and muscle cannot be preserved, mark out the incision directly over the orbital rim for 360°. The eyelids are then injected with 1% or 2% lidocaine in combination with epinephrine for hemostasis (Figure 53.22).
4. Place two 4-0 silk sutures through the lid margins to approximate them and act as traction sutures. If the eyelid tissue can be preserved, make a skin-muscle incision immediately above the lashes along the

Figure 53.22. The incision is outlined for an eyelid-sparing exenteration.

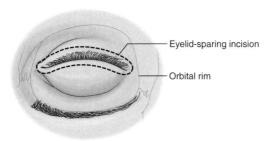

Eyelid-sparing incision

Orbital rim

marked-out line. A suborbicularis dissection plane is created and
maintained to the orbital rim for 360°. If the eyelid tissue cannot
be preserved, make the incision over the orbital rim and continue
through the orbicularis until the periosteum of the orbital rim is
exposed. Control bleeding with a wet-field bipolar cautery. A Colorado needle may also be used for the dissection and will also decrease
bleeding (Figures 53.23, 53.24).

5. Incise the periosteum with a No. 15 scalpel 2 to 3 mm outside the
   orbital rim. Continue this incision around the circumference of the
   orbital rim.
6. Elevate the periosteum away from the rim with the sharp end of a
   periosteal elevator (Figure 53.25). Tight adhesions of the periorbita
   to the bone will be encountered at the insertion of the trochlea, and
   the medial and lateral canthal attachments. Control bleeding from the

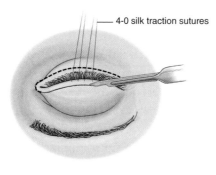

Figure 53.23. 4-0 silk sutures are placed
through the eyelid margins to approximate them
and act as traction sutures.

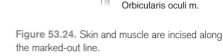

Figure 53.24. Skin and muscle are incised along
the marked-out line.

Figure 53.25. The periosteum is
elevated away from the rim with the
sharp end of a periosteal elevator.

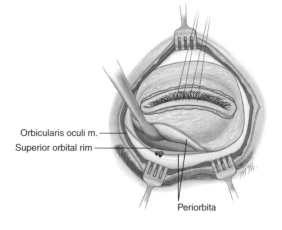

bone with bone wax or gently touching the boney bleeders with the Colorado needle tip.

7. Avoid inadvertent perforation of the bony walls as the periosteum is separated from them, especially the thin medial wall and the orbital floor. Perforations will often lead to persistent fistula tracts, which are difficult to close and create annoying crusting and discharge in the socket postoperatively. As the periosteum is lifted away, the major perforating vessels—including the anterior and posterior ethmoidal communicating vessels medially, the zygomatic vessels laterally, and the communicating branch of the infraorbital artery inferiorly— should be anticipated and cauterized followed by transection once encountered.

8. Identify the lacrimal sac within the lacrimal fossa in the inferior me- dial orbit. Separate the surrounding periorbita from the orbital wall until the sac is isolated. The dissection must be done carefully to avoid inadvertent perforation of the thin lacrimal bone. Once the sac has been isolated, it may then be transected with a No. 15 scalpel blade, Westcott scissors, or the Colorado needle (Figure 53.26A). The edges of the lacrimal sac can be sutured with 1 or 2 sutures (5-0 or 6-0 polyglactin) to close it and minimize the chance of fistula formation (Figure 53.26B).

9. Localize the inferior orbital fissure and carefully transect the tissues emanating from it posteriorly with the Colorado needle, or with a Westcott scissors and frequent application of bipolar cautery using a

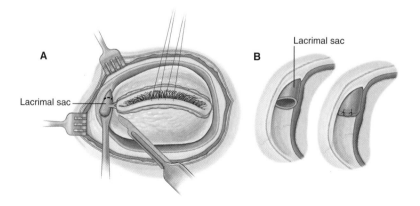

Figure 53.26. The lacrimal sac is identified and isolated. (A) The surrounding periorbita is separated from the orbital wall until the sac is isolated. (B) Once the sac has been isolated, it is transected and the edges of the lacrimal sac are sutured.

bayonet forceps. Perform the same type of dissection as the superior orbital fissure is encountered superotemporally.

10. Once the dissection has reached the apex, cross-clamp the apical tissues with a curved hemostat and then transect them with a curved enucleation scissors or an angled Beaver blade. If the space is tight, the hemostat may not fit in place and the apical transection should be completed without it (Figures 53.27, 53.28). Alternatively, an enucleation snare or tonsillar snare can be passed around the orbital contents from the temporal side, to avoid injury to the lamina papyracea. With upward traction on the 4-0 silk sutures on the eyelids, slowly constrict the snare as it is passed posteriorly (Figures 53.29A, 53.29B). Tighten the snare until it is compressing the apical tissues. It is left in this position for 5 minutes to provide hemostasis. Tighten the snare until the tissues are transected

Figure 53.27. The apex of the orbit is cut with enucleation scissors without placement of a hemostat if a hemostat cannot be placed because of space constraints.

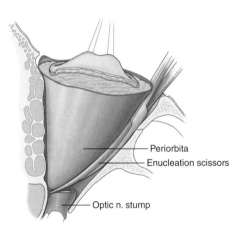

Periorbita
Enucleation scissors
Optic n. stump

Figure 53.28. The apex of the orbit is cut with a curved Beaver blade anterior to the placement of a hemostat. If the space is tight, the hemostat can be eliminated.

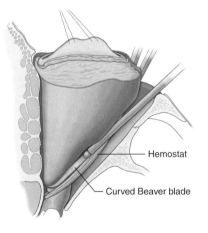

Hemostat
Curved Beaver blade

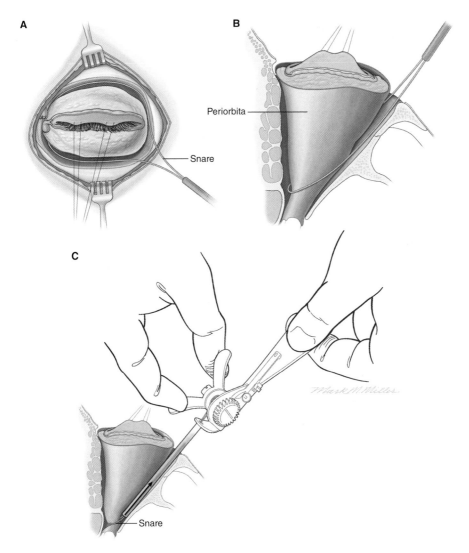

A

B

Periorbita

Snare

C

Snare

Figure 53.29. An enucleation snare is passed around the orbital contents from the temporal side: (A) Anterior view. (B) Sagittal view. (C) The enucleation snare is tightened until the orbital tissues are transected at the apex.

(Figure 53.29C). Once the orbital tissues are removed, control any oozing from the apical stump by direct pressure with a 4 × 4-inch gauze followed by cauterization with the bipolar cautery. Place several small pieces of oxidized cellulose (Surgicel) over the apex to further enhance hemostasis. If apical tumor extension is suspected, additional biopsies of the stump may be taken and sent for frozen sections.

11. If an eyelid-sparing exenteration has been performed, suture the orbicularis muscle together with a 5-0 absorbable suture followed by

Figure 53.30. Sagittal appearance of
an eyelid-sparing exenteration following
closure of the orbicularis muscle and the
skin.

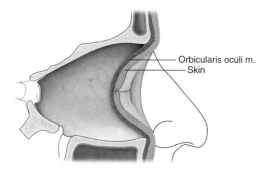

Orbicularis oculi m.
Skin

skin closure with a 6-0 plain suture (Figure 53.30). Unravel a 4 × 4-inch
gauze sponge and gently place it into the socket, pushing the eyelids
posteriorly, covered by 2 eye patches. The eyelids will not line the entire space at this stage, but over the next several weeks, they will stretch
and eventually conform to the orbital walls avoiding the need for a skin
graft. The dead space gradually becomes obliterated as the skin adheres
to the bony orbital surface.

12. If a split-thickness skin graft is required, harvest it from a non-hair-
    bearing region, such as the inner surface of the upper thigh (see
    Chapter 51).

13. Pass the skin graft through a 1:1 ratio mesher. Meshing the graft allows it
    to cover a greater surface area and facilitates drainage of the serosanguine-
    ous fluid from the orbital tissues (Figure 53.31). Suture the graft to the
    skin edges with 5-0 chromic interrupted sutures. It is not necessary to
    trim the graft to fit, as it will conform to the contour of the orbit. Place
    a Telfa pad over the skin graft in the socket. Unravel several 4 × 4-inch
    gauze sponges and place them into the socket, followed by 2 to 3
    eye patches on top to gently apply pressure to the graft. As an alterna-
    tive, wrap 2 or 3 sterile surgical scrub sponges (without the detergent)

Figure 53.31. An exenterated socket is lined with a
split thickness skin graft passed through a 1:1 ratio
mesher.

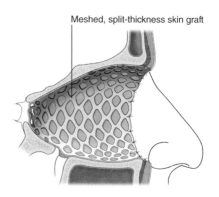

Meshed, split-thickness skin graft

in gauze and then place them into the eye socket. Hold the packing in place with several 4-0 silk sutures passed through the intact skin overlying the orbital rim. As the sponge expands beneath the gauze it will apply pressure to the skin graft lining the socket (Figures 53.32A, 53.32B).

14. If a skin graft has not been used and the socket is healing by spontaneous granulation, pack it loosely with 4 × 4-inch povidone-iodine soaked gauze sponges and antibiotic ointment followed by 2 or 3 eye patches.

Postoperative Care

1. Prescribe broad-spectrum antibiotics postoperatively for 5 to 7 days. The pressure dressing is removed in 5 days.

2. For patients undergoing an eyelid-sparing procedure, antibiotic ointment is applied to the sutures (eg, Polysporin) and the socket is re-packed with dry 4 × 4-inch gauze sponges, followed by 2 eye patches. Patients change the dressing every 2 to 3 days. This routine is continued for the first 2 to 3 weeks until the skin lines the socket well. Weekly visits are carried out to remove any dried discharge. Patients are referred to an ocularist for an orbital prosthesis once the socket is well healed.

3. For sockets with a skin graft, the healing process is more prolonged. Once the initial dressing is removed, wet-to-dry dressings are initiated. Topical antibiotic ointment is applied to the socket (eg, Polysporin) followed by unraveled 4 × 4-inch gauze sponges that have been soaked

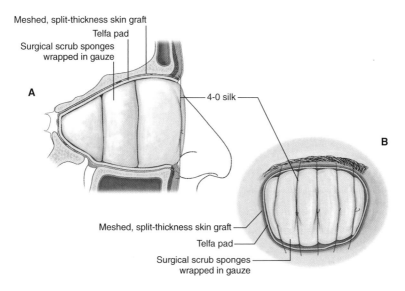

Figure 53.32. Surgical scrub sponges (without detergent) are wrapped in gauze and placed into an exenterated socket lined with a split thickness skin graft. (A) Sagittal view. (B) Anterior view.

in equal parts hydrogen peroxide and povidone-iodine (Betadine). The gauze is wrung out, unfolded, and loosely packed into the eye socket. All areas of the socket should be in contact with the gauze, which will serve to debride the socket of old blood and serous discharge that has dried. An eye patch may be placed on top of the dressing. Initially the dressings are changed twice daily; as the socket heals, the frequency is decreased to once daily. The patient should be seen weekly to remove any dried crust not debrided with the dressing changes. Once the socket is well epithelialized (2 to 3 months) the patient is referred to an ocularist for a custom-fit orbital prosthesis.

Complications

- Intraoperative bleeding
- Cerebrospinal fluid leakage
- Postoperative infection

The most common complication encountered during an orbital exenteration is intraoperative bleeding. Methods to avoid or minimize bleeding are (1) ensuring that the patient has stopped aspirin or any blood thinning medication prior to surgery, and (2) paying careful attention to hemostasis during the procedure by cauterizing the major vessels (the anterior and posterior ethmoidal arteries, and the zygomatic and communicating branches of the infraorbital artery).

Cerebrospinal fluid leakage is an uncommon but potentially serious complication because of the risk of meningitis in untreated or persistent cases. This complication occurs from inadvertent penetration of the dura, most commonly at the superior orbital fissure. A small leak may close spontaneously, but larger leaks require treatment (autogenous fat graft, temporalis pedicle flap, or repair by direct closure or dural graft). A simple, effective technique is the application of tissue adhesives (such as cyanoacrylate) to the area of leakage.

Postoperative infection is uncommon. Fistulae into the ethmoid or maxillary sinus result from bony defects in the floor or medial wall of the orbit; they are a nuisance as the socket often has discharge around a fistula. Furthermore, fistulae allow air/fluid entry into the socket, a problem if the patient wants to swim. Small asymptomatic fistulae do not require treatment but larger ones with chronic discharge may. Surgical closure is difficult, as vascularized tissue is required to cover the area but is in short supply due to the loss of tissue with the procedure. Recurrence of the fistula tract is not uncommon.

Chapter 54

Quickert Sutures for Involutional Entropion

Christopher K. Thiagarajah, MD
Robert Kersten, MD

Involutional entropion occurs when lower lid laxity and elongation of the lower lid retractors allow an overriding orbicularis to invert the tarsal plate, resulting in lashes abrading the cornea. Surgical procedures to correct this malposition usually involve horizontal tightening of the eyelid and some tightening of the lower lid retractors. The retractors can be tightened through an anterior approach, posterior approach, or placement of Quickert (full-thickness eyelid) sutures. Tightening the retractors in combination with horizontal tightening of the lower eyelid restores the tarsal plate to its normal position.

PREOPERATIVE STEPS

1. Document lid laxity and the position of the lid.
2. Note any corneal epitheliopathy.

INSTRUMENTATION AND SUPPLIES

- Straight iris scissors
- Wescott scissors
- Two-pronged skin hook
- Manhattan forceps
- Needle driver

- 5-0 chromic gut sutures, double-armed (3)
- Instrumentation as listed for the lateral tarsal strip procedure (Chapter 70).

SURGICAL PROCEDURE

1. Infiltrate the lower eyelid with 1% lidocaine with 1:100,000 epineph-rine (Figure 54.1).
2. Prep and drape the patient in a sterile manner.
3. Pass several double-armed 5-0 chromic gut sutures through the con-junctival fornix posteriorly, exiting anteriorly on the skin through the lower eyelid crease (Figure 54.2). Usually 3 sutures are sufficient: one each placed medially, centrally, and laterally. First, an arm of the su-ture is passed through the conjunctiva in the fornix and then brought up through the lower eyelid retractors, passing through the orbicularis and exiting the skin at the lower eyelid crease (about 4 mm inferior to the lash line). The other arm of the double-armed suture is then passed

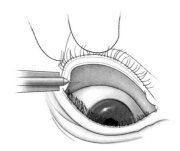

Figure 54.1. The lower eyelid is injected with local anesthetic.

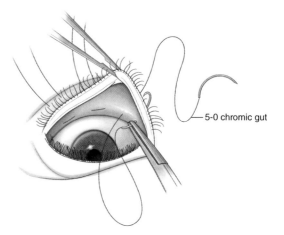

Figure 54.2. One needle of a double-armed 5-0 chromic suture enters the fornix of the conjunctiva.

5-0 chromic gut

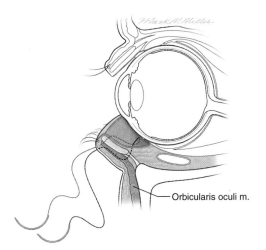

Figure 54.3. Sagittal view of the placement of each of the 3 Quickert sutures.

Orbicularis oculi m.

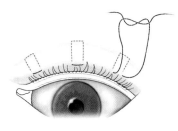

Figure 54.4. Sutures are cut and tied with eversion of the lower eyelid.

with approximately 4 mm of spacing, entering and exiting parallel to the first arm of the suture (Figure 54.3). This maneuver is repeated until all 3 sutures are placed (Figure 54.4). One arm of each suture is then cut and each suture is tied to itself directly onto the skin.

4. Perform a lateral tarsal strip procedure (Chapter 70).

COMPLICATIONS

- Suture failure
- Lid retraction
- Overcorrection (ie, ectropion)

If the Quickert sutures are not properly placed, they may fail to evert the eyelid. On the conjunctival side, placing the sutures high near the lid margin or exiting through the skin side of the eyelid too inferiorly will result in undercorrection of the rotation of the lid.

If the Quickert sutures exit the skin too close to the eyelid margin, tightening of the sutures may result in overcorrection and resulting ectropion.

Chapter 55

Repair of Lower Eyelid Involutional Entropion and Ectropion

Christopher K. Thiagarajah, MD
Robert Kersten, MD

Involutional entropion occurs when horizontal lower lid laxity and elongation of the lower lid retractors allow an overriding orbicularis to invert the tarsal plate, so that the eyelid margin lies against the globe. By horizontally tightening the lower eyelid and reinserting the lower lid retractors, the tarsal plate can be everted away from the globe into its normal anatomic position.

Full-thickness eyelid (or "Quickert") sutures combined with a lateral tarsal strip procedure (Chapter 70), as well as the technique described in this chapter can both be used to treat involutional entropion. Quickert sutures are easier to place and less time consuming, and are also a good choice for patients who must have a procedure at the bedside or who are unable to undergo a more invasive procedure. Published series report a greater than 90% success rate for curing involutional entropion with Quickert sutures and a lateral tarsal strip procedure; however, many surgeons feel that with a longer follow-up period, the rate of recurrence using Quickert sutures (which indirectly tightens the lower lid retractors) is greater than when using techniques that directly tighten the retractors, such as described below. Both techniques are therefore important components of a surgeon's armamentarium.

Involutional tarsal ectropion also results when lower lid laxity is accompanied by disinsertion of the lower lid retractors from the inferior border of the tarsal plate. Laxity of the lower eyelid allows the lower lid tarsal plate to rotate forward. If there is accompanying disinsertion of the lower eyelid retractors from their normal insertion on the inferior border of the tarsal plate, the lower lid may completely evert so that the inferior border of the tarsal plate migrates

332

superiorly and the entire tarsal plate is everted and exposed (so-called *tarsal ectropion*.) Reinserting the lower eyelid retractors pulls the inferior edge of the tarsal plate back into the cul-de-sac, allowing the tarsal plate to be rotated back into proper position. The remaining lower eyelid laxity is addressed by the tarsal strip tightening procedure.

PREOPERATIVE STEPS

1. Document lower eyelid laxity and the position of the lid.
2. Note any corneal epitheliopathy.

INSTRUMENTATION AND SUPPLIES

- Straight iris scissors
- Wescott scissors
- Two-pronged skin hook
- Manhattan forceps
- 6-0 mild chromic suture
- Needle driver
- Instrumentation for the lateral tarsal strip procedure (Chapter 70)

SURGICAL PROCEDURE

1. Infiltrate the lower eyelid with 1% lidocaine with 1:100,000 epinephrine.
2. Prep and drape the patient in a sterile manner.
3. Complete a lateral canthotomy and inferior cantholysis with a straight iris scissors (Figures 55.1, 55.2).

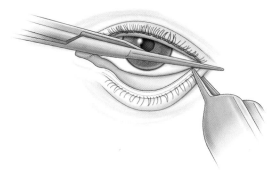

Figure 55.1. A lateral canthotomy is performed with a straight iris scissors.

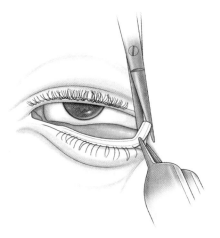

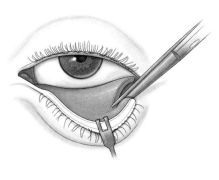

Figure 55.2. The straight iris scissors are directed inferiorly to complete the inferior cantholysis.

Figure 55.3. The conjunctiva and lower eyelid retractors are incised for 5 mm at the lateral portion of the lower eyelid.

4. Distract the lower eyelid with a 2-pronged skin hook.

5. Use Wescott scissors to dissect through the conjunctiva and the lower eyelid retractors at the inferior border of the lateral tarsus for approximately 5 mm (Figure 55.3). Once the conjunctival and retractor incision is begun laterally, the incision is carried medially for the full length of the lower eyelid (Figures 55.4A, 55.4B, and 55.4C).

6. Excise 4 mm of distal retractor and conjunctiva from the conjunctival and retractor flap that has been elevated in the fornix (Figure 55.5).

7. Reattach the cut edge of the conjunctiva and the lower lid retractors to the inferior border of the tarsal plate using a 6-0 mild chromic gut running suture (Figure 55.6).

8. Close the lateral canthal angle as described in Chapter 70.

COMPLICATIONS

- Lid retraction
- Overcorrection
- Bleeding
- Infection

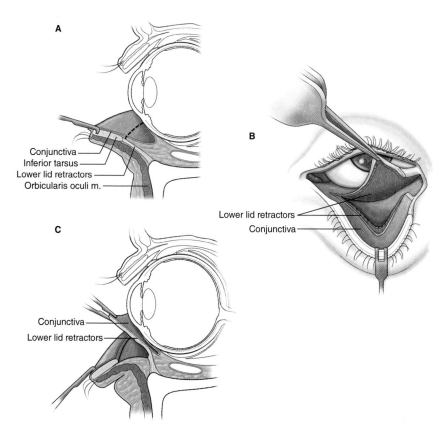

Figure 55.4. The lower lid retractors and conjunctiva are separated from the inferior border across the length of the lower lid. (A) Sagittal view of the incision line. Complete separation of the lower eyelid retractors and conjunctiva from the inferior border of the tarsus is viewed anteriorly (B) and sagittally (C).

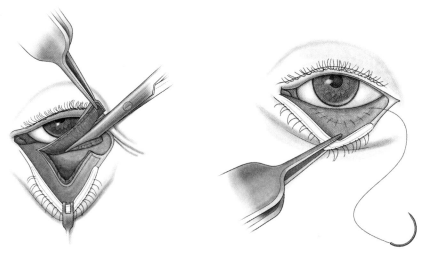

.Figure 55.5. The retractors and conjunctiva are resected.

Figure 55.6. The retractors and conjunctiva are reattached to the inferior border of the tarsus.

Chapter 56

Tarsotomy for Cicatricial Entropion

Christopher K. Thiagarajah, MD
Robert Kersten, MD

Cicatricial changes in the tarsal plate may result in inversion of the distal lid margin causing lashes to rub against the globe. Transverse tarsotomy with rotation sutures allows eversion of the distal tarsal plate, restoring the position of the eyelid margin and its normal apposition to the globe.

PREOPERATIVE STEPS

1. Document cicatricial changes.
2. Document the position of the eyelid.

INSTRUMENTATION AND SUPPLIES

- Straight iris scissors
- Wescott scissors
- Manhattan forceps
- Gentian violet marker
- Needle driver
- 4-0 silk suture
- No. 75 Beaver blade
- 6-0 polyglactin (Vicryl) suture, double armed (4)

SURGICAL PROCEDURE

1. Infiltrate the lower eyelid with 1% lidocaine with 1:100,000 epinephrine.
2. Prep and drape the patient in a sterile manner.
3. Place a 4-0 silk retraction suture through the eyelid margin and clamp the suture to the drape, everting the lid.
4. Use gentian violet to make a transverse line on the tarsal conjunctiva 3 mm proximal to the lid margin. Extend this marking 3 mm medial and lateral to the involved portion of the eyelid.
5. Use a No. 75 Beaver blade to make an incision through the tarsal plate along the entire previously marked line. Take care not to penetrate deep to the tarsus into the underlying orbicularis muscle (Figures 56.1A, 56.1B). Alternately, once the incision has been started, Wescott scissors may be introduced to complete the tarsotomy. It may be easier to meticulously control the position of the tarsotomy with Wescott scissors.
6. After the incision is complete, Wescott scissors may be used to make small, vertical relaxing incisions transecting the lid margin at the medial and lateral end of the tarsotomy. These relaxing incisions allow the distal tarsal fragment to be rotated freely away from the globe.
7. Pass a double-armed 6-0 polyglactin suture in a lamellar fashion in the proximal cut edge of the tarsus. After exiting the proximal cut edge of the tarsus, the suture traverses through orbicularis to exit the skin just below the lashes. Repeat this step with multiple 6-0 polyglactin sutures until the full length of the involved area of the lid is addressed (Figure 56.2).

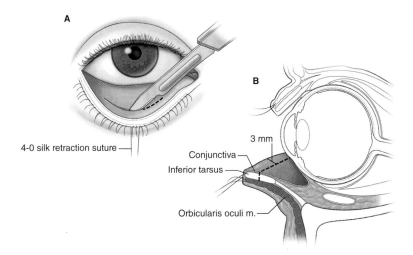

Figure 56.1. (A) A horizontal incision is made on the tarsal plate with a No. 75 eye knife. (B) A sagittal view of the placement and depth of the eyelid incision.

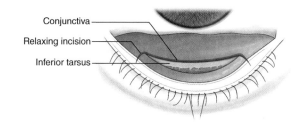

Figure 56.2. Vertical relaxing incisions are made at the medial and lateral ends of the tarsotomy to facilitate rotation of the involved segment.

Conjunctiva

Relaxing incision

Inferior tarsus

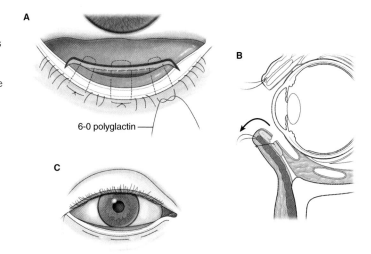

Figure 56.3. The tarsotomy is completed. (A) Sutures are tied and cut. (B) The tarsus is rotated after suture placement. (C) Appearance of the eyelid and sutures at the completion of the procedure.

A

B

6-0 polyglactin

C

8. Tie the sutures, bringing the distal lid margin to eversion. Moderate overcorrection is desired, as the lid will tend to invert as it heals (Figures 56.3A, 56.3B, 56.3C). Tightly tying the sutures may cause some undulation of the lid margin. This irregularity tends to smooth out over time.

COMPLICATIONS

- Entropion
- Persistent overcorrection
- Bleeding
- Infection
- Distortion of the lid margin

Recurrent entropion may occur if cicatricial forces cause contracture of the relaxing incision.

The lid margin may distort if the sutures exit the skin too close to the lid margin resulting in buckling of the distal fragment of the tarsus. This deformity usually gradually improves over time during the postoperative period.

Chapter 57

Medial Spindle for Punctal Ectropion

Christopher K. Thiagarajah, MD
Robert Kersten, MD

Involutional ectropion occurs when lower lid laxity and elongation of the lower lid retractors allow the lower lid to evert away from the globe. Laxity-related ectropion tends to begin medially, so that only the medial portion of the lower eyelid may be ectropic. When this malposition occurs, the lower lid punctum may not be properly aligned against the tear film and may be a cause of epiphora. A lid-tightening procedure such as a lateral tarsal strip (Chapter 70) combined with a medial spindle will tighten the medial portion of the lower lid and rotate the punctum into proper alignment.

PREOPERATIVE STEPS

1. Document lower eyelid laxity.
2. Document the position of the lower eyelid.

INSTRUMENTATION AND SUPPLIES

- Straight iris scissors
- Wescott scissors
- Two-pronged skin hook
- Manhattan forceps
- 6-0 mild chromic sutures

- Needle driver
- Instrumentation as listed for the lateral tarsal strip procedure (Chapter 70)

SURGICAL PROCEDURE

1. Prep and drape the patient in a sterile manner.
2. Infiltrate the lower eyelid with 1% lidocaine with 1:100,000 epinephrine.
3. Use Manhattan forceps to grasp the conjunctiva and the lower eyelid, retractors approximately 2 mm below the lower lid punctum. Use Wescott scissors to excise a diamond-shaped wedge of conjunctiva and underlying retractors with an apex 2 mm beneath the lower lid punctum. The diamond-shaped excision is approximately 4 mm high and 8 mm wide (Figures 57.1A, 57.1B).
4. Place 1 double-armed, 6-0 mild chromic suture to close the diamond excision. First, an arm is placed through the conjunctiva at the edge of the lateral portion of the lower apex of the diamond and out through the inside of the diamond excision. The same needle is then passed through the inside of the lateral side of the superior apex of the diamond excision out through the conjunctiva. Finally, the needle is brought back to the lateral portion of the inferior apex through the conjunctiva and passed out through the skin. Repeat this step on the other (ie, medial) side of the diamond excision with the other arm of the 6-0 mild chromic suture. Cut and tie the suture to itself directly on the skin (Figures 57.2A, 57.2B, 57.2C, 57.2D).
5. If significant lower lid laxity exists, the medial spindle procedure should be combined with a horizontal lid-tightening procedure such as a lateral tarsal strip (Chapter 70).

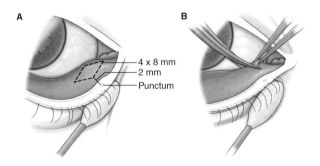

Figure 57.1. A diamond wedge of conjunctiva and lower eyelid retractors is resected for a medial spindle. (A) The dimensions and location of the medial spindle. (B) Westcott scissors are used to excise the spindle.

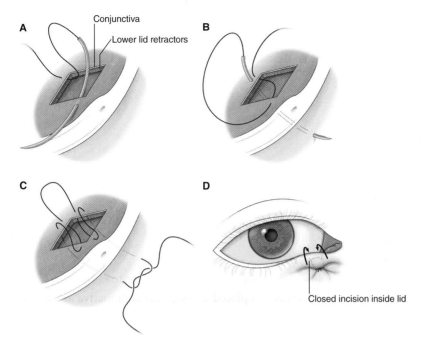

Figure 57.2. Medial spindle. (A, B) Placement of suture for medial spindle. (C) Diagram showing final suture placement. Suture is cut and tied directly onto the skin, rotating the medial portion of the lid into position. (D) Appearance of suture and eyelid at the completion of procedure.

COMPLICATIONS

- Failure
- Overcorrection
- Infection or suture abscess

Failure may be due to severity of ectropion, cicatricial anterior lamella shortening, or residual horizontal laxity.

Overcorrection is often due to over-resection of the lower lid retractors and can be repaired by release of the suture and replacement.

Chapter 58

External Levator Aponeurotic Resection

Yasaman Mohadjer, MD
John B. Holds, MD

Ptosis is a common cause of superior visual field obstruction. Generally, ptosis becomes visually significant when the margin reflex distance one (MRD-1), the distance from the superior eyelid margin to the pupillary light reflex, is ≤2 mm. Ptosis may be congenital or acquired, due to mechanical, neurogenic, aponeurotic, or traumatic causes. The most common form of ptosis is acquired, involutional, associated with a dehiscent or rarified levator aponeurosis (Figure 58.1) with normal levator function (12 mm or more).

External levator aponeurotic resection is performed on patients with normal levator function. Unlike the Putterman (conjunctivomullerectomy) or Fasanella-Servat procedures (Chapters 60 and 61), it can also be performed on patients with diminished levator function, achieving good result with as little as 4 or 5 mm of levator function. Patients with poor levator function (<4 mm),

Figure 58.1. Patient preoperatively showing bilateral severe aponeurotic ptosis.

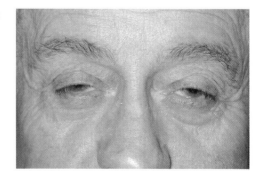

especially when the condition is bilateral, generally undergo a frontalis sling procedure (Chapter 59).

In addition, ptosis repair may be performed for purely aesthetic reasons if the superior visual field is not obstructed but the patient desires an improvement in appearance.

PREOPERATIVE STEPS

1. Obtain a detailed history. Patients with dry eyes or photophobia may have an exacerbation of these conditions postoperatively following otherwise successful ptosis repair. A history of previous eyelid surgery or use of rigid gas-permeable (RGP) lenses should be noted, as these factors may increase the risk of postoperative recurrence of ptosis. A history of diplopia or variability in eyelid position may alert the clinician to the presence of myasthenia gravis or other neurologic condition, such as a third cranial nerve palsy.

2. Perform a careful examination, measuring margin reflex distance one (MRD-1) and levator function and checking for lagophthalmos or keratopathy. A basic Schirmer's test may reveal decreased aqueous tear secretion. A patient with a significantly dry eye or poor protective mechanisms requires additional evaluation and counseling preoperatively, as ptosis repair may predispose the patient to significant ongoing or worsening exposure keratopathy.

3. The amount of levator aponeurosis to be resected depends upon the levator function as well as the degree of ptosis. In general, a levator with normal function will need to be resected approximately 2 to 3 mm for every millimeter of desired elevation. A levator with less-than-normal function will require a larger resection (up to 7 mm) for every millimeter of desired elevation. The exact amount to resect is fine-tuned by means of direct observation during the procedure.

INSTRUMENTATION AND SUPPLIES

- Anesthetic eye drop
- 2% lidocaine with epinephrine
- Small-gauge needle (27 or 30 gauge)
- Protective eye shield
- No. 15c blade

- Toothed forceps
- Sharp Westcott scissors
- Bipolar cautery
- 5-0 polyglactin (Vicryl) suture on spatulated needle (S-14 Ethicon)
- 7-0 polypropylene suture on small cutting needle (P-1 Ethicon)

SURGICAL PROCEDURE

1. Mark the central upper eyelid crease (Figure 58.2).
2. Place 1 drop of topical anesthetic on the eye, then infiltrate the eyelid crease with approximately 0.5 mL of anesthetic. An external levator aponeurotic resection may be performed under local anesthetic alone, but often it is performed in the operating room with monitored anesthesia care.
3. Prep and drape the patient's face, leaving the entire face exposed in the sterile field.
4. Place corneal shields in both eyes.
5. Incise the skin through the premarked central eyelid crease for 8 to 20 mm with the No. 15c blade (Figure 58.3). Experienced surgeons

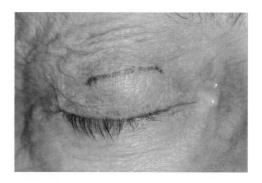

Figure 58.2. Right upper eyelid incision marked.

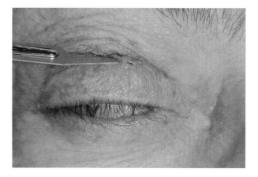

Figure 58.3. An incision is made with a No. 15c blade scalpel.

treating aponeurotic ptosis may tend toward the shorter incisions, with
the longer incision useful for novice surgeons or cases requiring large
aponeurotic resections (congenital ptosis or other myopathic ptosis).

6. Dissect through the full thickness of the orbicularis muscle with Westcott scissors (Figure 58.4) and open the central septum (Figure 58.5).

7. Maintain strict hemostasis with cautery.

8. Expose the superior edge of the tarsus with Westcott scissors by resecting several millimeters of the levator aponeurosis with a horizontal
   incision (Figure 58.6). This maneuver also creates a free edge of the
   levator aponeurosis.

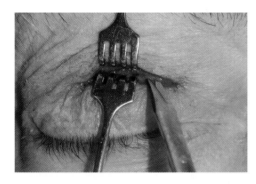

Figure 58.4. Sharp dissection is performed through the orbicularis muscle plane with Westcott scissors.

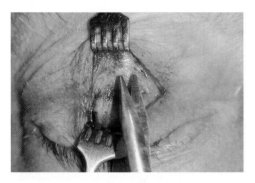

Figure 58.5. The orbital septum is opened to access the levator aponeurosis.

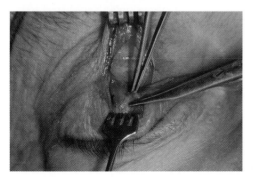

Figure 58.6. The inferior levator aponeurosis is resected, exposing the upper tarsus.

9. Using the 5-0 polyglactin suture, attach the levator aponeurosis to superior tarsus with 2 to 3 interrupted, partial-thickness tarsal bites that pass through the tarsus in its superior third and exit the inferior edge of the levator aponeurosis (Figure 58.7). Secure the sutures with slipknots. The distance from the inferior edge of the levator aponeurosis to the point through which the suture is passed (ie, the amount of levator aponeurosis resected) is greater with greater degrees of ptosis.

10. Observe the eyelid height, contour, and symmetry with the opposing side, both in the supine and upright positions, with the slipknots in place. In bilateral cases, symmetry in the height and contour of the upper eyelids is the goal (Figure 58.8). In unilateral cases, a 1 mm overcorrection of lid height in the upright position is generally desirable. If any area of the eyelid is lower than desired, untie the corresponding slipknot, remove the needle and suture from the aponeurosis, perform a larger resection (ie, take a "bigger bite"), and retie the slipknot. If any area of the eyelid is too high, untie the slipknot, remove the needle and suture from the aponeurosis, perform a smaller resection (ie, take a "smaller bite"), and retie the slipknot.

11. After achieving the desired height and contour, tie the slipknots without changing tension (Figure 58.9).

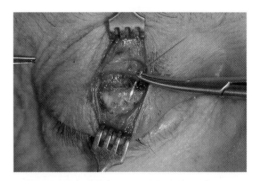

Figure 58.7. The levator aponeurosis is sutured to the upper tarsus with 5-0 polyglactin suture.

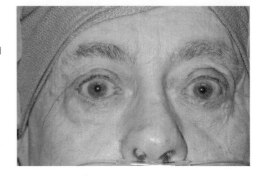

Figure 58.8. The eyelid height is checked intraoperatively in the upright position after completing left aponeurotic ptosis repair. The overcorrection of the eyelid height noted here will settle postoperatively.

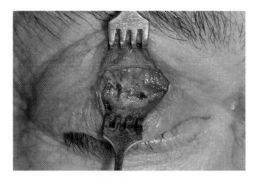

Figure 58.9. Two aponeurotic sutures are tied down in place.

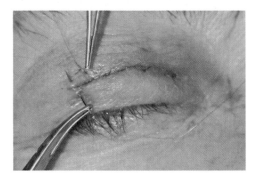

Figure 58.10. The skin is closed with a simple running suture.

12. Close the skin with a running polypropylene suture (Figure 58.10).
13. Apply antibiotic ointment to the wound.

COMPLICATIONS

- Undercorrection, overcorrection, or asymmetry
- Recurrence
- Lagophthalmos

Undercorrection, overcorrection, or asymmetry may require in-office adjustment. It is preferable to adjust the eyelid height within 2 weeks of the original surgery, before significant healing occurs. Within this time window, it is possible to bluntly pull the wound open and replace or remove an aponeurotic suture to raise or lower the eyelid height with minimal anesthesia and generally no cautery.

If ptosis recurs, rule out myasthenia gravis in appropriate patients.

Lagophthalmos should be treated with aggressive lubrication in the early postoperative period. If lagophthalmos persists and causes significant keratopathy, the upper eyelid may need to be lowered.

Chapter 59

Frontalis Sling

Yasaman Mohadjer, MD
John B. Holds, MD

Ptosis with poor levator function (ie, excursion of the eyelid of 4 mm or less) has many causes. Most commonly, it is seen in congenital ptosis as a result of poor or absent development of the levator muscle. Other causes of poor levator function include trauma to the levator muscle or neurologic disorders such as chronic progressive external ophthalmoplegia or oculopharyngeal dystrophy.

If the patient has adequate frontalis muscle function, a ptotic upper eyelid with poor levator function can be attached to the forehead musculature by means of a frontalis sling, so that elevation of the eyebrow will concurrently elevate the eyelid. A variety of materials have successfully been used as sling material, including banked or autologous fascia lata, silicone rods, and various sutures including polypropylene, Supramid, and Gore-Tex. The use of silicone rods is described below, though the procedure is performed virtually identically when using other sling materials.

PREOPERATIVE STEPS

1. Obtain a careful history and perform a thorough examination, measuring margin reflex distance one (MRD-1), levator function, and eyelid crease position or absence.
2. Evaluate ocular motility to rule out other neurologic disease processes, and ensure that adequate frontalis function (brow elevation) is present.

3. Have a frank discussion with the patient (or the parents if the patient is a child) regarding the appearance and function of the eyelids post-operatively and the potential for nocturnal lagophthalmos, and the possible need for topical lubricating ointment, perhaps indefinitely.
4. Note the presence or absence of lagophthalmos and keratopathy and discuss the potential for postoperative exacerbation. In children, assess for amblyopia and evaluate refractive status.

INSTRUMENTATION AND SUPPLIES

- Anesthetic eye drops
- 2% lidocaine with epinephrine
- Small-gauge needle (27 or 30 gauge)
- Protective eye shield
- No. 15c blade
- Toothed forceps
- Sharp Westcott scissors
- Hemostat
- Bipolar cautery
- Silicone sling with attached needle and sleeve
- Wright needle
- 6-0 plain gut suture
- 5-0 polypropylene suture

SURGICAL PROCEDURE

1. Mark the patient's upper eyelid and forehead in a pentagonal fashion to indicate the points where stab incisions are to be made (Figure 59.1).

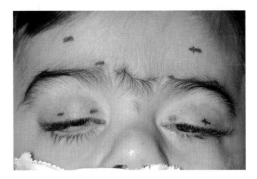

Figure 59.1. Patient with bilateral con-genital ptosis marked for frontalis sling in pentagonal pattern. (Courtesy of Morris E. Hartstein, MD)

Two marks are placed 2 to 3 mm above the eyelashes in the upper eye-lid: medially and laterally.

- Numerous patterns of incisions on the eyelids and forehead for placing the sling material have been described, such as a pentagon, double rhomboid, and classic Crawford pattern. The exact pattern used depends on the surgeon's preference, training, and personal experience.

2. This procedure may be performed under monitored sedation or gen-eral anesthesia. The marked areas and paths of the sling material are infiltrated with local anesthetic if performed with monitored sedation.

3. Prep and drape the patient's face, leaving the entire face exposed in the sterile field.

4. Place metallic eyelid shields in both eyes.

5. Make stab incisions in all 5 marks with the No. 15c blade; these inci-sions should extend down to the level of the tarsus in the eyelid and through dermis and muscle in the forehead.

6. Grasp a needle attached to the silicone rod with a hemostat and pass it horizontally across the eyelid incisions, retrieving it through the medial incision (Figure 59.2). The depth of these passes should be just anterior to the tarsus.

7. Grasp the medial needle and pass it superiorly, exiting through the medial brow incision (Figure 59.3). The lateral arm of the suture is passed similarly through the lateral brow incision. These passes should be made in a deep plane, posterior to the septum, but take care not to pass the needle through the full thickness of the eyelid.

8. Pass both the lateral and medial arms superiorly, deep to the dermis, exiting through the central brow incision.

9. Close the upper eyelid incisions with 6-0 plain gut suture prior to elevating the upper eyelids.

Figure 59.2. The needle is passed hori-zontally across the lid in the pretarsal plane. (Courtesy of Morris E. Hartstein, MD)

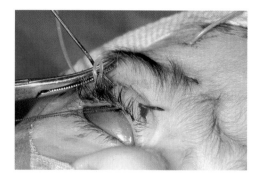

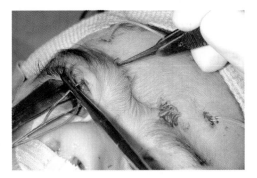

Figure 59.3. The needle is passed superiorly through the brow incision. (Courtesy of Morris E. Hartstein, MD)

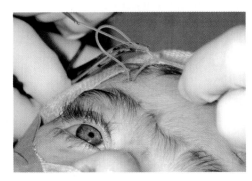

Figure 59.4. After the sling is passed through the forehead incision, the sleeve is placed over silicone rods and the tension in the rods is adjusted. The sleeve is locked with polypropylene sutures, and the ends of the rods are buried. (Courtesy of Morris E. Hartstein, MD)

10. Pass the silicone rods through the silicone sleeve and tighten them, adjusting the tension in the rods to achieve the desired upper eyelid position and contour (Figure 59.4).
11. Suture each end of the sleeve to the silicone with 5-0 polypropylene suture to prevent slippage.
12. Cut the silicone ends, leaving approximately 6 mm of excess.
13. Bury the exposed silicone and its sleeve bluntly in a deep pocket, beneath the frontalis muscle, using a needle holder.
14. Close the brow incisions with 5-0 polypropylene suture.
15. Place antibiotic ointment on the incisions and in the eye.

COMPLICATIONS

- Undercorrection, overcorrection, or asymmetry
- Exposure keratopathy (routine in the first few weeks after surgery)
- Sling breakage
- Inflammation or granuloma formation

Undercorrection, overcorrection, asymmetry: the use of silicone rods as sling material affords the advantage of easier postoperative adjustment if necessary; the central forehead incision can be opened, the sleeve located, and adjustment made after removing the locking polypropylene sutures.

Exposure keratopathy may follow excess tightening of the sling. All patients require lubricant drops and ointment in the first 1 to 2 weeks after surgery. Frequently, these must be continued to a moderate degree, even indefinitely. If necessary, the sling can be loosened as described above to lessen unacceptable exposure keratopathy.

Sling breakage is best prevented by avoiding nicking or otherwise damaging the sling material during implantation. Occasional breakages will necessitate a repeat sling procedure.

Inflammation or granuloma formation is usually due to poor technique, with superficial placement of the sling material or failure to place all permanent sutures and sling material firmly into a subdermal plane. Sling removal or replacement may be required.

Chapter 60

Müller Muscle Resection

Steven C. Dresner, MD
Alan W. McInnes, MD

Patients with minimal ptosis (1 to 2.5 mm) and a positive phenylephrine test are candidates for the Müller muscle conjunctival resection procedure. This procedure is quick, precise, reproducible, and requires no intraoperative patient cooperation.

PREOPERATIVE STEPS

1. For both eyes, measure and document interpalpebral fissures, the margin to reflex distance one (MRD-1), and levator excursions. Take photos and document the visual fields if required.
2. Place 2 drops of 2.5% phenylephrine in the ptotic eye or eyes.
3. Measure and document the margin to reflex distance post-phenylephrine (MRD-P). An elevation of 1.5 mm or greater is considered a positive test.
4. With a positive test, plan 4 mm of Müller muscle resection for every 1 mm of ptosis.

INSTRUMENTATION AND SUPPLIES

- Caliper
- Marking pen
- Müller muscle-conjunctiva clamp
- Desmarres retractor

- Toothed forceps (eg, Paufique)
- Needle holder
- No. 15 blade scalpel
- Suture scissors

SURGICAL PROCEDURE

1. Mark the central upper eyelid position while the patient is in an upright position.
2. Place topical tetracaine on the conjunctival surface. Place a subcutaneous eyelid block below the brow, using 2% lidocaine with 1:100,000 epinephrine and 200 USP units hyaluronidase per 20 cc of anesthetic (Figure 60.1).
3. Prep and drape the patient in a sterile manner.
4. Place a 4-0 silk suture in the upper eyelid margin at the previously marked area of the upper lid (Figure 60.2).
5. Reflect the eyelid over a Desmarres retractor.
6. Mark the palpebral conjunctiva medially, laterally, and centrally at the halfway point of resection, measured from the superior tarsal edge (eg, 4 mm from the superior tarsal edge for an 8-mm resection, Figure 60.3).
7. Make a mark centrally at the full resection point (eg, 8 mm for an 8-mm resection).
8. Place three 4-0 silk traction sutures at the halfway point through conjunctiva and Müller muscle: 1 pass through the center pupil mark and 1 pass on either side (Figure 60.4).
9. Elevate the sutures in 2 bundles and apply traction to free the Müller muscle from the underlying levator muscle (Figure 60.5), then place the clamp on the tissues, using the central full resection mark for reference (Figure 60.6).

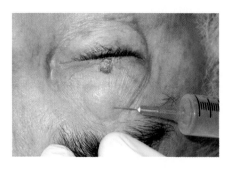

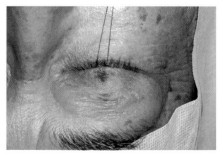

Figure 60.1. Local anesthetic is placed below the brow.

Figure 60.2. Lid margin traction suture is placed at the pupillary axis mark.

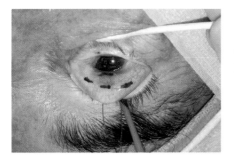

Figure 60.3. The conjunctiva is marked.

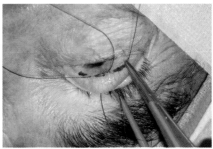

Figure 60.4. Traction sutures are placed in Müller muscle and conjunctiva.

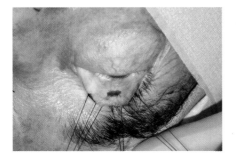

Figure 60.5. Traction sutures tent Müller muscle and conjunctiva.

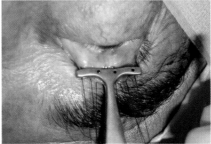

Figure 60.6. The clamp is placed at the central mark.

10. Pass a 6-0 polypropylene suture full thickness through the pre-tarsal eyelid at 1 end of the clamp, entering the skin and exiting the conjunctiva, and then pass the suture under the clamp in a running horizontal mattress fashion. At the opposite end of the clamp, "exteriorize" the suture (ie, pass the suture externally, back through the eyelid skin), Figure 60.7.

11. Amputate the clamped tissues with a No. 15 blade scalpel cutting between the clamp and polypropylene suture (Figure 60.8).

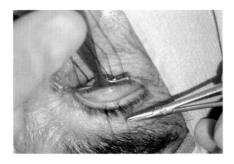

Figure 60.7. The suture is externalized.

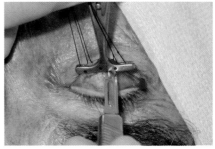

Figure 60.8. Müller muscle and conjunctiva are resected with a No. 15 blade scalpel.

Figure 60.9. The suture is tied on the external surface of the lid.

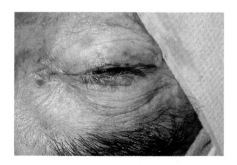

12. Remove the Desmarres retractor and return the eyelid to its anatomic position.
13. Tie the polypropylene suture to itself in the pretarsal area (Figure 60.9).
14. Remove the silk traction suture.
15. Place antibiotic ointment on the ocular surface.

POSTOPERATIVE CARE

1. Use antibiotic drops for 1 week.
2. Remove the suture in 5 to 7 days.

COMPLICATIONS

- Overcorrection
- Undercorrection

For overcorrection, once the suture is removed, digital massage can be used to lower the eyelid.

Undercorrection requires additional surgery, usually a Fasanella-Servat procedure.

Chapter 61

Fasanella-Servat Procedure

Steven C. Dresner, MD
Alan McInnes, MD

The Fasanella-Servat procedure is suited for patients with minimal ptosis (1 to 2.5 mm), a normal eyelid contour, and a negative phenylephrine test. This procedure is also helpful in patients with undercorrection after a Müller muscle conjunctiva resection or levator advancement surgery.

PREOPERATIVE STEPS

1. Measure and document in both eyes the interpalpebral fissures and the upper eyelid margin to corneal light reflex distance (MRD-1).
2. Take photographs and document the visual fields as required.

INSTRUMENTATION AND SUPPLIES

- Marking pen
- Caliper
- Desmarres retractor
- Fasanella-Müller's clamp
- Toothed forceps (eg, Paufique)
- Needle holder
- No. 15 blade scalpel

SURGICAL PROCEDURE

1. Mark the upper eyelid margin in the pupillary axis with the patient in an upright sitting position.
2. Apply topical tetracaine drops to the conjunctival surface. Inject 2% lidocaine with 1:100,000 epinephrine and 200 USP units hyaluronidase per 20 cc of anesthetic through the superior cul-de-sac.
3. Evert the eyelid over a Desmarres retractor.
4. Using the calipers and a pen, mark the location on the tarsal conjunctival surface at the pupillary axis, inferior to the superior tarsal margin, that delineates the amount of resection to be performed; 2 mm of tarsus is excised for every 1 mm of ptosis (Figure 61.1).
5. Pass a 4-0 silk suture through the superior tarsal margin medially and laterally.
6. Remove the Desmarres retractor.
7. Elevate the tissues with the traction sutures (Figure 61.2).
8. Place the clamp over the tissues, extending the superior edge of the clamp to the central mark (Figure 61.3).

Figure 61.1. The tarsal conjunctiva is marked for clamp placement.

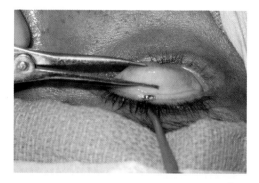

Figure 61.2. Silk traction suture is placed at the superior tarsal margin.

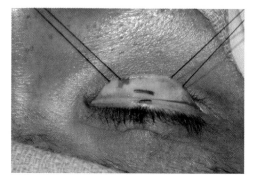

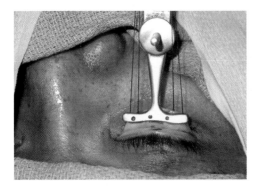

Figure 61.3. The Müller muscle (Dresner-Uzcategui) clamp is placed.

9. Pass a 6-0 polypropylene suture full thickness through the pre-tarsal eyelid at one end of the clamp, entering the skin and exiting the conjunctival surface, and then pass the suture under the clamp in a running mattress fashion. At the opposite end of the clamp, "exteriorize" the suture (ie, pass it back through the eyelid, exiting the skin surface), Figures 61.4, 61.5.

10. Excise the clamped tissues between the clamp and sutures (Figure 61.6).

11. Reflect the eyelid back to the anatomic position.

12. Tie the polypropylene suture to itself in the pre-tarsal area (Figure 61.7).

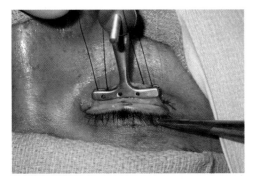

Figure 61.4. The polypropylene suture is passed through the skin to the conjunctival surface.

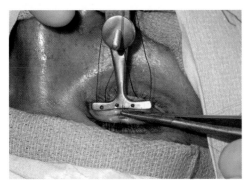

Figure 61.5. The suture is run in a horizontal mattress fashion.

Figure 61.6. The conjunctiva and tarsus are resected.

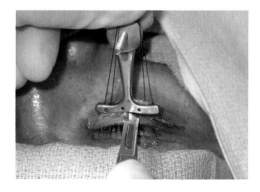

Figure 61.7. The externalized ends of the suture are tied.

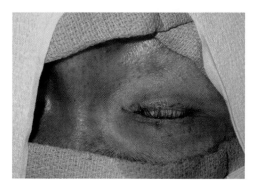

POSTOPERATIVE CARE

1. Use antibiotic drops for 1 week.
2. Remove the suture in 5 to 7 days.

COMPLICATIONS

- Overcorrection
- Undercorrection
- Foreign body sensation
- Contour abnormality

Overcorrection is managed by digital massage after the suture is removed in 5 to 7 days. More-complex recession may be required later.

Undercorrection is managed by levator aponeurosis resection via an external approach at a later date.

Foreign body sensation may be seen rarely when an absorbable suture is passed and tied internally. Contour abnormalities are more common when a hemostat is used to clamp the tissues. Foreign body sensation and contour abnormalities are exceedingly rare when a polypropylene suture is externalized and the Müller muscle-conjunctiva clamp is used.

Chapter 62

Eyelid Tumor Excision and Full-Thickness Reconstruction of Eyelid Defects

Rhonda V. Barrett, MD
Dale R. Meyer, MD, FACS

This chapter covers the technique for full-thickness excision of eyelid tumors and also the various techniques for reconstruction that may be utilized by the ophthalmic surgeon. The relationship between the eyelid defect size and the method of reconstruction is discussed.

EYELID TUMOR EXCISION (FULL-THICKNESS PENTAGONAL WEDGE EXCISION)

Suspicious eyelid lesions should be biopsied and evaluated for pathologic diagnosis. If a malignancy is confirmed, definitive tumor excision with reconstruction should be arranged. Removal of eyelid lesions can be performed by the ophthalmologist or a specialist skilled in Mohs micrographic surgery. The first priority should be total removal of the lesion, facilitated by "margin evaluation," which in many cases can be performed by intraoperative pathologic evaluation via frozen sections.

Preoperative Steps

1. Obtain preoperative medical clearance by the patient's primary physician for patients requiring parenteral anesthesia.
2. Discontinue aspirin 10 to 14 days prior to surgery, Coumadin 5 days prior, and nonsteroidal anti-inflammatory drugs 3 days prior, if allowed by the patient's primary physician.

3. Preoperative blood pressure control is necessary to limit intraoperative bleeding.

4. Make arrangements for eyelid reconstruction following full-thickness tumor excision. It should be emphasized that the final defect size may be much larger than the visible lesion, and it is important that the surgeon be skilled in appropriate reconstructive techniques as outlined below.

5. Counsel the patient that the reconstructive technique will be guided by the size of the defect, and flaps or grafts from adjacent or more distant sites may be required. The patient should be prepared for the possibility of a lid-sharing procedure for larger defects, with possible occlusion of the eye for 2 to 6 weeks postoperatively and the need for a second-stage operation.

Instrumentation and Supplies

- Local anesthetic: 2% lidocaine with epinephrine 1:100,000
- Stevens scissors
- Toothed forceps
- Electrocautery or handheld thermal cautery
- Needle holder
- 5-0 polyglactin (Vicryl) suture for the deep layer
- 6-0 fast-absorbing gut suture or 6-0 silk for the superficial layer

Surgical Procedure

1. Using a sterile marking pen, outline the proposed medial and lateral incision sites. These incision sites should be perpendicular to the lid margin. Be sure to include 1 to 2 mm of normal-appearing tissue on either side (Figure 62.1).

2. Using a 27-gauge needle, infiltrate anesthesia into the eyelid, including the margin in the area of the lesion.

3. Using Stevens scissors, incise along the outlined skin markings extending the full extent of the tarsus, making sure to stay perpendicular to the lid margin. Once reaching the distal end of the tarsus, angle the incision to a point in order to create a pentagon (Figure 62.2).

4. Provide hemostasis by direct pressure. Minimal cautery should be used.

5. The specimen may be sent to pathology for frozen sections. Additional tissue resection should be performed until the margins are tumor-free.

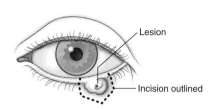

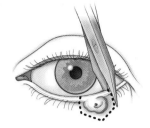

Figure 62.1. The proposed full-thickness pentagonal wedge to be excised is outlined incorporating the lesion with 1 to 2 mm of normal-appearing tissue on either side.

Figure 62.2. The full-thickness pentagonal wedge is excised.

6. The size and location of the defect and the degree of lid laxity determine the type of closure. The individual methods of eyelid reconstruction are described later in this chapter.
   - Small defect (<33%): direct closure (if the cut edges can be reapproximated without significant tension) or canthotomy and cantholysis with advancement
   - Moderate defect (33% to 50%): semicircular flap (Tenzel flap)
   - Large defect (>50%): tarsal-conjunctival advancement flap (Hughes flap) for a lower lid defect, or Cutler-Beard bridge flap for an upper lid defect
7. Once reconstruction has been completed, prophylactic antibiotic ointment may be applied to the wound 4 times daily. This treatment will also allow skin sutures to dissolve appropriately. If sutures are placed that require removal, the ointment should be applied for 3 to 4 more days following removal.

Complications

- Bleeding
- Failure
- Involvement of the lacrimal system

Bleeding is reduced by using local anesthetic with epinephrine. Control with gentle pressure and light electrocautery.

Despite intraoperative pathologic evaluation, residual microscopic tumor cells may remain necessitating future surgical procedures.

If the lacrimal system is involved in the tumor, then it must be removed in order to obtain tumor-free margins. Surgical repair of such a defect should be performed at a later time once no malignancy has been shown to recur. This approach will decrease the risk of allowing spread of a malignancy into the sinuses or nasal mucosa.

CANTHOTOMY AND CANTHOLYSIS WITH ADVANCEMENT

Following tumor excision, eyelid reconstruction is performed to optimize the final appearance and symmetry while maintaining functionality. Priorities in eyelid reconstruction include providing adequate eyelid closure, a stable lid margin, adequate vertical lid height, and a smooth, epithelialized internal eyelid surface.

When repair of a defect by direct closure cannot be achieved without placing undue tension on the wound, a lateral canthotomy and cantholysis may provide enough relaxation to allow for adequate closure. This procedure is performed when a gap of about 3 mm or less exists between the cut edges of the wound on attempted reapproximation. This procedure can be performed for upper or lower eyelid reconstruction.

Preoperative Steps

1. Precede reconstruction with removal of the lesion with tumor-free margins.
2. Obtain preoperative medical clearance by the patient's primary physician for patients requiring parenteral anesthesia.
3. Discontinue aspirin 10 to 14 days prior, Coumadin 5 days prior, and nonsteroidal anti-inflammatory drugs 3 days prior if allowed by the patient's primary physician.
4. Preoperative blood pressure control is necessary to limit intraoperative bleeding.

Instrumentation and Supplies

See instrumentation for "Eyelid Tumor Excision" above. Additional instrumentation includes a hemostat.

Surgical Procedure

1. Using a 27-gauge needle, infiltrate anesthesia into the lateral canthus and lateral portion of the involved eyelid.

2. Incise the skin and superficial orbicularis muscle at the lateral canthus using Stevens scissors. Extend the incision for 5 to 7 mm lateral to the lateral canthal angle (Figure 62.3).

3. Using Stevens scissors, bluntly dissect to the inner aspect of the lateral orbital rim.

4. Grasp the lid at the cut margin using toothed forceps, pulling slightly medially to place medial traction on the wound. This maneuver will allow the surgeon to identify when lysis of the lateral canthal tendon has been achieved.

5. Strum the lateral canthal tendon with the Stevens scissors and cut inferiorly through the tendon (Figure 62.4). Avoid cutting through conjunctiva if possible. When the tendon has been appropriately lysed, the lid will have several millimeters of medial movement, allowing for closure of the eyelid wound.

6. Perform closure of the full-thickness eyelid wound using the techniques outlined in Chapter 74.

7. Using a 5-0 polyglactin suture, reattach the new lateral eyelid margin to the periorbita on the inner aspect of the lateral orbital rim (Figure 62.5A, 62.5B).

8. Perform a gray line closure using a 6-0 fast-absorbing gut suture. Place this suture by first passing the suture through the gray line on the lower lid and out through the cut eyelid margin, entering 1 to 2 mm from the tissue edge. Next, pass the suture through the cut margin of the upper lid and out through the gray line (Figure 62.6). The suture may be tied and cut with the knot falling between the eyelids in the lateral canthal angle (Figure 62.6).

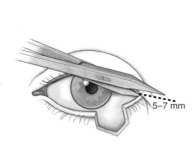

Figure 62.3. The lateral canthal skin and superficial orbicularis (canthotomy) are incised.

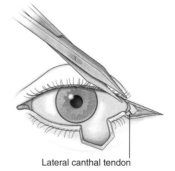

Lateral canthal tendon

Figure 62.4. The inferior crus of the lateral canthal tendon is lysed (cantholysis).

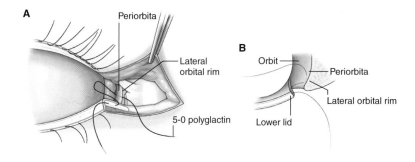

Figure 62.5. (A) and (B). The newly advanced lower eyelid is resuspended to the periosteum just inside the lateral orbital rim.

Figure 62.6. A gray line closure is performed.

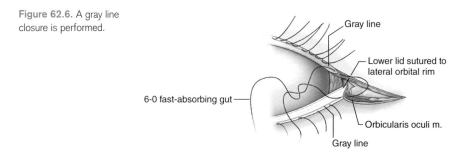

Figure 62.7. Postoperative appearance after lower-eyelid, full-thickness wedge excision with lateral canthotomy and cantholysis with advancement.

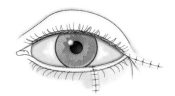

9. Close the skin using interrupted 6-0 fast-absorbing gut suture or 6-0 silk, incorporating a small amount of the orbicularis muscle into the suture bites (Figure 62.7).

10. Prophylactic antibiotic ointment may be placed on the incision site at the close of the procedure and 4 times daily until the skin sutures dissolve.

Complications

- Bleeding
- Wound dehiscence
- Other

Bleeding is be reduced by using local anesthetic with epinephrine. Control with gentle pressure or light cautery.

If undue tension remains on the wound, dehiscence may occur.

Rounding of the lateral canthal angle, droopiness of the lid, or ectropion can occur if a firm reattachment of the lid to the periorbita is not achieved.

SEMICIRCULAR FLAP (TENZEL FLAP)

Following eyelid tumor resection, grasp the cut edges of the wound and attempt to reapproximate the wound margins. If a gap of more than about 3 mm exists, a Tenzel semicircular flap may be necessary to provide enough tissue for closure. A Tenzel flap is usually fashioned if direct closure or closure utilizing a lateral canthotomy and cantholysis is not feasible due to undue tension on the wound.

The Tenzel semicircular flap may be used for reconstruction of the upper or lower eyelid.

Ideal wounds amenable to closure using this technique involve up to 30% to 50% of the eyelid, and occasionally larger defects.

Preoperative Steps

See the preoperative steps for "Canthotomy and Cantholysis With Advancement" in this chapter.

Instrumentation and Supplies

See instrumentation and supplies for "Eyelid Tumor Excision" in this chapter. Additional instrumentation includes a hemostat and sterile marking pen.

Surgical Procedure for Lower Eyelid Defects

1. Outline a superiorly directed semicircle at the lateral canthus.
2. Using a 27-gauge needle, infiltrate anesthesia into the lateral canthus and the lateral portion of the involved eyelid.
3. Using Stevens scissors, incise the skin and underlying muscle along the outlined skin incision (Figure 62.8). A lateral canthotomy and cantholysis of the lower branch of the lateral canthal tendon should be performed (Figure 62.9). The lateral skin incision, however, should

Figure 62.8. Superiorly directed semicircular lateral canthal incision for Tenzel flap
eyelid reconstruction.

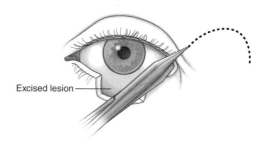

Excised lesion

Figure 62.9. Incision of the inferior crus
of the lateral canthal tendon is performed
once the skin and orbicularis have been undermined under the lateral semicircular flap.

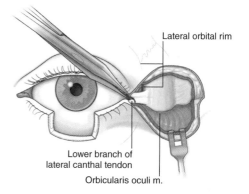

Lateral orbital rim

Lower branch of
lateral canthal tendon

Orbicularis oculi m.

not extend straight laterally, but should extend along the superiorly
directed outlined semicircle.

4. Maintain hemostasis using cautery.

5. Undermine the laterally based musculocutaneous flap using blunt dissection with Stevens scissors. This maneuver should provide adequate
laxity of the remaining portion of the lower eyelid and adjacent flap to
allow reapproximation of the wound margins.

6. Perform closure of the full-thickness eyelid wound using the techniques
outlined in the Chapter 74.

7. Following reapproximation of the full-thickness eyelid wound
margins, the lateral canthus is reconstituted. Use a single interrupted 5-0 polyglactin suture to reattach the deep lateral edge of
the flap to the periorbita on the inner aspect of the lateral orbital
rim. The lateral portion of the orbicularis muscle and underlying
fascia in the rotated flap can be reattached to pre-zygomatic fascia
using deep and interrupted 5-0 polyglactin sutures to further reduce any tension on the eyelid wound (Figure 62.10).

8. Complete the lateral canthal angle repair by passing a 6-0 fast-absorbing gut suture through the gray line of the opposite intact eyelid, out

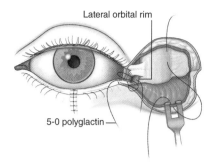

Lateral orbital rim

5-0 polyglactin

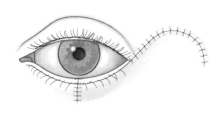

Figure 62.10. The newly advanced eyelid margin is resuspended to the inner aspect of the lateral orbital rim. The deep edge of the lateral aspect of the Tenzel flap is also resuspended by attachment to the pre-zygomatic fascia.

Figure 62.11. Postoperative appearance after eyelid reconstruction with Tenzel semicircular flap.

of the cut wound edge, and through the corresponding portion of the flap. [Note: there will not be a gray line on the lateral position of the flap.] Each pass should enter 1 to 2 mm from the tissue edge. The suture may then be tied and cut, allowing the knot to fall within the lateral canthal angle.

9. Close the skin using interrupted 6-0 fast-absorbing gut suture incorporating a small amount of the orbicularis muscle into the suture bites (Figure 62.11).

10. If a "dog ear" is discovered at the most lateral portion of the flap during wound closure, excise a small lateral triangle of tissue.

11. Prophylactic antibiotic ointment may be placed on the incision site at the close of the procedure and 4 times daily until the sutures dissolve.

Surgical Procedure: Semicircular Flap for Upper Eyelid Defects

The procedure should be performed as outlined in "Lower Lid Defects" in this chapter, with the semicircle extending inferiorly at the lateral canthal angle instead of superiorly. In addition, when performing the lateral cantholysis, the surgeon should lyse the upper crus of the tendon to provide laxity of the remaining lateral portion of the upper eyelid.

Complications

- Bleeding
- Wound dehiscence
- Other

Bleeding is reduced by using local anesthetic with epinephrine. Control with gentle pressure and light cautery.

If undue tension remains on the wound, dehiscence may occur.

The lower lid and soft issue should be firmly reattached to the periorbita and pre-zygomatic fascia in order to prevent drooping of the eyelid or ectropion following lower eyelid reconstruction.

Some tightening of the upper eyelid may occur with reconstruction of upper eyelid defects, inducing some degree of ptosis. It is best to avoid undue tension if possible, but in some cases, this cannot be avoided. Some improvement of the ptosis can be expected with time, however.

Rounding of the lateral canthal angle can occur if a firm reattachment of the lid to the periorbita is not achieved.

TARSAL-CONJUNCTIVAL ADVANCEMENT FLAP (HUGHES FLAP) FOR LOWER EYELID RECONSTRUCTION

When the previously described techniques for reconstruction are not feasible, a Hughes flap can be performed for lower eyelid defects. Hughes flaps are ideal for full-thickness defects involving >50% of the lower eyelid margin, particularly those in the more central portion of the eyelid. It is important to note that the Hughes flap is an "eyelid-sharing" procedure. This type of flap is generally used when other local flaps are not adequate, given the requirement for eyelid closure and therefore an induced monocular status until the eyelids heal sufficiently, allowing for a second procedure to open the eyelids.

Preoperative Steps

See the preoperative procedure for "Canthotomy and Cantholysis With Advancement" in this chapter. Additional consideration: counsel the patient on the postoperative course including eyelid closure for several weeks and the need for a second-stage operation.

Instrumentation and Supplies

See instrumentation for "Eyelid Tumor Excision" in this chapter. Additional instrumentation includes Desmarres retractor and No. 15 Bard-Parker blade.

Surgical Procedure

1. Using a 27-gauge needle, infiltrate anesthesia into the upper and lower eyelids.
2. Using a Desmarres retractor, evert the upper eyelid.
3. Incise the conjunctiva and tarsus using a No. 15 Bard-Parker blade. This incision should begin 3 to 4 mm above the eyelid margin and extend parallel to the upper eyelid margin. The length is determined by the horizontal extent of the lower lid defect to be repaired (Figure 62.12).
4. Using Stevens scissors, make vertical cuts superiorly extending to the superior edge of tarsus on both sides of the original incision.
5. Elevate the flap using Stevens scissors and blunt dissection in order to separate the tarsal-conjunctival flap from the underlying tissues (Figure 62.13).
6. Use Stevens scissors to extend the conjunctival incision to the superior fornix, dissecting Muller's muscle off of the conjunctiva as best as possible.
7. Remove the Desmarres retractor. Extend the mobilized tarsal-conjunctival flap inferiorly into the lower lid defect. The superior border of the tarsus should be flush with the remaining lower eyelid margins on either side.
8. Using 5-0 polyglactin or chromic gut sutures in an interrupted fashion, attach the tarsal-conjunctival flap to the remaining lower eyelid tarsus on either side and to the remaining lower eyelid retractors inferiorly (Figure 62.14).

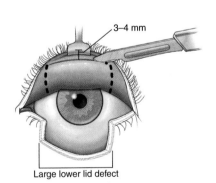

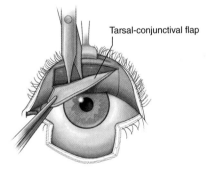

Figure 62.12. The superior conjunctiva and tarsus are incised with the horizontal extent equal to the horizontal extent of the lower eyelid defect.

Figure 62.13. The conjunctiva and tarsus are dissected superiorly, with special care taken to separate Müller's muscle from the conjunctiva to avoid lid retraction postoperatively.

Figure 62.14. The tarsal-conjunctival flap is transposed inferiorly into the lower eyelid defect and sewn into position.

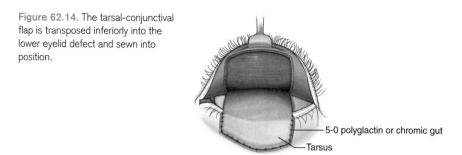

5-0 polyglactin or chromic gut

Tarsus

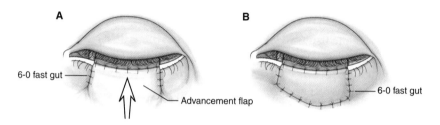

A

B

6-0 fast gut

Advancement flap

6-0 fast gut

Figure 62.15. Choices for anterior lamellar reconstruction. (A) Lower eyelid skin can be undermined and advanced superiorly. (B) A full-thickness skin graft can be used to cover the tarsal-conjunctival flap.

9. The anterior lamella of the lid can be created by:
   - An advancement flap if there is sufficient lid laxity (Figure 62.15A)
   - A transposition flap from the upper eyelid
   - A full-thickness skin graft using either postauricular, supraclavicular, or upper eyelid skin (Figure 62.15B)
10. Prophylactic antibiotic ointment may be placed on the incision site at the close of the procedure and 4 times daily until the sutures dissolve.

Postoperative Care

1. A patch is usually placed for several days.
2. Separation of the eyelids is then accomplished in 2 to 6 weeks by cutting across the flap at the level of the intended lower eyelid margin and suturing the edge of the conjunctival flap back into the upper eyelid.

Complications

- Bleeding
- Failure
- Lid laxity

- Ectropion
- Suture keratopathy
- Eyelid retraction
- Ptosis

Bleeding is reduced by using local anesthetic with epinephrine. Control with gentle pressure and light cautery.

A skin graft may fail due to the interruption of the original blood supply.

Lower lid laxity may be induced if the flap is too wide for the defect, causing the lower eyelid to not fit snugly against globe. To prevent postoperative laxity, use forceps to pull the lower lid wound edges together at the beginning of the case to measure the size of the defect in need of closure.

Ectropion may be induced by advancement flaps in younger patients without sufficient skin laxity.

Suture keratopathy can be avoided by ensuring that tarsal sutures are not full thickness, especially at the eyelid margin.

Prevent upper eyelid retraction by maintaining at least 3 to 4 mm of uninvolved tarsus in the upper eyelid margin and undermine the tissue to the superior fornix (dissecting Muller's muscle off the conjunctiva).

Careful dissection will avoid damage to the levator aponeurosis.

CUTLER-BEARD "BRIDGE" FLAP FOR UPPER EYELID RECONSTRUCTION

When the previously described techniques for reconstruction are not feasible and a large upper eyelid defect is present, a Cutler-Beard flap can be performed. Cutler-Beard flaps are ideal for full-thickness defects involving >60% of the upper eyelid margin. It is important to note that the Cutler-Beard flap, like the Hughes flap, is an "eyelid-sharing" procedure, generally only used when other local flaps are not adequate. Postoperatively, the eye is covered for 1 to 2 months, inducing a monocular status until the eyelids heal sufficiently to allow for a second procedure to separate the flap and open the eyelids.

Preoperative Steps

See the preoperative procedure for "Tarsal-Conjunctival Advancement Flap (Hughes Flap)" in this chapter.

Instrumentation and Supplies

See instrumentation for "Tarsal-Conjunctival Advancement Flap (Hughes Flap)" in this chapter. Additional instrumentation includes a protective corneal shield and a sterile marking pen.

Surgical Procedure

1. Using a 27-gauge needle, infiltrate anesthesia into the upper and lower eyelids.
2. Place a corneal protector on the operative eye.
3. Grasp the cut edges of the upper eyelid wound, and attempt to reapproximate the wound. Using a marking pen, translate the medial and lateral extent of the upper eyelid defect to the corresponding aspects of the lower eyelid. Connect the marks with a horizontally placed line 4 to 5 mm below the eyelid margin. This will allow preservation of the marginal arcade in the lower eyelid.
4. Using the marking pen, outline 2 vertical incisions drawn from each side of the horizontal incision extending toward the inferior orbital rim.
5. Incise the skin and orbicularis along the horizontal skin marking using a No. 15 Bard-Parker blade (Figure 62.16).
6. Evert the lower lid using a Desmarres retractor and incise the corresponding aspect of the conjunctiva using the No. 15 blade scalpel (Figure 62.17). Both the skin and conjunctival incisions should maintain a 4 to 5 mm distance from the lid margin.

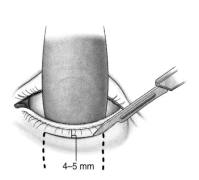

4–5 mm

Figure 62.16. The bridge flap is created by making a full-thickness eyelid incision 4 to 5 mm below the lid margin. Special care should be taken to protect the globe.

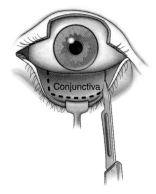

Conjunctiva

Figure 62.17. The corresponding aspect of the conjunctiva is incised using a No. 15 blade.

7. Stevens scissors may be used to complete a full-thickness blepharotomy.
   - The advancement flap should not contain tarsus. Autogenous cartilage (such as ear cartilage), banked tarsus, a free tarsal graft, or other posterior lamella substitute can be inserted on the posterior aspect of the flap for enhanced structural support. The "standard" Cutler-Beard procedure does not utilize this technique and therefore further discussion is not included in this text.
8. Using Stevens scissors, incise along the vertical relaxing incisions. Be sure that the base of the flap is slightly wider than the apex.
9. Remove the corneal protector.
10. Place the advancement flap under the intact lower lid margin (the "bridge") and advance to the superior aspect of the upper eyelid defect (Figure 62.18).
11. Using 5-0 polyglactin or chromic gut suture in an interrupted fashion, attach the conjunctiva and deep layer of the advancement flap to the remaining upper eyelid conjunctiva and deep layer, taking care to keep all knots facing anteriorly and minimizing exposed sutures toward the globe. Similarly, suture the deep superior portion of the flap (conjunctiva and capsulopalpebral fascia) to the remaining edge of the levator aponeurosis (Figure 62.19).

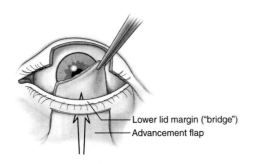

Figure 62.18. The Cutler-Beard flap is extended superiorly, passing underneath the lid margin "bridge."

Lower lid margin ("bridge")
Advancement flap

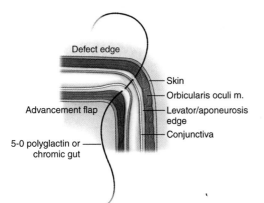

Figure 62.19. The flap is sewn into the upper lid defect with a tri-layered closure.

Defect edge

Skin
Orbicularis oculi m.
Levator/aponeurosis edge
Conjunctiva

Advancement flap

5-0 polyglactin or chromic gut

Figure 62.20. Postoperative appearance after reconstruction of upper eyelid with Cutler-Beard "bridge" flap.

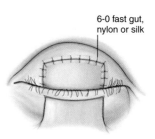

6-0 fast gut, nylon or silk

12. Close the skin using interrupted 6-0 fast-absorbing gut, nylon, or silk suture (Figure 62.20).

13. Utilizing a standard eyelid margin closure, suture the nasal and temporal eyelid margins to the flap. A patch is usually placed for several days. Three to 8 weeks later, the eyelids can be separated by incising the flap at the level of the desired new upper eyelid margin and suturing the extra skin/muscle flap back into the lower eyelid.

14. Prophylactic antibiotic ointment may be placed on the incision site at the close of the procedure and 4 times daily until the sutures dissolve.

Complications

- Bleeding
- Vascular compromise
- Suture keratopathy
- Entropion with trichiasis
- Eyelid retraction
- Ptosis

Bleeding is reduced by using local anesthetic with epinephrine. Control with gentle pressure and light cautery.

Adequate tissue should be mobilized inferiorly such that the flap is able to easily pass under the lower eyelid margin and into the upper eyelid defect. This maneuver will prevent vascular compromise of the flap and lower eyelid margin. In addition, the horizontal lower eyelid incision should maintain a 4 to 5 mm distance from the margin in order to preserve the vascular supply and prevent necrosis of the "bridge."

Suture keratopathy can be prevented by ensuring that conjunctival sutures are not full thickness, especially at the eyelid margin.

Upper eyelid entropion with trichiasis may occur following separation of the eyelids, as fine lanugo hairs present on the newly created upper eyelid margin can cause corneal irritation. This complication can be prevented during the second-stage procedure by beveling the incision such that the conjunctival edge is slightly more inferior than the skin edge.

If upper eyelid retraction occurs, the flap can be reunited and left in place for a few more weeks. Allowing an appropriate amount of time for healing before performing the second-stage procedure may also help to prevent this common complication.

Ptosis will usually improve as the tissue retracts with healing.

Chapter 63

Upper Blepharoplasty

Joseph A. Mauriello Jr, MD

Functional upper blepharoplasty can be performed to address the following problems:

- A subjective sense of heaviness of the upper lids affecting vision, evidenced by fatigue on sustained reading, watching television, or driving
- Mechanical ptosis with documented superior visual field defect that may be further supported by repeat visual field testing showing an improved superior field when the upper eyelids are taped open
- A new pseudo-eyelid margin created by excess skin overhanging the eyelid margin
- Dermatitis due to skin overlying skin, not responsive to medical treatment such as a short-term trial of a topical corticosteroid
- Frontal headache that progresses during the day due to constant use of the frontalis muscle to elevate the eyelids

Cosmetic upper blepharoplasty is performed to improve the appearance of the eyelids. Asymmetry of the upper eyelid creases, protrusion of orbital fat, and a relative lack of exposed pretarsal skin below the upper eyelid folds are among the many factors that may lead patients to consider aesthetic upper eyelid surgery.

PREOPERATIVE STEPS

1. Good communication between the surgeon and patient is especially important in aesthetic surgery. It is best to ask the patient, with a mirror in hand, to point out the specific problem. Assess the patient's goals and stress both the potential benefits and limitations of surgery.

2. An increased risk of dry eye occurs in patients following upper blepharoplasty, especially when combined with ptosis repair. A preoperative history of a dry eye, including symptoms of burning, intermittent dryness, or foreign body sensation may be contraindications for undergoing upper blepharoplasty. Evaluation of the tear film, including tear break-up time, Schirmer's testing with topical anesthetic, and examination of the level of the tear meniscus, may help identify patients at a greater risk of developing dry eye complications postoperatively. Other factors that may adversely affect the tear film—the presence of lower eyelid retraction, an incomplete blink, the presence of lagophthalmos, deficient corneal sensation, or a poor Bell's reflex—should be noted preoperatively and may be severe enough to contraindicate upper blepharoplasty.

3. Since refractive surgery can result in dry eye symptoms, upper blepharoplasty should not be performed until a minimum of 6 months after a corneal refractive procedure.

4. Counsel the patient that it is impossible to predict whether a patient with underlying dry eye will have problems after surgery; a conservative surgical approach will diminish risks significantly.

5. In many patients, upper blepharoplasty may have both functional and cosmetic components. In the great majority of patients, upper blepharoplasty is performed bilaterally.

INSTRUMENTATION AND SUPPLIES

- No. 15 blade scalpel
- Straight sharp iris scissors
- Castroviejo 0.5 forceps
- Monopolar cautery
- 6-0 plain gut suture

SURGICAL PROCEDURE

1. It is useful to post preoperative photographs in the operating room as a guide to the appropriate amount of surgery during the procedure.

2. Mark the desired amount of skin to be excised with a surgical marking pen or methylene blue. Initially, mark the eyelid crease medially to the level of the superior punctum and laterally to the level of the lateral canthus; it is important to follow the patient's crease and to not change

the crease unless the creases are asymmetric or the level of the crease is distinctly abnormal. The incision must then extend laterally to accommodate excision of redundant skin and muscle that extends beyond the lateral canthus; therefore, at the level of the lateral canthus, gently curve the mark obliquely, superiorly and laterally (Figure 63.1A).

3. To determine the placement of the superior incision—and the amount of skin to be removed—the "pinch" technique can be used. Grasp excess skin with toothed forceps at the eyelid crease. Gauge the appropriate amount of skin to be excised above the crease by ensuring that the upper eyelid margin is not excessively pulled upward to create lagophthalmos that may persist postoperatively. The level of the superior incision can then be marked on the eyelid above the forceps (Figures 63.1B, 63.1C, 63.1D).

4. Infiltrate a 1:1 mixture of 1% lidocaine with epinephrine and 0.50% bupivacaine while the patient is sedated. Avoid epinephrine if the patient has cardiovascular disease. (The author favors intravenous sedation administered by an anesthesiologist.)

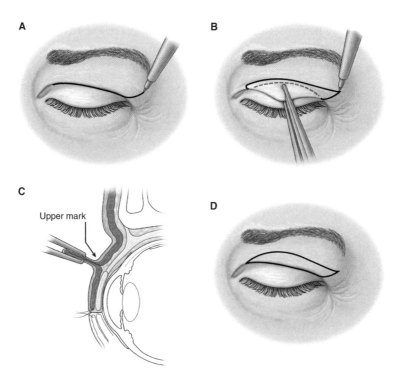

Figure 63.1. Creating the upper blepharoplasty mark. (A) The mark follows the skin crease from the level of the upper punctum to the lateral canthus. (B) The mark gently curves superotemporally. (C) View of the "pinch" technique employed to determine the amount of skin to excise without causing postoperative lagophthalmos. (D) Appearance of the final mark.

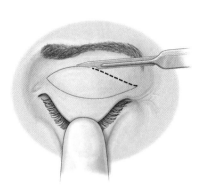

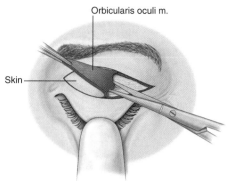

Figure 63.2. Skin markings are incised with a No. 15 blade.

Figure 63.3. The skin and underlying orbicularis muscle are excised in one piece.

5. Incise the skin markings with a No. 15 blade scalpel (Figure 63.2). Creating a defined incision is facilitated by stabilizing the upper eyelid tissues with the other hand. In patients with thin skin and a prominent globe, avoid incising too deeply through the underlying levator aponeurosis, which might create an iatrogenic levator dehiscence.

6. Excise the skin and the underlying orbicularis muscle together in one piece down to the level of the orbital septum with the iris scissors (Figure 63.3). Obtain hemostasis with cautery.

7. If fat prolapse is to be addressed, open the orbital septum with iris scissors (Figure 63.4).

8. Gently tease forward the preaponeurotic fat with blunt dissection, and inject it with the local anesthetic. The deep medial fat pocket has a whitish appearance while the central pre-aponeurotic fat is more yellow in color.

9. Resect prolapsed fat with a combination of scissors and cautery (Figure 63.5). Only the fat that readily presents itself should be

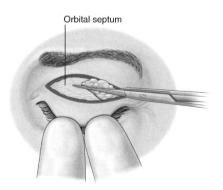

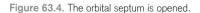

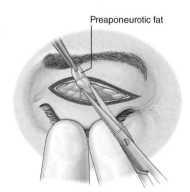

Figure 63.4. The orbital septum is opened.

Figure 63.5. The preaponeurotic fat is excised.

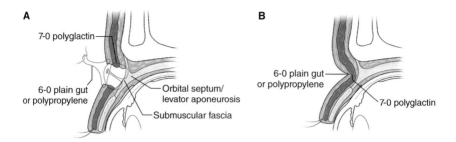

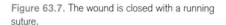

Figure 63.6. Creating a deeper, well-defined skin crease. (A) Deeper suture bites are placed through the submuscular fascia/levator complex with 7-0 polyglactin. (B) The appearance of the lid crease following skin closure.

Figure 63.7. The wound is closed with a running suture.

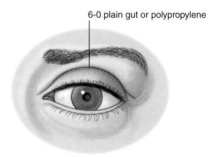

excised. Meticulous attention to hemostasis is important to avoid bleeding into the orbit postoperatively.

10. In patients with poor eyelid creases, deep intervening bites of submuscular fascia help re-create the eyelid crease. Deep buried sutures of 7-0 polyglactin may be taken through the dermal edge of the inferior skin muscle flap that is slightly undermined and advanced superiorly. Do so by taking a second bite through the submuscular fascia as well as the fused orbital septum and levator aponeurosis, sufficiently above the upper tarsal border to flatten the pretarsal skin platform (Figures 63.6A, 63.6B).

11. Close the incision with a running 6-0 plain gut or 6-0 polypropylene suture (Figure 63.7).

POSTOPERATIVE CARE

1. Advise the patient to apply ice pack compresses to the eyelids every 15 minutes at 1-hour intervals while awake. This is to be done for 4 days. For the compress, ice or frozen peas are placed in a plastic bag while sterile gauze is situated between the eyelid and ice pack.

2. Head elevation is preferred during sleep for the first week.

3. Topical antibiotics are prescribed for 1 week. Broad-spectrum oral antibiotics are generally prescribed for 4-lid blepharoplasty but not 2-lid surgeries.
4. The sixth day after surgery, hot sterile compresses can be started. Hot water that has been boiled first may be used and applied with a sterile gauze for 10 to 15 minutes 4 times a day.
5. Patients are instructed to avoid driving for at least 1 week, avoid exercise for 18 days, and avoid makeup to the wounds for 21 days.
6. Patients are requested to contact the surgeon if they note increased pain, swelling, mucous discharge, decreased vision, or evidence of hemorrhage develops.
7. Patients return for follow-up examination in 1 week and then again 2 weeks after surgery.

COMPLICATIONS

- Orbital hemorrhage
- Infection
- Undercorrection
- Overcorrection

If the septum is opened, bleeding from the orbicularis muscle or from the preaponeurotic fat can track into the orbit, causing an orbital hemorrhage with the potential for visual loss that may be permanent. In such cases, a lateral canthotomy and inferior cantholysis may be required, with evacuation of the hemorrhage necessary in severe cases.

Postoperative infection is rare and is usually treatable with a short course of oral antibiotics.

Not resecting enough tissue may lead to residual excess upper eyelid skin or bulging fat and asymmetry. Undercorrections generally do not necessitate revision surgery if mild. Undercorrections are relatively common and preferable to overcorrections.

Removal of too much fat will give the eyelid a "sunken" appearance. Excision of too much skin and muscle can lead to lid closure problems such as incomplete blinking or frank lagophthalmos. Eyelid closure problems may affect vision after blepharoplasty since the eyelids (especially the upper lid) clear the tear film, and blinking keeps the eyes moist. Dry eye may cause temporary blurred vision. Topical lubricating drops and conscious blinking over several days (or over months in rare cases) may improve the condition. In cases where symptomatic, chronic lagophthalmos is present, a skin graft to the upper lids may be required.

Chapter 64

Lower Blepharoplasty

Joseph A. Mauriello Jr, MD

Traditional lower blepharoplasty is a technically challenging procedure due to the following possible adverse results: cicatricial lower lid retraction, a hollowed-out lower lid appearance, and residual lower lid puffiness due to insufficient tightening or removal of skin, especially in patients with a hypoplastic maxilla and malar eminence. The traditional technique generally includes a subciliary incision across the entire lower eyelid that extends beyond the lateral commissure into the lateral canthal area combined with orbital fat excision. Transconjunctival fat removal diminishes the risk of postoperative lower lid retraction since the orbital septum is not violated, but fat removal alone does not address tightening of the anterior lamella. After fat removal, anterior lamellar wrinkling may in fact be exacerbated, somewhat analogous to deflating a balloon.

A lateral canthopexy or some other form of horizontal tightening of the lower eyelid that may involve a lateral canthoplasty has become quite popular in order to avoid the most common postoperative complication of traditional lower blepharoplasty, lower eyelid retraction, or even frank ectropion. A canthoplasty, by definition, combines incising the lateral canthal tissues with a cantholysis of the inferior crus (or superior crus) of the lateral canthal tendon; a canthopexy does not involve incising the lateral canthus. A lateral canthopexy raises the Lockwood suspensory ligament and provides support to the lateral canthus and lower eyelid. Exposure with resultant dry eye after lower eyelid surgery is more likely to develop in patients with lid laxity or poor orbicularis muscle tone.

384

In order to treat a hollow appearance of the lower eyelid, some surgeons employ transposition of orbital fat over the orbital rim. Temporary improvement of this problem has also been achieved with an off-label use of dermal fillers. Finally, attempts to effect tightening of residual lower eyelid skin popularized transconjunctival removal of fat combined with ablative laser skin resurfacing, most commonly with the carbon dioxide laser, in the mid-1990s.

Lower blepharoplasty is an evolving technique and the traditional blepharoplasty that includes an incision across the entire lower eyelid with simple fat excision and a lateral canthopexy or canthoplasty may not prevail over time.

Indications include the following:

- Lower blepharoplasty is virtually always considered a cosmetic rather than a functional procedure. Rarely, in downgaze, prolapsed lower eyelid fat or redundant lower lid tissue can obstruct vision or come in contact with eyeglasses to fog vision; in such cases, lower blepharoplasty may improve vision, especially when reading, and be considered functional.
- As with aesthetic upper eyelid surgery, good communication between the surgeon and patient is critical. It is best to ask the patient, with a mirror in hand, to point out the specific problems the patient wishes addressed. Assess the patient's goals and stress the limitations of surgery. Reinforce that undercorrection is preferable to overcorrection that may result in lower eyelid retraction and visual problems due to disruption of the tear film.

PREOPERATIVE STEPS

1. Evaluate the tear film including tear break-up time, Schirmer's testing with topical anesthetic, and level of tear meniscus on slit-lamp examination.
2. Assess other factors that may influence tear film after surgery: the presence of lower eyelid retraction, completeness of blink, the presence of lagophthalmos, intact corneal sensation, and Bell's reflex.
3. Emphasize to the patient that dry eye after lower lid surgery alone is unlikely unless an eyelid malposition such as lower lid retraction or frank ectropion develops.
4. Note the presence of malar hypoplasia that may predispose the patient to postoperative eyelid retraction.
5. Assess lower lid laxity. Orbicularis muscle tone is evaluated by the snap-back test: the surgeon gently pulls the lower lid away from

the globe in order to determine whether the lid resumes its previous normal position or displays ectropion that diminishes after blinking. The lid distraction test provides evidence of lid laxity when the lower lid is grasped and gently distracted 8 mm or more from the globe. In cases of poor orbicularis muscle tone or eyelid laxity, it may be prudent to perform a lower eyelid tightening procedure (such as a lateral tarsal strip [Chapter 70]) in conjunction with lower blepharoplasty to reduce the incidence of postoperative eyelid malposition.

6. Measure and record the amount of inferior scleral shown and the marginal reflex distance-2 (distance from center of pupil to the lower lid margin) in millimeters.

7. Assess the distance from the lower lid margin to the junction of the eyelid-cheek skin interface, since an increased distance may predispose the patient to lid retraction after lower blepharoplasty.

8. Assess the amount of redundant skin and excess fat.

9. Note the following features that may require surgical treatment:
    • Ptosis of the midface region
    • Festoons
    • Nasojugal depression
    • A diamond-shaped depression over the infraorbital foramen

10. Take standardized photographs that include frontal, lateral, and oblique views. Additional frontal views with the patient in up- and down gaze are helpful. The photographs should be taken utilizing the Frankfort horizontal plane (the plane that is parallel to the horizontal, extending from the cephalic edge of the tragus through the infraorbital rim).

SURGICAL PROCEDURES

Isolated Transconjunctival Blepharoplasty

This procedure is performed rarely in young patients with a large amount of anteriorly prolapsed orbital fat but minimal, if any, redundant skin and sagging orbicularis muscle.

1. Make an incision in the conjunctiva 3 mm below the tarsus in the inferior conjunctival cul-de-sac with Westcott scissors or monopolar electrocautery in the cutting mode. A scleral protective lens should be in place. The incision extends medially below the caruncle in order to address the large medial fat pad, and laterally almost to the lateral commissure parallel to the lower tarsal border (Figure 64.1).

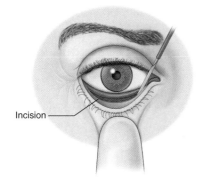

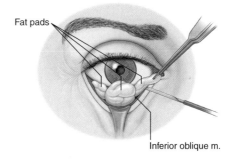

Figure 64.1. A transconjunctival incision is made across the entire lower lid below the tarsus.

Figure 64.2. Lower eyelid fat is excised conservatively down to the level of the orbital rim.

2. Excise fat conservatively from all 3 fat pads (medial, central, and lateral) only to the level of the orbital rim to prevent a hollowed-out appearance of the eyelids (Figure 64.2). Note that the inferior oblique separates the medial fat pad from the central fat pad. Gentle pressure on the globe demonstrates areas of excess fat.

3. A bulge in the central portion of the lower eyelid inferiorly is due to residual fat just anterior to the inferior oblique muscle. This fat pad should be bluntly dissected and excised, taking care to avoid injury to the inferior oblique muscle. A cotton-tipped applicator may be used to mobilize the fat away from the inferior oblique muscle. The muscle should not be incised or cauterized.

4. In order to avoid a hollow appearance to the lower lids, some surgeons do not excise fat. Instead, they employ judicious mobilization of orbital fat anteriorly over the inferior orbital rim and suture the fat to the suborbicularis oculi fat with absorbable sutures or even nonabsorbable sutures that are externalized and tied over cotton bolsters on the skin surface. (This author prefers to tighten the eyelid skin and, therefore diminish the hollow appearance under the eye rather than mobilize fat, as described below.)

5. Close the conjunctival wound with 2 or 3 interrupted 6-0 plain gut sutures to restore eyelid anatomy and possibly to support the globe and prevent pyogenic granuloma on the raw conjunctival edges (Figure 64.3). Some surgeons choose not to close the conjunctiva.

Traditional Lower Blepharoplasty With a Skin-Muscle Flap

This procedure is performed when redundant skin and sagging orbicularis muscle needs to be removed along with prolapsed fat.

Figure 64.3. The conjunctival wound is closed
with 2 interrupted absorbable sutures.

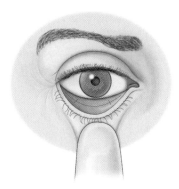

1. If necessary, transconjunctival fat removal is achieved without surgically violating the orbital septum as previously described. A skin
   approach to the orbital fat may induce orbital septal scarring and
   retraction of the lower eyelid postoperatively.
2. Make a subciliary skin incision just below the lash line with a No. 15
   Bard-Parker blade (Figure 64.4). Extend the incision from just below
   the punctum, across the lower eyelid, and beyond the lateral commissure into the lateral canthus for 5 to 8 mm.
3. Mobilize a skin-muscle flap inferiorly to just below the inferior orbital
   rim, with a portion of the malar fat pad attached to the flap. The dissection is accomplished with Stevens scissors (Figure 64.5).
4. As an alternative to the traditional technique, use of carbon dioxide
   laser for dissection facilitates judgment of the appropriate amount of

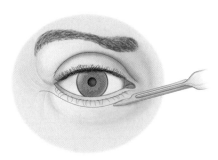

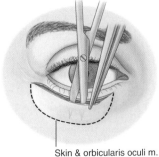

Skin & orbicularis oculi m.
undermined

Figure 64.4. A subciliary incision is made from
the level of the lower punctum extending beyond
the lateral commissure for 5 mm.

Figure 64.5. A skin-muscle flap is mobilized with
Stevens scissors.

redraping of tissues because bleeding and swelling during the procedure are minimized. (The laser as compared to the cold blade probably
does not reduce postoperative edema or ecchymosis.)

5. The lateral portion of the orbicularis oculi muscle may be treated under direct visualization with a defocused carbon dioxide laser (.2 mm)
   in the continuous mode (power setting of 4 to 6 watts) or with very
   light focal cautery using a monopolar Bovie cautery and Colorado
   needle. These modalities serve to tighten the orbicularis oculi muscle
   and overlying eyelid skin.
   - The procedure may be performed through a subciliary incision that
     straddles the lateral canthus 5 to 8 mm medially and lateral to the
     commissure depending on the amount of excess skin.
   - The carbon dioxide laser causes skin-orbicularis oculi muscle tight-
     ening that is observed intraoperatively but also gradually over 6 months
     after surgery.
   - The small-incision technique helps to avoid postoperative lower lid
     ectropion.

6. Treatment of horizontal eyelid laxity is based on preoperative assess-
   ment, and tightening of the orbicularis oculi muscle is performed.
   - If marked horizontal lower eyelid laxity is evident, a lateral tarsal
     strip (Chapter 70) may be performed.
   - If there is mild-to-moderate horizontal lower eyelid laxity, a can-
     thopexy may be performed with a double-armed 6-0 polypropylene
     (Prolene) suture. This suture is secured to the anterior aspect of
     the lateral edge of the tarsus. The two ends of the suture are then
     brought through the lateral ocular retinaculum (at the lateral orbital
     tubercle of Whitnall) to exit in the lateral aspect of the upper bleph-
     aroplasty wound or through a small buttonhole incision in the skin
     (of the lateral aspect of the upper eyelid) if an upper blepharoplasty
     is not performed (Figure 64.6).

Periosteum of lateral orbital rim

Figure 64.6. A lateral canthopexy is performed with a double-armed nonabsorbable suture.

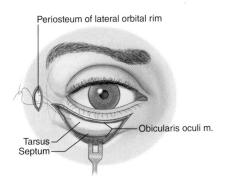

Obicularis oculi m.

Tarsus
Septum

7. The previously undermined flap consisting of skin-orbicularis oculi muscle and the attached malar fat pad complex are now mobilized superiorly by grasping the superior edge of the orbicularis oculi flap.

8. Take a horizontal bite of the orbicularis muscle from the superior edge of the flap with a 5-0 polyglactin (Vicryl) suture. The location of this bite is critical since its placement will properly resuspend the entire flap and smooth the skin surface of the entire lower lid.

9. The skin-muscle flap is suspended by a substantial bite of the periosteum at the appropriate position of the lateral canthus (Figure 64.7). When this suture is properly placed, the skin appears flattened with minimal tension. The positioning of this flap is again confirmed with the patient looking up and mouth opened. The suture is replaced if necessary.

10. Minimal excess skin and residual muscle are excised from the superior edge of the skin-muscle flap when the patient looks up with the mouth open (Figure 64.8).

11. Close the wound with 6-0 plain suture (Figure 64.9). Place Steri-Strips while the patient is recumbent and looks up in order to support the lower lid in a somewhat overcorrected position (Figure 64.10). The Steri-Strips effectively "dam" the fat back into the orbit, tamponade any postoperative edema, and maintain the lower lid and upper cheek in a relatively superior position for 7 to 10 days after surgery. Intravenous corticosteroids the day of surgery and oral corticosteroids (prednisone, 60 mg/day for 3 days after surgery) reduce edema and facial distortion.

12. Postoperative head elevation and liberal use of ice compresses allow the lateral canthus to heal in relatively upward position.

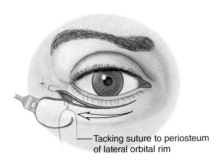

Tacking suture to periosteum of lateral orbital rim

Figure 64.7. The skin-muscle flap is suspended to the periosteum of the inferolateral orbital rim with 5-0 Vicryl.

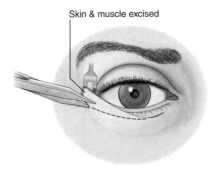

Skin & muscle excised

Figure 64.8. With the patient looking up and with the mouth open, excess skin and muscle are excised.

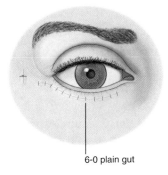

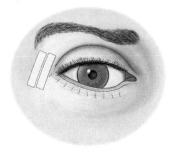

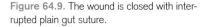
6-0 plain gut

Figure 64.9. The wound is closed with interrupted plain gut suture.

Figure 64.10. The wound is supported with
Steri-Strips in an overcorrected position.

POSTOPERATIVE CARE

1. Advise the patient to apply ice pack compresses to the eyelids every
   15 minutes at 1-hour intervals while awake. This is to be done for
   4 days. For the compress, ice or frozen peas are placed in a plastic bag
   while sterile gauze is situated between the eyelid and ice pack.
2. Head elevation is preferred during sleep for the first week.
3. Topical antibiotics are prescribed for 1 week. Broad-spectrum oral
   antibiotics are generally prescribed for 4-lid blepharoplasty but not
   2-lid surgeries.
4. The sixth day after surgery, hot sterile compresses can be started. Hot
   water that has been boiled first may be used and applied with a sterile
   gauze for 10 to 15 minutes 4 times a day.
5. Patients are instructed to avoid driving for at least 1 week, avoid exercise for 18 days, and avoid makeup to the wounds for 21 days.
6. Patients are requested to contact the surgeon if they note increased
   pain, swelling, mucous discharge, decreased vision, or evidence of
   hemorrhage develops.
7. Patients return for follow-up examination in 1 week and then again
   2 weeks after surgery.

COMPLICATIONS

- Ectropion
- Bilateral or asymmetric hollowing out of lower lids

- Entropion and lower lid retraction
- Residual bags and fat
- Scarring
- Dry eye and conjunctival chemosis
- Double vision

Ectropion due to insufficient horizontal tightening may require revision after conservative treatment, with upward massage of the lower lid for several weeks along with upward taping of the lower lid at bedtime.

Bilateral or asymmetric hollowing-out of lower lids with or without mild lid retraction: this complication is avoided when the surgeon attempts to undercorrect the condition.

Entropion and lower lid retraction may result. This complication is prevented by careful suturing of the conjunctival surfaces after transconjunctival removal of fat.

Residual malar bags and residual lower lid fat may require surgical revision 6 to 12 months after the initial surgery.

Scarring and postoperative wrinkling of thin lower lid skin similarly may require surgical revision.

Dry eye and conjunctival chemosis with minimal or no lid malposition may require topical lubricating drops, Restasis, or punctal plugs.

Double vision due to inferior oblique muscle injury may require prisms or strabismus surgery.

Chapter 65

Lacrimal Surgery:
Three-Snip Punctoplasty

Jed T. Poll, MD
Michael T. Yen, MD

Tearing is a common complaint. Excessive tearing can be frustrating for patients and interfere with optimal vision. Tearing can result from overproduction of tears or from impaired tear drainage. A careful clinician can distinguish between the myriad causes of tearing and choose the appropriate treatment.

Impairment of tear drainage can occur at all levels in the lacrimal system: the punctum, canaliculus, lacrimal sac, and nasolacrimal duct. Three-snip punctoplasty is an effective procedure in addressing epiphora resulting from punctal stenosis.

PREOPERATIVE STEPS

1. Take a history and conduct the ocular exam with attention to the ocular surface and eyelid position. Determine if tearing is due to hypersecretion or impaired drainage of tears. Rule out eyelid malposition.
2. Evaluate the lacrimal system, including punctal probing and irrigation, and the level of the obstruction.

INSTRUMENTATION AND SUPPLIES

- Anesthetic eye drops
- 2% lidocaine with epinephrine

- Small-gauge needle (27 or 30 gauge)
- Betadine swabs
- Punctal dilator
- Toothed forceps
- Sharp Westcott scissors

SURGICAL PROCEDURE

1. Appy 1 drop of topical anesthetic and infiltrate the palpebral conjunctiva near the punctum to be snipped.
2. Prep the site with a Betadine swab.
3. Dilate the punctum with a punctal dilator.
4. Engage the tarsus with toothed forceps.
5. Insert sharp Westcott scissors into the punctum and excise the posterior wall of the punctum as follows:
   - Make a vertical incision on the conjunctival side of the lid through the nasal side of the punctum (Figure 65.1).
   - Make a vertical incision on the conjunctival side of the lid through the temporal side of the punctum (Figure 65.2).
6. Connect the 2 vertical snips at the base with a third horizontal snip (Figure 65.3).
7. Achieve hemostasis with "hot temp" cautery (usually minimal bleeding is encountered with adequate local anesthetic with epinephrine).
8. Apply a prophylactic antibiotic-corticosteroid ointment.

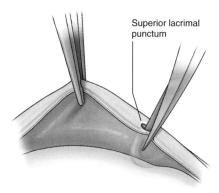

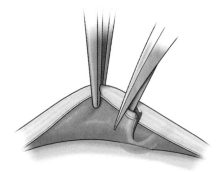

Figure 65.1. A vertical snip is created in the nasal punctum.

Figure 65.2. A second vertical snip is created in the temporal punctum.

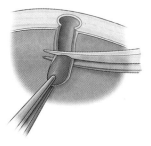

Figure 65.3. A horizontal snip completes the punctoplasty.

COMPLICATIONS

- Failure
- Bleeding
- Dry eye due to excessive tear drainage

Failure may occur secondary to scarring at the surgical site or previously undiagnosed obstruction more distal in the lacrimal system (ie, canaliculus or nasolacrimal duct). A more distal obstruction may require placement of a silicone stent, or additional procedures such as dacryocystorhinostomy (Chapter 67) or Jones tube placement.

Chapter 66

Lacrimal Surgery: Probing and Intubation

Jed T. Poll, MD
Michael T. Yen, MD

Congenital tearing is a common problem encountered in children. As with adults, a careful examination will often reveal the cause for the tearing. While congenital nasolacrimal duct obstruction (NLDO) predominates as a cause of pediatric tearing, the clinician must evaluate each patient for other potential causes such as lid malposition, trichiasis, ocular surface abnormalities, or congenital glaucoma.

Managed conservatively, congenital NLDO resolves without intervention in the vast majority of children within the first year of life. Patients with persistent NLDO after age 1, or beyond 4 months associated with frequent dacryocystitis, should undergo lacrimal probing. Simple probing is often curative; however, bicanalicular or monocanalicular silicone stents are frequently placed at the time of probing.

PREOPERATIVE STEPS

1. Perform a careful ocular examination with attention to the lacrimal system.
2. Check for patency of the puncta; attempt to express contents of the lacrimal sac using digital massage.

INSTRUMENTATION AND SUPPLIES

- Lacrimal dilator and probes (eg, Bowman probes)
- Silicone tubes
- Grooved director
- Nasal speculum
- 4-0 polyglactin (Vicryl) suture

SURGICAL PROCEDURE

1. General anesthesia is preferred.
2. Use a lacrimal probe to probe the superior punctum as follows:
   - Pass the probe vertically into the punctum for 2 mm (Figure 66.1).
   - With lateral tension on the eyelid, advance the probe horizontally toward the nose until reaching a bony stop, about 8 to 10 mm from the punctum (Figure 66.2).
   - Redirecting the exposed portion of the probe superiorly above the patient's brow (while maintaining the contact between the probe

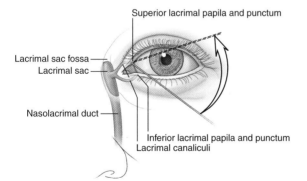

Superior lacrimal papila and punctum

Lacrimal sac fossa

Lacrimal sac

Nasolacrimal duct

Inferior lacrimal papilla and punctum
Lacrimal canaliculi

Figure 66.1. The superior punctum and the canaliculus are probed.

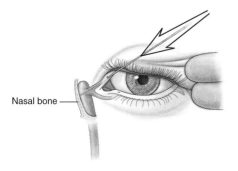

Nasal bone

Figure 66.2. The probe is advanced into the lacrimal sac to a hard, bony stop.

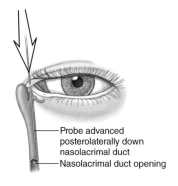

Probe advanced
posterolaterally down
nasolacrimal duct
Nasolacrimal duct opening

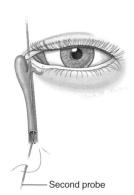

Second probe

Figure 66.3. The probe is reoriented vertically, down the nasolacrimal duct.

Figure 66.4. Probe placement is confirmed with metal-on-metal contact.

and the lacrimal bone), advance the probe inferiorly and slightly posterolaterally down the nasolacrimal duct (20 mm). At the end of the duct, a small "pop" may be felt if a stenosis or membrane is passed (Figure 66.3).

3. Check the position of the probe; the correct position is most easily ascertained by inserting another lacrimal probe into the nasal cavity under the inferior turbinate to elicit metal-on-metal contact (Figure 66.4). Alternatively, one can check placement of the probe with direct visualization using a headlight and nasal speculum.

4. Repeat probing through the inferior punctum.

5. Intubate the superior and inferior canaliculus with silicone tubes (stents). The same series of steps as described above is performed, but using the metal rods attached to lacrimal tubes instead of lacrimal probes (eg, Crawford lacrimal stents). The metal rods can be extracted from the nasal cavity with the aid of a grooved director, and when both metal ends of the stent are extracted, the metal rods are removed from the tubes and the 2 ends of the tubing tied with 1 tight square knot (ie, 2 throws).

6. Secure the knot to the nasal ala inside the nose with 4-0 polyglactin suture to prevent tube prolapse.

POSTOPERATIVE CARE

1. Leave the tubes in for 3 to 6 months before removal. Typically by this time the polyglactin suture would have dissolved, allowing for instrument-free removal of the tubes if they were not tied.
2. If the tubes were tied, either the palpebral or the nasal side may be cut for removal through the nose or out the canaliculus, respectively.

COMPLICATIONS

- Failure
- False passage
- Bleeding

Probing with intubation is successful in greater than 90% of cases of congenital nasolacrimal duct obstruction. The failure rate can be reduced by inferior turbinate medialization, or infracturing, to enlarge the inferior meatus; by prolonged silicone intubation; or by balloon dacryoplasty (generally reserved for difficult cases and prior probing failures).

False passage can be incurred during probing; care must be taken during probing to avoid making a false passage when resistance is encountered.

Bleeding can be minimized by preoperative packing of the nose with nasal decongestant.

Chapter 67

Lacrimal Surgery: External Dacryocystorhinostomy

Jed T. Poll, MD
Michael T. Yen, MD

Nasolacrimal duct obstruction (NLDO) is a common cause of epiphora in the pediatric and adult populations. In children, NLDO is usually secondary to membranous occlusion distally at the valve of Hasner. Spontaneous resolution by age 1 is common. Generally, persistent cases are treated successfully with probing and silicone tube intubation.

Conversely, NLDO in the adult population usually occurs as a result of involutional stenosis of the interosseus nasolacrimal duct; however, it may also result from recurrent dacryocystitis, chronic sinusitis, or granulomatous diseases. Standard probing and intubation procedures are frequently ineffective in providing adequate tear drainage in adult patients. External dacryocystorhinostomy (DCR) creates a new opening from the lacrimal sac through the nasal bone into the nasal cavity, thus bypassing the NLDO.

PREOPERATIVE STEPS

1. Carefully examine the lacrimal system, including probing and irrigation, to identify the site of the obstruction.
2. Identify and treat predisposing conditions if present; if NLDO is complicated by acute to dacryocystitis, DCR should be delayed until acute infection resolves.

INSTRUMENTATION AND SUPPLIES

- Local anesthetic: 2% lidocaine with 1:100,000 epinephrine, nasal decongestant, or cocaine for nasal packing
- Nasal speculum
- Halogen head lamp
- Cotton pledgets
- No. 11 and No. 15 Bard-Parker blades
- Westcott scissors
- Freer periosteal elevator
- Lacrimal probes
- Mosquito clamp
- Needle holder
- Small rake retractors
- Bone rongeurs
- Silicone tubes
- 4-0 polyglactin (Vicryl) suture
- 6-0 silk suture
- Tissue adhesive or absorbable suture (plain gut) for skin closure

SURGICAL PROCEDURE

1. The procedure is usually performed with local infiltrative anesthesia and intranasal packing, though general anesthesia may be preferred in select patients. Infiltrate the area inferonasal to the medial canthal tendon and pack the nose with pledgets soaked with anesthetic (cocaine or other nasal anesthetic). This also promotes hemostasis of the nasal mucosa.
2. Use the No. 15 blade scalpel for incision medial to the medial canthal angle, starting at the level of the medial canthal tendon and extending inferiorly and laterally for approximately 1 to 1.5 cm (Figure 67.1).
3. Dissect bluntly down to the anterior lacrimal crest. Utilize rake retractors to enhance visualization; be sure to identify the angular artery.
4. Expose the nasal bone and anterior lacrimal crest with a Freer elevator, and reflect the lacrimal sac out of the lacrimal sac fossa.
5. Create a bony osteotomy in the lacrimal bone using a small, curved mosquito clamp.
6. Enlarge the osteotomy with Kerrison bone rongeurs; the osteotomy must be of adequate size and in the proper position. Extend the

Figure 67.1. The skin incision for external dacryocystorhinostomy is made up to the level of the medial canthal tendon.

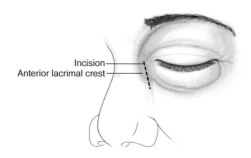

Incision
Anterior lacrimal crest

osteotomy superiorly to the level of the sac fundus, anteriorly to include the anterior lacrimal crest and a portion of the nasal bone, and inferiorly to include the superior few millimeters of the bony nasolacrimal duct.

7. Check the position of the osteotomy by intubating the inferior punctum with the lacrimal probe and tenting the lacrimal sac to ensure the osteotomy is adjacent to the nasolacrimal sac (Figure 67.2).

8. Incise the lacrimal sac with an H-shaped incision using a No. 11 blade, creating anterior and posterior lacrimal sac mucosal flaps. Take care to ensure that the entire lacrimal sac is opened superiorly to inferiorly. The posterior flap may be excised.

9. Inject the nasal mucosa using 2% lidocaine with 1:100,000 epinephrine, through the bony osteotomy, to enhance hemostasis.

10. Create a flap of the nasal mucosa using a No. 11 blade. A rectangular U-shaped incision will create a large anteriorly based nasal mucosal flap.

11. Remove nasal packing from the nose.

12. Intubate the inferior and superior puncta using silicone tubing (Figure 67.3), withdrawing the metal ends of the stents from the nose with the aid of a grooved director.

13. Tie a silk suture around the tubes approximately 3 mm from the internal common punctum, near the bony osteotomy site; this suture

Figure 67.2. The osteotomy is created adjacent to the lacrimal sac; incisions in the lacrimal sac and the nasal mucosa create flaps for the anastomosis.

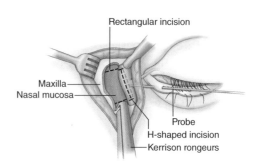

Rectangular incision

Maxilla
Nasal mucosa

Probe
H-shaped incision
Kerrison rongeurs

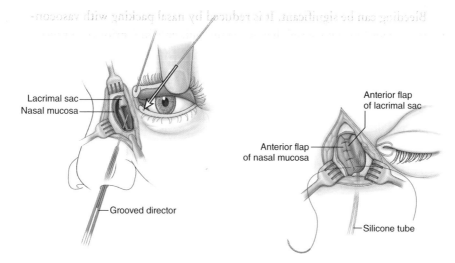

Figure 67.3. Intubation is performed with bicanalicular stents.

Figure 67.4. The anterior nasal and lacrimal sac flaps are sutured.

will keep the tubes together, preventing prolapse from the palpebral aperture.

14. Suture the anterior flap of the lacrimal sac to the anterior flap of the nasal mucosa using 4-0 polyglactin (Figure 67.4).
15. Tie and cut silicone tubes at the end of the naris and allow tubes to retract slightly inside the nose.
16. Approximate subcuticular soft tissues with 5-0 polyglactin suture.
17. Close the skin with absorbable suture (such as 6-0 plain gut) or tissue adhesive. Steri-Strips may be applied over the wound.
18. Apply an antibiotic-corticosteroid ointment.

POSTOPERATIVE CARE

1. Wait at least 3 months before removing silicone tubes.

COMPLICATIONS

- Bleeding
- Failure
- Infection

Bleeding can be significant. It is reduced by nasal packing with vasoconstricting agent (cocaine, nasal decongestant, epinephrine) prior to surgery; avoiding the angular artery with careful dissection; and intranasal packing intraoperatively or postoperatively if necessary.

Failure commonly occurs secondary to fibrosis at the osteotomy site or poor osteotomy location and size. Repeat DCR has a lower success rate. Failure may also be due to so-called "sump syndrome." In this condition, the failure to completely fillet open the lacrimal sac may lead to a small remnant of sac remaining inferiorly that collects tears and becomes infected. This complication may be prevented by opening the entire sac vertically from the sac fundus down to the bony entrance of the nasolacrimal duct.

The failure rate can be reduced by intranasal corticosteroids to reduce postoperative inflammation and scarring; intraoperative silicone intubation; appropriate osteotomy size and location; and adequate treatment of pre-existing dacryocystitis. Also consider using antimetabolites (mitomycin C) topically for re-operations to reduce scarring at the ostomy site.

Postoperative infections are uncommon and typically respond well to oral antibiotics.

Chapter 68

Temporal Artery Biopsy

M. Reza Vagefi, MD
John D. McCann, MD, PhD

Giant cell arteritis (GCA) is a medium- to large-sized vessel granulomatous vasculopathy that typically occurs in adults over 50 years of age. Symptoms may include the following:

- Ocular symptoms: decreased vision, transient or sustained loss of vision, or diplopia
- Other systemic complaints: headache, scalp or temple tenderness, pain with mastication, neck pain, fever, malaise, loss of appetite, weight loss, night sweats, or fatigue
- Ophthalmic findings: anterior ischemic optic neuropathy, central retinal artery occlusion, or palsies involving cranial nerves III, IV, or VI.
- Systemic findings: polymyalgia rheumatica, anemia, temporal artery tenderness, or stroke

   Clinical suspicion of GCA merits laboratory testing of acute phase reactants including platelets, erythrocyte sedimentation rate, and C-reactive protein levels for elevated levels. Fundus fluorescein angiography (FA) may demonstrate patchy or generalized filling defects affecting the choroid. Superficial temporal artery biopsy can provide the definitive diagnosis. If clinical suspicion is high, corticosteroid treatment should be commenced immediately to prevent vision loss, contralateral eye involvement, and other sequelae. Temporal artery biopsy must be performed within 10 days of beginning corticosteroid therapy.

PREOPERATIVE STEPS

1. A careful history as well as physical and ophthalmic examination can aid in ascertaining the diagnostic likelihood of GCA. Laboratory evaluation and FA can help raise or decrease clinical suspicion.
2. Duplex ultrasound or positron emission tomography may have a role in the diagnosis of GCA.
3. Steroid treatment should be begun if clinical suspicion is high.
4. Ideally, the patient should have discontinued anticoagulants, if clinically appropriate, for the proper amount of time prior to biopsy. This is often not possible given the urgent nature of the biopsy.

INSTRUMENTATION AND SUPPLIES

- Surgical marking pen
- Razor blade
- 2% lidocaine with epinephrine 1:100,000
- 1.5-inch, 27-gauge needle
- Povidone-iodine swabs
- Bipolar or monopolar cautery
- No. 15 blade
- Scalpel handle
- Stevens tenotomy scissors or Wescott scissors
- Paufique forceps
- Castroviejo needle driver
- Lacrimal rakes or skin hooks
- 4-0 silk ties
- 4-0 chromic suture
- Specimen cup with formaldehyde

SURGICAL PROCEDURE

1. Palpate the superficial temporal artery as it courses from anterior to the tragus over the temporalis muscle and onto the forehead (Figure 68.1). Ultrasound may assist in identifying the course of the vessel if the artery is small.
2. Mark the course of the vessel with a surgical marking pen.
3. The hair over the temporal area may be shaved or braided.

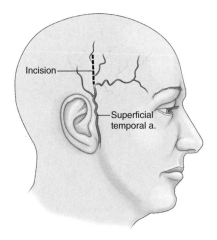

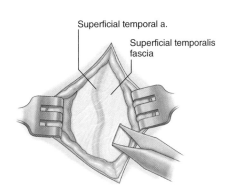

Figure 68.1. The superficial temporal artery can be palpated over the temporalis muscle.

Figure 68.2. The superficial temporal artery courses through the superficial temporal fascia.

4. Inject local anesthetic. Take care to not puncture the temporal artery or to administer too much anesthetic as the epinephrine can cause constriction of the artery, making its identification more difficult.

5. Prep the area with povidone-iodine swabs and drape appropriately.

6. Use the No. 15 blade scalpel to make a skin incision over the temporal area 4 cm in length.

7. Achieve hemostasis with cautery.

8. An assistant aids with retraction by placing the lacrimal rakes or skin hooks to part the incision site.

9. Perform blunt dissection with scissors and forceps to identify the superficial temporal artery that courses on the same plane as the superficial temporalis fascia (Figure 68.2). Take care to not proceed too anteriorly as the risk for facial nerve damage increases.

10. Isolate a 3-cm length of artery.

11. Pass 4-0 silk ties beneath the proximal and distal ends of the artery and tie tight with surgeon's knots using the needle driver (Figure 68.3). Two sets of suture ties may be placed to ensure that it is adequately tied off.

12. Use scissors to cut the artery, then cauterize the cut ends (Figure 68.4).

13. Note the measurement of the specimen and place the biopsy in the specimen cup.

14. Close the skin using 4-0 chromic suture. Some surgeons prefer separate closure of the deep tissues with 5-0 polyglactin sutures and skin closure with 6-0 plain gut.

15. Dress the wound with antibiotic ointment and a head dressing.

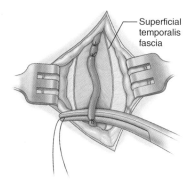

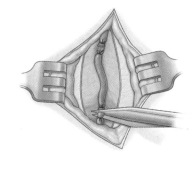

Figure 68.3. Silk ties are passed beneath the artery.

Figure 68.4. The artery is tied, then cut.

COMPLICATIONS

- Bleeding
- Temporal hematoma
- Wound infection
- Facial nerve trauma
- Scalp necrosis
- False negatives

Bleeding from the superficial temporal artery or its branches may occur during the procedure. Care must be taken to assure adequate hemostasis and tying of sutures around the artery.

A temporal hematoma may occur after closure, especially with postoperative blood pressure elevation. A hematoma may require drainage and re-exploration with cautery of the bleeding vessel. Take care during the procedure to assure adequate hemostasis. Once the procedure is complete, a head dressing may be used, and the patient should be placed in an upright position.

Wound infection may occur, requiring oral antibiotics.

Facial nerve trauma may occur with vigorous or misdirected dissection, resulting in prolonged or permanent facial paralysis of the temporal or zygomatic branches of the facial nerve.

Scalp necrosis may occur from inadequate collateral circulation.

A false negative result may occur from an inadequate specimen due to "skip lesions." A negative result, therefore, does not exclude the diagnosis of GCA. A biopsy of the contralateral side may be considered; some surgeons recommend routinely performing bilateral surgery to reduce the incidence of a "false-negative" biopsy.

Chapter 69

Orbital Decompression Surgery

M. Reza Vagefi, MD
John D. McCann, MD, PhD

Graves orbitopathy, also known as thyroid-related ophthalmopathy (TRO), is an autoimmune disorder in which antibodies created against the thyroid gland are believed to activate fibroblasts and myoblasts in the soft tissues of the orbit. Activation of these cell types leads to expansion of orbital fat and the extraocular muscles. Disease can occur in any thyroid state but is most common with hyperthyroidism. Ocular symptoms include eye irritation, dry eye, redness, double vision, decreased color vision, or decreased visual acuity. Ophthalmic evaluation may reveal eyelid retraction, conjunctival injection, chemosis, lagophthalmos, keratopathy, restrictive myopathy, proptosis, elevated intraocular pressure (IOP), choroidal folds, or compressive optic neuropathy. In adults, TRO is the most common cause of unilateral or bilateral proptosis and the most common cause of diplopia.

Two types of disease presentation may be noted. Type 1 TRO demonstrates expansion of orbital fat with little muscle involvement. Type 2 TRO demonstrates enlargement of the extraocular muscles with possible crowding of the apex and compression of the optic nerve. Orbital decompression is considered once TRO is stable and proptosis results in significant anterior segment pathology that cannot be clinically controlled or because of an unacceptable aesthetic appearance. Decompression is considered acutely when active disease results in significant proptosis and eyelid retraction with corneal compromise or in compressive optic neuropathy with acute vision loss.

PREOPERATIVE STEPS

1. A careful history as well as physical and ophthalmic examination can aid in ascertaining TRO severity and activity. Laboratory evaluation of thyroid-stimulating hormone, free T4, and thyroid-related immunoglobulins should be performed. Evaluation includes clinical assessment of eyelid position, the anterior segment, ocular motility, proptosis with Hertel exophthalmometry, IOP, and optic nerve including ophthalmoscopy, pupil, color vision, and visual field testing.
2. Obtain orbital imaging, usually in the form of computed tomography, to assess muscle size, fat expansion, optic nerve compression, and orbital anatomy for planning of decompression.
3. If compressive optic neuropathy is found, oral or intravenous corticosteroid treatment can be begun immediately to preserve nerve function and quiet the disease process until decompression can be performed.
4. Ideally, the patient should have discontinued anticoagulants for the appropriate amount of time prior to decompression. Stopping anticoagulants may not be possible if decompression is being urgently performed for corneal decompensation or optic neuropathy.

INSTRUMENTATION AND SUPPLIES

- Surgical marking pen
- 2% lidocaine hydrochloride with epinephrine 1:100,000
- 1.5-inch, 27-gauge needle
- Betadine prep
- Bipolar or monopolar cautery
- No. 15 blade
- Scalpel handle
- Stevens tenotomy scissors
- Paufique forceps
- Tenzel elevator, Freer elevator, and chisel
- Frazier suction tip
- 3.5 mm coarse diamond burr drill bit
- High-speed (>40,000 RPM) neurosurgical drill
- Desmarres and malleable retractors
- Glasgow forceps, Takahashi forceps, and Kerrison rongeurs
- Castroviejo needle driver

- 4-0 polyglactin (Vicryl) suture
- 6-0 plain gut suture

SURGICAL PROCEDURES

Decompression surgery can be approached in several ways (Figure 69.1). The best techniques must take into consideration the patient's clinical presentation, the risk of inducing postoperative diplopia, and the surgeon's experience. For compressive optic neuropathy in Type 2 TRO, the apex can best be relieved from a medial wall approach. In patients with disfiguring proptosis but relatively normal extraocular movements, a lateral approach is often taken, as this is associated with a low incidence of postoperative diplopia. Most would agree that patients with Type 1 TRO benefit from fat removal.

Medial Wall Decompression

1. General anesthesia is used. Local anesthesia with epinephrine is injected in the medial upper and lower eyelids and caruncular area to assist with hemostasis.
2. Prep and drape the patient in a sterile manner.
3. Make a conjunctival incision at the junction of the caruncle and semilunar fold (Figure 69.2).
4. Extend the conjunctival incision into the medial portion of the superior and inferior fornix.
5. With Stevens scissors, dissect down to the level of the periorbita of the posterior lacrimal crest and incise the periorbita (Figure 69.3). Extend

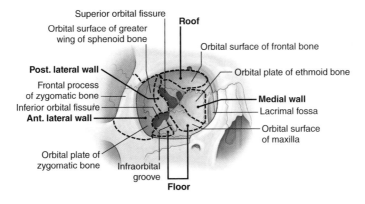

Figure 69.1. Various portions of the bony orbit can be removed [dotted lines] to achieve decompression.

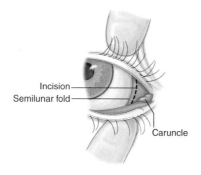

Figure 69.2. A conjunctival incision is made at the junction of the caruncle and semilunar fold.

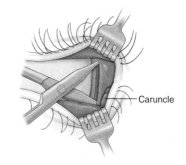

Figure 69.3. Dissection is carried down to the posterior lacrimal crest.

the periosteal incision from the medial orbital roof to the medial orbital floor, then lift the periosteum off the bone using a Freer elevator.

6. Carry out dissection posteriorly to identify the anterior and posterior ethmoidal arteries, which are cauterized and cut. Take care when cauterizing the posterior ethmoid artery, as it is approximately 6 mm from the optic nerve.

7. Further expose the medial wall and floor with elevators, using a malleable retractor to hold the tissues laterally.

8. Enter the medial wall posterior to the lacrimal crest and remove it in piecemeal fashion using the Takahashi front-biting forceps and Frazier suction tip (Figure 69.4). Proceed with bone removal almost to the medial optic strut, exposing the posterior ethmoid air cells. Take care not to proceed superior to the ethmoidal suture and breach the fovea

Figure 69.4. Takahashi front-biting forceps are used to remove the ethmoid air cells.

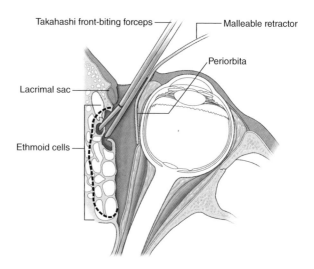

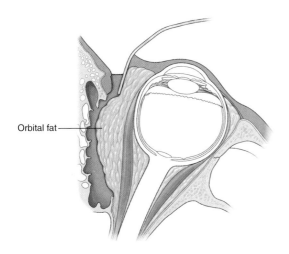

Figure 69.5. After the periosteum is cut, orbital fat herniates into the decompressed ethmoid sinus.

Orbital fat

ethmoidalis and cribriform plate. Direct forces inferiorly or toward the orbit to avoid entering the anterior cranial fossa.

9. In some cases, it may be desirable to remove the posterior third of the strut separating the ethmoid and maxillary sinus. This maneuver is accomplished with Kerrison rongeurs.

10. Incision of the periorbita can then be performed to release orbital fat (Figure 69.5). Exposed orbital fat may be excised to provide further decompression or allowed to herniate into the ethmoid sinus.

11. Perform closure with a single 6-0 plain gut suture reapproximating the conjunctiva to the caruncle.

Lateral Wall Decompression

1. General anesthesia is used. Local anesthesia with epinephrine is injected into the lateral portion of the upper eyelid to assist with hemostasis.

2. Prep and drape the patient in a sterile manner.

3. Make a lateral upper eyelid skin incision using a No. 15 blade scalpel (Figure 69.6).

4. Using Stevens scissors and Paufique forceps, dissect down to the level of the frontozygomatic process (Figure 69.7). Use a Desmarres retractor to lift the eyelid superolaterally.

5. Incise the periosteum 3 to 4 mm posterior to the lateral orbital margin with a scalpel, cutting cautery, or cutting elevator (Figure 69.8). The periosteal incision should be parallel to the orbital rim and extend from the lateral canthal tendon to the superior lateral rim. The periosteum is then lifted to the arcus marginalis.

Figure 69.6. An extended upper eyelid skin crease incision is created.

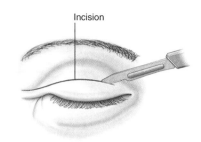

Incision

Figure 69.7. Dissection is carried down to the frontozygomatic process.

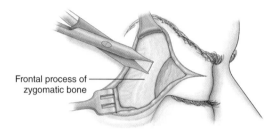

Frontal process of zygomatic bone

Figure 69.8. The periosteum of the lateral orbital rim is incised.

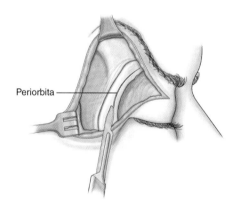

Periorbita

6. Release the arcus marginalis and carry dissection into the orbit. Identify and cauterize the zygomaticotemporal and zygomaticofacial vessels and nerves, using malleable retractors to assist with visualization.
7. Carry out dissection until the superior and inferior orbital fissures are reached, exposing the greater sphenoid wall in its entirety. For adequate exposure inferiorly, it is imperative that all the soft tissues be released over Whitnall's tubercle.
8. Begin decompression by drilling along the anterior orbital rim over the lacrimal fossa to create a keyhole for visualization of the deep orbit.
9. Drilling of the greater sphenoid wall is commenced just inferior and anterior to the superior orbital fissure and is carried to the inner table of bone (Figure 69.9). Take care to not breach dura. Continue drilling

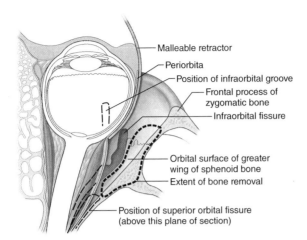

Figure 69.9. Dotted lines indicate the portion of the lateral wall that is drilled out.

Malleable retractor
Periorbita
Position of infraorbital groove
Frontal process of zygomatic bone
Infraorbital fissure
Orbital surface of greater wing of sphenoid bone
Extent of bone removal
Position of superior orbital fissure (above this plane of section)

between the superior and inferior orbital fissure until the posterior two-thirds of the greater sphenoid has been shaved down. Irrigation is used to cool the drill bit.

10. Open the periorbita in the inferotemporal quadrant axially between the lateral and inferior rectus muscles, using tenotomy scissors. Take care to retract the lateral rectus muscle away from the incision site using Desmarres and malleable retractors.

11. Exposed fat can be excised or allowed to sit in the decompressed area of the greater sphenoid wall.

12. Reapproximate the periosteum at the superolateral orbital rim with interrupted 4-0 polyglactin suture.

13. Close the skin using 6-0 plain gut suture.

COMPLICATIONS

- Bleeding
- Muscle cut
- Infraorbital nerve dysfunction
- Burn
- CSF leakage
- Bulbar chemosis, eyelid edema
- Wound dehiscence
- Diplopia
- Inferomedial dislocation of the globe
- Hemorrhage or swelling
- Reactivation of TRO
- Residual proptosis

Bleeding from the ethmoidal or zygomatic arteries may occur during the procedure if they are not properly identified and cauterized. Care must be taken as excessive cautery deep in the apex can result in thermal injury to the optic nerve.

The adjacent extraocular muscle may be cut when the periorbita is opened if care is not taken to appropriately retract it and may require repair.

Infraorbital nerve dysfunction may occur after removal of the inferomedial wall. Sensation typically recovers in 6 to 8 months.

The drill may burn the skin if attention is not taken of its direction, causing the drill shaft to make contact with the skin incision.

A CSF leak may be encountered if the dura is breached with drilling during lateral wall decompression, or if the fovea ethmoidalis is penetrated during medial wall decompression. These may self-seal or require patching. Subarachnoid hemorrhage and stroke can happen if vessels are disrupted or brain tissue is removed.

Bulbar chemosis and eyelid edema may persist after decompression, possibly related to the chronic inflammatory state in TRO. They may resolve with a short course of oral or topical corticosteroids.

Wound dehiscence may occur because of severe edema and will require repair once the orbital congestion has resolved. Also, wound infection may occur, requiring oral antibiotics and debridement.

Diplopia is a common complaint following decompression surgery. Double vision resulting from edema and contusion of the extraocular muscles will resolve as orbital congestion clears. Diplopia that persists can be a result of entrapment of extraocular muscles from excessive prolapse of orbital tissue and may require orbital reconstruction. TRO patients often need strabismus surgery for ocular misalignment.

Inferomedial dislocation of the globe may occur with too aggressive a decompression requiring orbital reconstruction. Preservation of the anterior strut between the medial wall and floor can prevent this complication.

Retrobulbar hemorrhage or severe orbital swelling can lead to further compressive optic neuropathy, requiring intravenous corticosteroids and possible further emergent surgery for evacuation of blood or decompression.

Reactivation of TRO is possible and necessitates prompt treatment with corticosteroids or other immune suppressants.

The patient may continue to have residual proptosis once recuperation from surgery is complete. This may reflect inadequate decompression or reactivation of TRO. Follow-up imaging should be obtained and repeat decompression can be considered.

Chapter 70

Lateral Canthoplasty (Lateral Tarsal Strip)

Paul D. Langer, MD, FACS

The lateral tarsal strip (also commonly called "the tarsal strip") is one of the most frequently performed procedures in all of ophthalmic plastic surgery. The lateral tarsal strip tightens the inferior crus of the lateral canthal tendon, thereby decreasing the horizontal laxity of the lower eyelid. It is often performed in isolation to raise a lower eyelid that is retracted due to laxity, but it is also commonly performed in conjunction with lower lid retractor plication surgery to treat involutional entropion or ectropion, or in addition to lower eyelid skin grafting to treat cicatricial lower eyelid retraction. Tarsal strips are also employed to "reattach" the lower eyelid at the conclusion of an orbital procedure in which a canthotomy and cantholysis have been performed to gain access to the inferior orbital space.

INSTRUMENTATION AND SUPPLIES

- Sharp iris scissors
- Castroviejo 0.5 forceps
- Locking Castroviejo needle holder
- 5-0 polyglactin (Vicryl) suture with P-2 needle
- 6-0 plain gut suture
- Monopolar or bipolar cautery

SURGICAL PROCEDURE

1. Infiltrate the lateral canthus using 1% lidocaine with epinephrine 1:100,000. The depth of the injection should begin just beneath the skin but ultimately extend down to the bony lateral orbital rim.
2. Perform a lateral canthotomy with iris scissors.
   - The 2 blades of the scissors are placed to "straddle" the lateral commissure, with a blade anterior to the skin and a blade in the lateral fornix, and the lateral canthus is then split by the scissors.
   - Take care to ensure that the angle of the scissors follows an imaginary line through the medial and lateral canthi, so that the canthotomy incision is not created in a downward or upward slant (Figure 70.1).
3. Sever the inferior crus of the lateral canthal tendon with the iris scissors (ie, perform an inferior "cantholysis"). The inferior crus can be palpated or "strummed" with the blades of the scissors as a band that attaches the most lateral portion of the inferior tarsus to the lateral orbital rim. When cutting the inferior crus, the blades of the scissors should be directed inferiorly, perpendicular to the original canthotomy incision (Figure 70.2). After the cantholysis is performed, the lower eyelid will no longer be attached laterally to the orbital rim.
4. Obtain hemostasis with cautery.
5. With the iris scissors, divide the lateral, exposed portion of the lower eyelid at the level of the gray line to separate the anterior and posterior lamellae for approximately 5 mm (Figure 70.3).
6. Obtain hemostasis with cautery.
7. Remove the strip of epithelium from the superior surface of the separated posterior lamella with the iris scissors (Figure 70.4). Then make a 3- to 4-mm incision into the conjunctiva with the iris scissors,

Figure 70.1. A lateral canthotomy is performed.

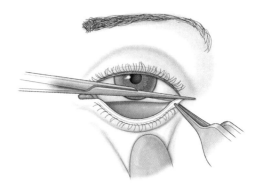

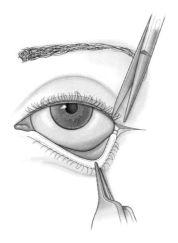

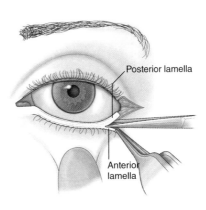

Figure 70.2. An inferior cantholysis is created by directing the scissors perpendicular to the original incision.

Figure 70.3. The gray line is incised with scissors to separate the anterior and posterior lamellae.

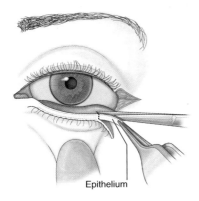

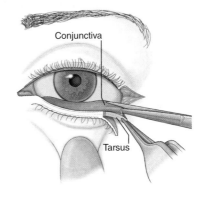

Figure 70.4. The surface epithelium is removed from the posterior lamella.

Figure 70.5. A conjunctival incision is created to create a de-epithelialized tarsal strip.

parallel to the lid margin, just beneath the tarsus (Figure 70.5). These maneuvers create a de-epithelialized strip of tarsus.

8. Reattach the tarsal strip to the periosteum of the lateral orbital rim with a horizontal mattress 4-0 polyglactin suture on a P-2 (half-circle) needle (Figure 70.6). The horizontal mattress suture will promote a posterior vector to the lateral part of the lower eyelid so that it follows the curvature of the globe; the half circle P-2 needle is extremely useful to place the suture in the tight confines of the lateral canthus. If the surgery is performed under local anesthesia, the patient can be sat

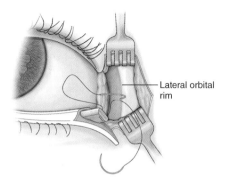

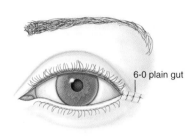

Figure 70.6. The tarsal strip is attached to the periosteum of the lateral orbital rim with a horizontal mattress suture.

Figure 70.7. The wound is closed, taking care to reform a sharp lateral canthal angle.

upright to check the position of the lateral canthus, to ensure that the lower eyelid has not been reattached too high or too low.

9. In cases where the lower eyelid is extremely lax, the tarsal strip itself can be shortened with a scissors to increase the tightening effect of the procedure.

10. Close the skin with 6-0 plain gut suture, taking care to re-create a sharp lateral canthal angle (Figure 70.7).

COMPLICATIONS

- Wound dehiscence
- Lower eyelid retraction
- Lateral canthal dystopia

Wound dehiscence usually occurs when the tarsal strip has excessively tightened the lower eyelid. Surgical reapproximation is usually necessary.

If the tarsal strip has not adequately tightened the lower eyelid, especially in cases where there is significant laxity preoperatively, the lower lid may continue to droop postoperatively. Further shortening of the tarsal strip may be required.

If the tarsal strip is placed too high or too low on the lateral orbital rim, clinically significant canthal dystopia may result. If severe, the tarsal strip may need to be taken down and the polyglactin suture attaching the tarsal strip to the orbital rim may need to be replaced at a more appropriate level.

Chapter 71

Anterior Orbitotomy

Roger E. Turbin, MD, FACS

The technical approach to orbital surgery is guided by the location of the lesion, the expected lesion type (based on the tissue involved and radiographic characteristics), and the goal of surgery (incisional biopsy versus complete lesion removal).

In general, the anterior orbitotomy is most useful for obtaining surgical access to lesions within the anterior half of the orbit, and is used to obtain access to intraconal, extraconal, or extraperiosteal lesions. Although typically performed using general anesthesia, it is performed in some centers using local or regional blocks as an alternative. The combination of multiple approaches is a common practice. For example, a transcaruncular approach may be combined with an inferior transconjunctival incision, with or without a canthotomy and cantholysis to improve exposure, and a lateral orbitotomy with bone removal may be combined with a medial orbitotomy to provide more space within the orbit in which to dissect a medial or intraconal lesion.

Incisional procedures are used to obtain a representative biopsy (inflammatory, lymphoproliferative, diffuse infiltrative, or in preparation for a more radical procedure) whereas excisional procedures seek gross total excision (such as for a lacrimal pleomorphic adenoma—Chapter 72).

General principles are similar for most transconjunctival approaches (eg, inferior, transcaruncular, and medial incisions) and for transeptal approaches (eg, sub-brow, upper eyelid crease, superior-medial, subciliary, and lower eyelid crease incisions). A surgical assistant is useful and often necessary in many of the approaches to the orbit.

PREOPERATIVE STEPS

1. Localize the expected lesion site by analyzing the vector of displacement of the globe and palpation of periorbital and septal abnormalities. Additional information about a lesion can be gained from deeper palpation after the patient is anesthetized.

2. Order appropriate imaging studies and review with radiologists and collaborating surgical services. Consider orbital, sinus, or brain CT and MRI studies (with contrast as necessary), and occasionally angiographic studies. Some centers utilize intraoperative navigational radiographic techniques, although these techniques are most useful for deeper procedures with complex sino-orbito-cranial disease, as well as bone-removing decompression.

3. Design the surgical approach, balancing cosmetic expectations of the patient with the risk of damaging or seeding tumor in adjacent tissues. Malignant lesions, for example, should be approached with an incision that most directly reaches the abnormality via the surface projection of the lesion in order to minimize tumor seeding.

4. Obtain preoperative informed consent, which in orbital surgery should routinely include a discussion of the risk of orbital hemorrhage, double vision, periorbital numbness, dry eye, eyelid malposition, pupil and accommodative damage, and ipsilateral blindness. Other potential complications are specific to the surgical approach and listed below.

5. If cessation of antithrombotic agents for systemic disease is necessary, this should be carried out under the guidance of a general medical doctor or an internist. A discussion of the risk and benefit ratio for cessation of anticoagulation is necessary in selected cases.

INSTRUMENTATION AND SUPPLIES

- Headlight, surgical loupes, operating microscope with longer focal length (greater than 220 mm provides clearance between surgical field and scope for orbital instruments)
- Forceps: 0.3 mm and 0.5 mm Castroviejo, Bishop-Harmon, fine-toothed Adson
- Retractors: Senn double-ended, malleable, orbital Sewell, Desmarres eyelid retractors, small rakes, single- and double-pronged skin hooks, self-retaining retractors

- Scissors: assorted (blunt, sharp, straight, curved) Stevens, Westcott, Iris, and Metzenbaum
- Clamps: mosquito, Kelly, and Serrefine
- Needle holders: Webster, Castroviejo
- Bard-Parker knife handle and Nos. 11, 12, and 15 blades; MVR blade, disposable sickle blade
- Freer periosteal elevator
- Suction catheters: assortment of Frazier tips of varying sizes
- Local anesthetic of choice (1% to 2% lidocaine with epinephrine, bupivacaine 0.25% to 0.75%), topical tetracaine ophthalmic
- Prothrombotic agents: absorbable cellulose mesh (Surgicel) or purified porcine skin gelatin sponge (Gelfoam), thrombin
- Shielded bipolar cautery, monopolar needle-tip cautery
- Corneal protective shield, surgical cottonoids
- Muscle hooks: Jameson, Gass (helpful for slinging muscles)
- Lacrimal instruments: punctal dilator, Bowman probes
- Grasping instruments for sampling: pituitary rongeur, Takahashi rongeur, Blakesley
- Cryoprobe

SURGICAL PROCEDURES

Transseptal Anterior (Superior and Inferior) Orbitotomy

1. Palpate the mass (before and after induction), confirm the location, and mark the operative site. It may be helpful to mark a superior incision while the patient is awake. Similarly, prior to injecting anesthetic, a subciliary incision should be drawn 1 to 2 mm beneath the lash line (Figure 71.1).
2. After induction or sedation, inject the operative site with lidocaine (1% to 2%) or bupivacaine (0.20% to 0.75%) with epinephrine 1:100,000. Some surgeons use a combination to maximize rapid onset (lidocaine) with increased duration (bupivacaine) with or without hyaluronidase.
3. Place traction sutures into the eyelid margin as necessary to aid in retraction, using a 4-0 to 6-0 nylon or silk suture. Place protective corneal shield.
4. Incise skin using a No. 15 scalpel. Grasp the orbicularis with forceps, and buttonhole muscular tissue. Open medially and laterally along the direction of orbicularis fibers (Figure 71.2).

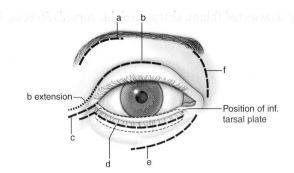

Figure 71.1. The sub-brow incision (a) should be created immediately inferior to the eyebrow, sparing the lash follicles. An eyelid crease incision (b) may be extended laterally (beyond the vertical hash mark) for increased exposure. A lateral canthotomy incision (c) is effective with lateral, superior lateral, and inferior lateral lesions. The subciliary incision (d) is created 2 mm below the eyelid margin, and is associated with a relatively high incidence of postoperative lower eyelid retraction. The lower crease incision (e) is cosmetically poor and has fallen out of favor. Although the modified Lynch incision (f) leaves a visible scar, it provides wide access to the deep medial and extraperiosteal space. It was frequently employed by ENT surgeons to perform external ethmoidectomy before endoscopic ethmoidectomy found widespread use. Care should be taken to avoid angular vessels along the lateral nasal wall.

Figure 71.2. The orbicularis is tented up, tunneled, and incised parallel to the direction of the muscle fibers.

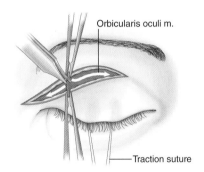

5. Obtain hemostasis with needle-point cautery.

6. Perform blunt dissection to isolate the orbital septum, and open with Westcott scissors or needle-point cautery. Deep orbital fat pads visualized through the orbital septum are a helpful guide to isolate the variable and often attenuated orbital septum (Figure 71.3).

7. If an extraocular muscle is present within the surgical field, it may be helpful to protect the muscle with a traction suture (4-0 silk), or neurosurgical cottonoid. Orbital fat may be resected or cauterized to cause shrinkage using monopolar cautery. Do not allow bleeding orbital fat to retract posteriorly as it increases the risk of orbital hemorrhage (Figure 71.4).

8. Using a combination of blunt and sharp dissection, isolate the lesion and dissect appropriate exposure (depending on whether total

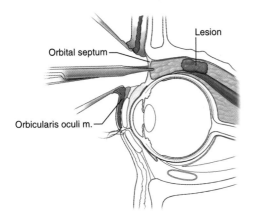

Figure 71.3. An extraconal (in this diagram) mass is accessed by incising orbital septum and approaching the appropriate surgical space. Intraconal lesions will require avoiding the relevant extraocular muscle or levator palpebrae.

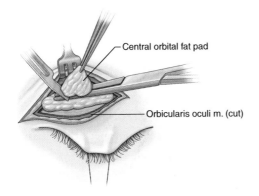

Figure 71.4. A fat pad is teased out with blunt dissection after incising orbital septum. Fat is clamped, cut, and cauterized to prevent a bleeding fat pad from retracting in an uncontrolled fashion into the orbit.

resection versus incisional biopsy is indicated). The lesion may be removed via a piecemeal dissection with grasping and cutting forceps (pituitary rongeur, Takahashi rongeur, Blakesley), or as a complete resection by dissecting in an anterior-to-posterior circumferential plane around the lesion. This approach is facilitated by using a combination of bipolar cautery and small incisions with Westcott scissors in the cauterized plane when lesions are adherent to orbital tissue. A skilled surgical assistant is indispensable. Finally, some lesions may be grasped and coupled using a cryoprobe, or alternatively "deflated" in order to aid removal. Dermoids should be removed without disrupting the capsule to prevent inflammatory tissue reaction (Figure 71.5).

9. Take care not to disrupt the levator palpebrae superioris, superior oblique tendon and muscle body, superior-ophthalmic vein, or other neurovascular structures in the upper eyelid. Similarly, avoid damage to lower eyelid retractors, inferior rectus, and inferior oblique in the lower eyelid. In addition, it is important to relax retraction of the

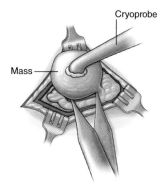

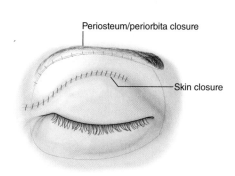

Figure 71.5. A lesion is obtained behind the orbital septum. Well-circumscribed, nonadherent lesions can be coupled to a cryoprobe and extracted.

Figure 71.6. After the periosteum is reapproximated with absorbable suture, the wound is carefully closed with interrupted or running sutures.

globe or tight orbital tissues on a routine basis to avoid vascular occlusive damage.

10. After adequate hemostasis is obtained, remove excess hemostatic material. Shielded bipolar cautery should be used in deeper orbital tissue to prevent damage to vital structures.

11. Consider drain placement in appropriate cases with known infection or difficult hemostasis. A 1/4-inch Penrose drain, sterile rubber band, or vascular retracting loop make effective drains.

12. Reapproximate subcutaneous tissues with 5-0 absorbable suture.

13. Close the skin with interrupted or running absorbable 6-0 plain gut, or nonabsorbable nylon or polypropylene suture (Figure 71.6).

14. Fix the drain, if present, to the skin. Apply benzoin tincture and adhesive strips. Remove the traction sutures and corneal shield.

Extraperiosteal Anterior (Superior, Medial, or Inferior) Orbitotomy

1. Confirm the location of the lesion and mark the operative site. It may be helpful to mark the incision while patient is awake to delineate a lid crease incision. The superior rim is easily obtained via a sub-brow or eyelid crease incision. The medial rim may be reached by a modified Lynch, or transconjunctival approach. The inferior rim is best obtained via a transconjunctival incision with or without a canthotomy/cantholysis, but may be approached via a subciliary incision. The lower eyelid crease incision is cosmetically inferior and has fallen out of favor (see Figure 71.1).

2. After induction or sedation, inject the operative site with lidocaine (1% to 2%) or bupivacaine (0.25% to 0.75%) with epinephrine 1:100,000.

3. Place traction sutures into the eyelid margin as necessary to aid in retraction, using a 5-0 nylon or silk suture.

4. Incise the skin using a No. 15 scalpel. Grasp the orbicularis with forceps, and buttonhole muscular tissue. Open medially and laterally along the direction of orbicularis fibers (see Figure 71.2).

5. Obtain hemostasis with needle-point cautery.

6. Perform a combination of blunt and sharp dissection to isolate the bony orbital rim (Figure 71.7).

7. It is useful to compress the fascial tissues against the orbital rim with a malleable retractor and expose the periosteal covered bone with a needle point cautery (Figure 71.8).

8. If an extraperiosteal approach is necessary (extraperiosteal abscess or hematoma, fracture, dermoid, or cholesterol granuloma) the periosteum should be isolated and incised 1 to 2 mm outside of the rim in a circumferential fashion with radial relaxing incisions. Elevate the periosteum with a Freer or periosteal elevator (Figure 71.9). Periosteum is most firmly adherent at the orbital rim (arcus marginalis). The

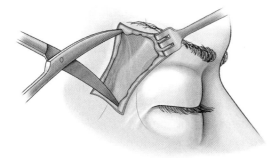

Figure 71.7. Stevens scissors are used to bluntly separate tissues down to the periosteum overlying the orbital rim.

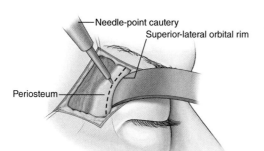

Needle-point cautery
Superior-lateral orbital rim
Periosteum

Figure 71.8. The periosteum is opened with needle point cautery.

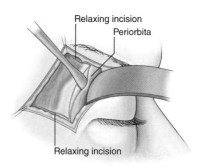

Figure 71.9. The periosteum is dissected off of the orbital rim with a Freer elevator.

Relaxing incision
Periorbita

Relaxing incision

periosteum is more easily dissected interior to the orbital rim. Areas of firm adherence typically mark perforating vessels, which should be cauterized prior to division.

9. Take care not to damage neurovascular structures along the upper eyelid and orbital margin. Similarly, avoid damage to the inferior rectus and inferior oblique in the lower eyelid and along the inferior-medial orbital wall. Along the medial wall, it is recommended that dissection be performed inferior to the line joining the anterior and posterior ethmoidal arteries to remain below the fovea ethmoidalis (the roof of the ethmoid sinuses), Figures 71.10, 71.11. In addition, it is important to relax retraction of the globe or tight orbital tissues on a routine basis to avoid vascular occlusive damage.

10. Consider drain placement in appropriate cases with known infection or difficult hemostasis. A 1/4-inch Penrose drain, sterile rubber band, or vascular retracting loop make effective drains.

11. Reapproximate the periosteum with 5-0 polyglactin (Vicryl) suture on a spatulated needle.

12. Reapproximate subcutaneous tissues with 5-0 absorbable suture.

13. Close the skin with interrupted or running absorbable 6-0 plain gut, or nonabsorbable nylon or polypropylene suture.

14. The drain, if present, is fixed to the skin. Benzoin tincture and adhesive strips are applied.

Transconjunctival Inferior Orbitotomy

1. Confirm the location of the lesion and mark the operative site.

2. After induction or sedation, inject the operative site using lidocaine (1% to 2%) or bupivacaine (0.20% to 0.75%) with epinephrine 1:100,000. In fornix-based incisions, tumescent conjunctival injection augments dissection and hemostasis.

3. Place traction sutures into the lower eyelid margin using a 5-0 nylon or silk suture. Place a protective corneal shield as necessary.

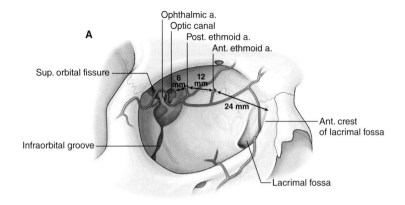

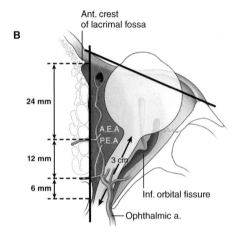

Figure 71.10. (A) Important anatomic landmarks in orbital surgery. The line joining the anterior and posterior ethmoidal arteries marks an important safety landmark above which the orbital surgeon should not stray, as it marks the inferior limit of the skull base defined by the fronto-ethmoidal suture adjacent to the fovea ethmoidalis, or roof of the ethmoid sinus. (B) The anterior ethmoidal artery is located 24 mm behind the anterior lacrimal crest; 12 mm posterior to the anterior ethmoidal artery lies the posterior ethmoidal artery, and an additional 6 mm posteriorly lies the optical canal (24-12-6).

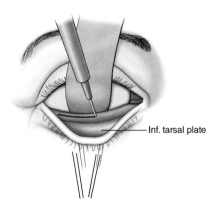

Figure 71.11. The lower transconjunctival incision can be made just below the tarsal plate, as well as deeper in the fornix, allowing one to reach the inferior orbital rim by compressing the tissues against the orbital rim with a malleable retractor and cauterizing deeply.

4. If the lower eyelid is tight, or the dissection requires additional exposure, perform a full-thickness lateral canthotomy using a straight scissors. Distract the lower eyelid and strum the inferior canthal tendon to determine the appropriate tissue to incise to create an inferior cantholysis. Moderate bleeding is encountered by transection of the marginal arcade laterally. Quickly obtain hemostasis with monopolar or bipolar cautery.

5. The fornix incision and dissection may be approached via direct sharp dissection with a scalpel or needle-point cautery fashioned 1 to 2 mm below the inferior border of the inferior tarsal plate (see Figure 71.11). Deeper fornix incisions are also possible.

6. Another elegant approach minimizes lower eyelid retraction by bluntly dissecting the orbicularis muscle off of the underlying orbital septum. After the conjunctiva and lower eyelid retractors are cut from the inferior border of the tarsus, they are placed on traction with 5-0 silk sutures clamped superiorly to the head drape (Figure 71.12; see also Chapter 76). Blunt dissection is then performed with a cotton-tipped applicator in the preseptal plane inferiorly, down to the orbital rim, while applying anterior-inferior traction to the eyelid with a Desmarres retractor. The septum or periosteum can then be incised to reach the inferior extraconal, intraconal, or extraperiosteal spaces. (Figure 71.13).

7. After the procedure is completed, close the periosteum with 5-0 absorbable suture. Consider drain placement in appropriate cases with known infection or difficult hemostasis. A 1/4-inch Penrose drain, sterile rubber band, or vascular retracting loop make effective drains.

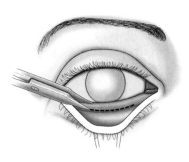

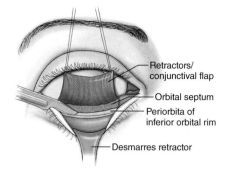

Figure 71.12. After the lower lid retractors and conjunctiva are dissected off of the orbital septum, they are clamped to the head drape superiorly (see also Figure 76.3).

Figure 71.13. This schematic diagram shows the relevant surgical planes to reach the extraperiosteal space. Modifications can be made to reach the extraconal supraperiosteal space and the intraconal space.

8. Close the inferior transconjunctival incision with 3 or 4 interrupted 6-0 gut sutures.
9. Close the canthotomy by reapproximating the lower eyelid to the orbital rim or upper eyelid using a 4-0 polyglactin (Vicryl) suture on a P-2 needle (see Chapter 70).
10. Remove the traction sutures and the corneal protective shield.

Transcaruncular Medial Orbitotomy

1. Confirm the location of the lesion and mark the operative site.
2. Inject the medial orbital tissue and upper and lower eyelid using lidocaine (1% to 2%) or bupivacaine (0.25% to 0.75%) with epinephrine 1:100,000.
3. Create a curvilinear 12-mm conjunctival incision just lateral to the caruncle (Figure 71.14). The incision may be extended superiorly and inferiorly, but care must be taken to avoid the superior and inferior canaliculus, which may be avoided by pre-placing a lacrimal Bowman probe.
4. With Stevens scissors, dissect through the thickened connective tissue adjacent to the caruncle, extending posteriorly and medially to the posterior lacrimal crest (Figure 71.15). Place a malleable retractor in this plane against the medial orbital wall to guide further dissection medially and posteriorly.
5. Open the periosteum deep to the posterior lacrimal crest with the Stevens scissors while the malleable retractor protects the lacrimal sac.
6. The extraperiosteal plane can now be dissected (Figure 71.16).

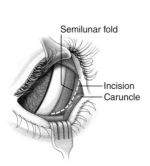
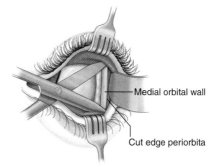

Figure 71.14. A 12 to 15 mm curvilinear incision is created just lateral to the caruncle.

Figure 71.15. Dissection is performed medially and posteriorly, through the thickened underlying fibrous layer, directed toward the posterior lacrimal crest.

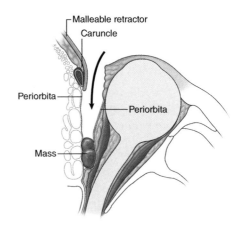

Figure 71.16. This surgical plane is developed after inserting a small malleable retractor against the medial orbital wall posteriorly to locate the posterior lacrimal crest. The dissection should remain posterior to this retractor to protect the lacrimal sac.

7. Consider drain placement in appropriate cases with known infection or difficult hemostasis. A 1/4-inch Penrose drain, sterile rubber band, or vascular retracting loop make effective drains.

8. Close the wound with several simple 6-0 gut sutures medially.

POSTOPERATIVE CARE

1. With extensive orbital dissection, overnight observation for vision monitoring, pain, and emesis control may be considered. It is a reasonable practice to ensure the patient has form vision in the few hours following deep orbital dissection. The patient is typically evaluated on postoperative day 1. Serial pupil and intraocular pressure assessment in the immediate postoperative period are occasionally indicated.

2. An icing regimen to the orbit is an important component to postoperative care.

3. Administer systemic postoperative antibiotics or corticosteroids in selected cases.

4. Some surgeons prefer to avoid an occlusive patch because it may mask visual loss in the immediate postoperative period, although it may be necessary to prevent wound leakage when an orbital drain is placed.

5. Instruct the patient to avoid straining (Valsalva) or applying pressure (especially during sleep) to the eye.

COMPLICATIONS

- Infection
- Hemorrhage

- Diplopia or strabismus
- Visual loss or blindness
- Eyelid malposition
- Sensory hypoesthesia
- Dry eye
- Pupillary or accomodative damage
- Orbital compartment syndrome

Steps to avoid infection include systemic intravenous antibiotic infusion immediately before the incision. Intraoperative irrigation of a bacitracin and polymyxin solution in dirty wounds is appropriate. If postoperative antibiotic coverage is necessary, it should be directed toward the suspected pathogen.

To minimize hemorrhage, use meticulous hemostasis. Techniques can include temporary intraoperative packing with surgical gauze or a variety of pro-thrombotic cellulose materials. It is appropriate to irrigate out and remove this material to prevent mass effect and postoperative compartment syndrome. We have seen cases in which retained absorbable hemostatic agents have swelled, leading to mass effect, raised intraorbital pressure, visual loss, and even orbital necrosis.

To minimize the chance of diplopia (neurogenic, myopathic, or restrictive strabismus), careful attention to the dissection plane is important. Most myopathic and incomplete neuropathic injury will typically recover, and further surgical intervention should be delayed at least 6 months. Temporize with prism application or occlusive patching.

Visual loss or blindness is an unusual complication that most likely occurs from postoperative swelling, bleeding, or vasospasm. Postoperative visual loss may require immediate sight-saving decompression and evacuation of a hematoma. Arterial disruption causing central retinal or ophthalmic artery occlusion is rare.

Eyelid retraction is not uncommon with inferior approaches (especially subciliary) and is minimized with transconjunctival techniques. Ptosis in upper eyelid surgery is usually temporary.

Mild pupil distortion may be detected intraoperatively, and dissection redirected away from a sensitive area. If damage to the long ciliary nerve is minor, the patient may experience anisocoria, pupillary irregularity, and ipsilateral loss of accommodation. If the damage is more complete or affects the lateral ciliary ganglion, the findings will be more permanent and simulate an Adie pupil. More often, intraoperative pupillary dilation is secondary to epinephrine effect.

Chapter 72

Lateral Orbitotomy

Roger E. Turbin, MD, FACS

The technical approach to orbital surgery is guided by location of the lesion, the expected lesion type (based on tissue involved and radiographic characteristic), and the goal of surgery (incisional biopsy versus excisional lesion removal). See further discussion in Chapter 71.

The lateral orbitotomy is used to access lacrimal lesions requiring complete lacrimal gland removal, such as pleomorphic adenoma; to access middle and posterior orbital lesions; to improve access to larger medial lesions if access would be limited via an anterior orbitotomy; or to provide additional space for dissection and displacement of the globe combined with another anterior technique. Lateral approaches utilize a variety of surface incisions; variations include the Stallard-Wright incision, the lateral canthal splitting incision that may release upper and lower canthal tendons (Berke-Reese), the extended eyelid crease incision for superior lesions, or a "hockey stick" incision that respects the lateral aspect of the upper lid crease and the lateral canthal lines of facial expression. The deeper posterior orbit may also require endoscopic transnasal or transmaxillary assistance as well as orbito-cranial techniques.

PREOPERATIVE STEPS

1. Localize the expected lesion location by analyzing the vector of displacement of the globe and palpation of periorbital and septal abnormalities. Additional information about a lesion can be gained from deeper palpation after the patient is anesthetized.

2. Order appropriate imaging studies, and review them with radiologists and collaborating surgical services.

3. Consider orbital, sinus, or brain CT and MRI studies (with contrast as necessary), and occasionally angiographic studies. Some centers utilize intraoperative navigational radiographic techniques, although these techniques are most useful for deeper procedures with complex sino-orbito-cranial disease, as well as bone-removing decompression.

4. Obtain preoperative informed consent, which in orbital surgery should routinely include a discussion of the risk of orbital hemorrhage, double vision, periorbital numbness, dry eye, eyelid malposition, pupil or accommodative damage, and ipsilateral blindness. Other potential complications are specific to the surgical approach and listed below.

5. If cessation of antithrombotic agents for systemic disease is necessary, this should be carried out under the guidance of a general medical doctor or an internist. A discussion of the risk/benefit ratio for cessation of anticoagulation is necessary in selected cases.

INSTRUMENTATION AND SUPPLIES

- Headlight, surgical loupes, operating microscope with longer focal length (greater than 220 mm provides clearance between surgical field and scope for orbital instruments)
- Forceps: 0.3-mm and 0.5-mm Castroviejo, Bishop-Harmon, fine-toothed Adson
- Retractors: Senn double-ended, malleable, orbital Sewell retractors, Desmarres lid retractors, small rakes, single- and double-pronged skin hooks, self-retaining retractors
- Scissors: assorted (blunt, sharp, straight, curved) Stevens, Westcott, Iris, Metzenbaum
- Clamps: mosquito, Kelly, Serrefine
- Needle holders: Webster, Castroviejo
- Bard-Parker knife handle with Nos. 11, 12, and 15 blades
- Freer periosteal elevator
- Suction catheters: assortment of Frazier tips of varying sizes
- Local anesthetic of choice (1% to 2% lidocaine with epinephrine, bupivacaine 0.25% to 0.75%), topical tetracaine ophthalmic
- Prothrombotic agents: absorbable cellulose mesh (Surgicel) or skin gelatin sponge (Gelfoam), thrombin
- Shielded bipolar cautery, monopolar needle-tip cautery

- Corneal protective shield, surgical cottonoids
- Also available as necessary:
  - Muscle hooks: Jameson, Gass (helpful for slinging muscles)
  - Lacrimal instruments: punctal dilator, Bowman probes
  - Bone cutters/rongeurs: oscillating saw, drill, assorted Kerrison rongeurs, Luer double-action rongeur, pituitary rongeur, Takahashi rongeur, Blakesley rongeur
  - Cryoprobe

SURGICAL PROCEDURE

1. Palpate the mass (before and after induction), confirm the location, and mark the operative site. A variety of cutaneous incisions have been described (Figure 72.1).
2. After induction or sedation, inject the operative site using lidocaine (1% to 2%) or bupivacaine (0.20% to 0.75%) with epinephrine 1:100,000. Some surgeons use a combination to maximize rapid onset (lidocaine) with increased duration (bupivacaine) with or without hyaluronidase in sedated patients. Place a protective corneal shield.
3. Incise skin using a No. 15 scalpel. Grasp the orbicularis with forceps, and buttonhole muscular tissue when dissecting in the lateral eyelid. Carry the inferior temporal dissection along the lateral orbit with a spreading blunt dissection initially using a Stevens or larger scissors. Continue dissection inferiorly to expose the temporalis muscle and temporalis fascia (Figure 72.2).
4. Obtain superficial hemostasis with needle-point cautery. Design and incise a flap using a bovie or needle-point cautery in the temporalis muscle and temporalis fascia, with the base located temporally

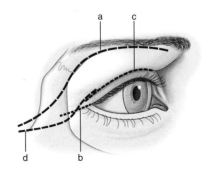

Figure 72.1. The lateral orbital area can be obtained through (a) the Stallard-Wright incision; (b) a lateral canthal splitting incision with or without release of upper and lower canthal tendons (Berke-Reese); (c) an extended lid crease incision for superior lesions; or (d) a hockey stick incision (see Figure 72.2).

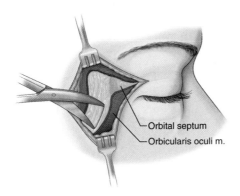

Figure 72.2. The hockey stick incision is a blend of the Stallard-Wright incision and an eyelid crease incision, limiting the dissection of the eyelid to its lateral half. It provides a more pleasing aesthetic result by "hiding" the resulting scar in the natural folds of facial expression. The more extended Stallard-Wright provides a great deal of exposure superiorly for larger tumors, as well as excision of the entire lacrimal gland en bloc.

Orbital septum
Orbicularis oculi m.

(Figure 72.3). This will expose the underlying orbital rim and intact periosteum.

5. After incising the anterior temporalis muscle and fascia, perform sharp dissection through periosteum in a curvilinear fashion with radial relaxing incisions to facilitate posterior-lateral and internal dissection. The incision should be placed 2 mm lateral to the orbital rim, extending superior to the zygomatico-temporal suture and inferior to the superior border of the zygomatic arch. The periosteum overlying the orbital rim is thereby reflected medially (Figure 72.4).

6. Free the posterior-lateral surface of the lateral orbital wall using blunt dissection with a periosteal elevator and monopolar cautery, or by forcefully and bluntly dissecting the temporalis posteriorly using a combination of a periosteal elevator and digital manipulation (Figure 72.5). This maneuver will require the surgeon to cauterize the zygomaticotemporal and zygomaticofacial arteries where they penetrate the periorbita from

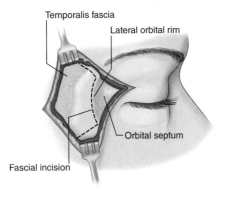

Temporalis fascia
Lateral orbital rim
Orbital septum
Fascial incision

Figure 72.3. The temporalis muscle is reflected, creating a circumferential incision with relaxing incisions created with either bovie or needle point dissection. Some surgeons prefer to create a T-shape on its side.

Figure 72.4. The periosteum is stripped from the zygoma medially, superiorly, and inferiorly. The periosteum is incised 2 mm outside of the rim to leave a surface for closure with relaxing wing incisions to obtain the inner surface of the lateral wall. This step can also be performed prior to or after the disinsertion of the temporalis muscle from the external lateral orbital wall.

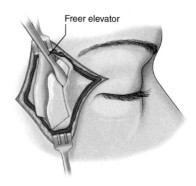

Figure 72.5. All surfaces of the lateral orbital wall are eventually freed, in preparation for the osteotomies and removal of the wall. This exposure is performed by stripping the temporalis from the outer surface of the zygoma along the external lateral orbital wall. Brisk bleeding can be encountered. The temporalis may be freed with bovie cautery or blunt dissection as shown.

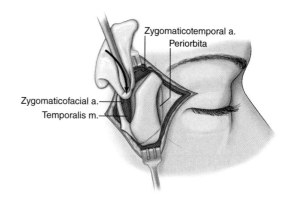

the lateral orbital wall. Bone wax application is effective at controlling bleeding from bone, but excess wax should be removed.

7. Expose the surface of the lateral orbital rim to the superior and inferior extent defined in Step 8 to allow for an adequate sized osteotomy (Figure 72.6).

Figure 72.6. The interior surface of the lateral orbital wall should be stripped of the periosteum.

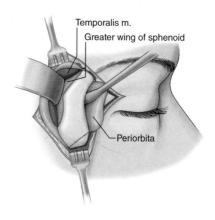

8. Premark the superior and inferior lines of the osteotomy with a sterile surgical marking pen or monopolar cautery. The superior and inferior extent of the osteotomy is adjusted to the size of the lesion; however, care should be taken at the superior extent to avoid entering the anterior cranial fossa above the zygomatico-frontal suture. The inferior osteotomy is most typically placed just superior to the junction of the orbital rim with the zygomatic arch.

9. Protect soft tissue with malleable retractors as the osteotomies are created with the oscillating saw (Figure 72.7).

10. Pre-place drill holes above and below each of the 2 osteotomy sites (Figure 72.8).

11. Outfracture the orbital rim using a large double-action Luer or Bull-nose rongeur. Store the bone fragment in a saline-soaked gauze for future replacement (see Figure 72.8).

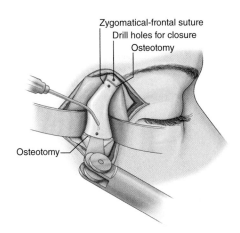

Zygomatical-frontal suture
Drill holes for closure
Osteotomy

Osteotomy

Figure 72.7. The osteotomies are created such that the superior and inferior cuts point slightly toward each other on the medial side. This prevents medial dislocation of the fragment, and keeps it from sliding after closure.

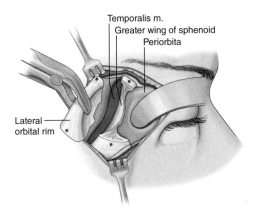

Temporalis m.
Greater wing of sphenoid
Periorbita

Lateral orbital rim

Figure 72.8. Pre-placement of drill holes before outfracture allows for "self-fixation of the fragment." The rim is grasped with a large bullnose or double-action Luer rongeur and outfractured. This requires a moderate degree of force, with care not to injure the orbital contents. Cauterize any remaining attachments and bleeders as the rim is pulled from its bed. Further dissection of the lateral orbital rim can be made with rongeurs, or diamond drill bit, which provides bone hemostasis.

12. Additional lateral orbital wall may be removed with a 3 to 4 mm drill or rongeur. Drilling provides bone hemostasis. Additional hemostatic control within cancellous bone and the marrow of the sphenoid is easily obtained using bone wax.

13. The lateral periorbita is incised over the palpated lesion, and if an extraocular muscle is present within the surgical field, it may be helpful to protect the muscle with a traction suture (4-0 silk) or a neurosurgical cottonoid (Figure 72.9). Orbital fat may be resected or cauterized to cause shrinkage using monopolar cautery. Do not allow bleeding orbital fat to retract posteriorly as it increases the risk of orbital hemorrhage. If a pleomorphic adenoma or adenoid cystic carcinoma of the lacrimal gland is suspected, the periosteum and lacrimal gland with or without the lateral orbital wall hinged to the periosteum may be removed en bloc (Figure 72.10).

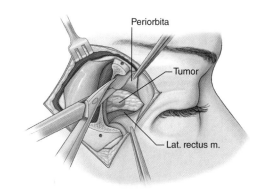

Figure 72.9. The periosteum can then be opened if necessary to obtain the lesion. The lateral rectus can be retracted with traction sutures or protected with surgical cottonoids.

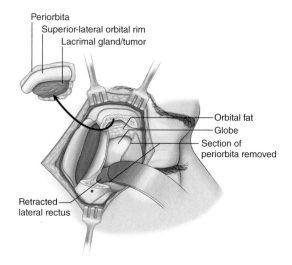

Figure 72.10. If it is anticipated that a lesion requires en bloc removal along with the bony rim, the periosteum between the rim and lesion can be left intact as a hinge to allow undisturbed en bloc removal. This maneuver is shown in the case of a lacrimal gland pleomorphic adenoma.

14. Using a combination of blunt and sharp dissection, isolate the lesion and create appropriate exposure (depending on whether a total resection versus incisional biopsy is indicated). A skilled surgical assistant is indispensable. The lesion may be removed via a piecemeal dissection with grasping forceps, or as a complete resection by dissecting in an anterior-to-posterior circumferential plane around the lesion. This approach is facilitated by using a combination of bipolar cautery and small incisions with Westcott scissors in the cauterized plane when lesions are adherent to orbital tissue. Finally, some lesions may be grasped using a cryoprobe, or "deflated" in order to aid removal (see Figure 71.5).

15. When adequate hemostasis is obtained, the periorbita may be loosely reapproximated with a 4-0 absorbable suture, after a drain is place as necessary.

16. Replace the lateral orbital wall fragment after adequate bulb irrigation. Using 4-0 nonabsorbable braided nylon or polypropylene sutures through the pre-placed drill holes is adequate to fixate the lateral orbital wall; avoid palpable wire sutures or plates on the orbital rim (Figure 72.11). The suture knot may be rotated into the drill holes placed in the rim to prevent a palpable defect.

17. Close the periorbita with 4-0 absorbable suture.

18. Reapproximate the temporalis fascia with 4-0 absorbable suture, and orbicularis muscle with 5-0 absorbable suture.

19. The skin may be closed with interrupted or running absorbable 6-0 plain gut, or nonabsorbable nylon or polypropylene suture.

20. The drain, if present, is fixed to the skin. Benzoin tincture and adhesive strips are applied.

21. Traction sutures and corneal shield are removed.

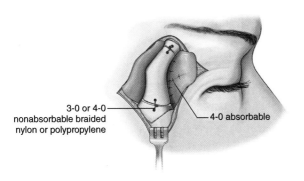

Figure 72.11. The rim can be fastened with a larger nonabsorbable suture and the knot rotated internally inside the predrilled hole.

3-0 or 4-0 nonabsorbable braided nylon or polypropylene

4-0 absorbable

POSTOPERATIVE CARE

1. With extensive orbital dissection, overnight observation for vision monitoring, pain, and emesis control may be considered. It is a reasonable practice to ensure the patient has form vision in the few hours following deep orbital dissection. The patient is typically evaluated on postoperative day 1. Serial pupil and intraocular pressure assessment in the immediate postoperative period are occasionally indicated.
2. An icing regimen to the orbit is an important component of postoperative care.
3. Administer systemic postoperative antibiotics or corticosteroids in selected cases.
4. Some surgeons prefer to avoid an occlusive patch because it may mask visual loss in the immediate postoperative period, although it may be necessary to prevent wound leakage when an orbital drain is placed.
5. Instruct the patient to avoid straining (Valsalva) or applying pressure (especially during sleep) to the eye.

COMPLICATIONS

- Infection
- Hemorrhage
- Diplopia or strabismus
- Visual loss or blindness
- Eyelid malposition
- Sensory hypoesthesia (regional or incision site)
- Dry eye
- Pupillary or accommodative paresis
- Cerebrospinal fluid (CSF) leakage
- Orbital compartment syndrome

Steps to avoid infection including systemic intravenous antibiotic infusion immediately before incision as well as intraoperative irrigation of bacitracin/polymyxin solution into dirty wounds. Antibiotic coverage should be directed toward the suspected pathogen (eg, penicillin with *Actinomyces*).

To minimize hemorrhage, use meticulous hemostasis, which can include temporary intraoperative packing with surgical gauze or a variety of prothrombotic cellulose materials. Electro-cautery or bone wax application is effective at controlling bleeding from bone. It is appropriate to irrigate out and remove this material to prevent mass effect and postoperative compartment syndrome. We have seen cases in which retained absorbable hemostatic agents have swelled, leading to mass effect, raised intraorbital pressure, visual loss, and even orbital necrosis.

To minimize diplopia (neurogenic, myopathic, or restrictive strabismus), careful attention to the dissection plane is important. Most myopathic and incomplete neuropathic injury will typically recover, and further surgical intervention should be delayed at least 6 months. Temporize with prism application or occlusive patching if necessary.

Visual loss or blindness is an unusual complication that most likely occurs from postoperative swelling or bleeding. Postoperative visual loss may require immediate sight-saving decompression and evacuation of hematoma. Arterial disruption causing central retinal or ophthalmic artery occlusion is rare.

Eyelid retraction is not uncommon with inferior approaches (especially subciliary) and is minimized with transconjunctival techniques. Ptosis in upper eyelid surgery is usually temporary.

Mild pupil distortion may be detected intraoperatively, and dissection can be redirected away from a sensitive area. If damage to the long ciliary nerve is minor, the patient may experience anisocoria, pupillary irregularity, and ipsilateral loss of accommodation. If the damage is more complete or affects the lateral ciliary ganglion, the findings will be more permanent and simulate an Adie pupil. More often, intraoperative pupillary dilation is secondary to epinephrine effect.

Evaluation, management, and repair of a CSF leak is beyond the scope of this discussion. Intraoperative neurosurgical consultation may be appropriate.

Chapter 73

Optic Nerve Sheath Fenestration

Roger E. Turbin, MD, FACS

Optic nerve sheath fenestration is the procedure of choice in patients with visual loss due to elevated intracranial pressure who are not candidates for other shunting procedures (idiopathic intracranial hypertension, cryptococcal meningitis, others), as well as in patients with visual loss related to anterior optic nerve sheath hematoma. The medial transconjunctival incision is a standard approach to access the optic nerve, but both a lateral and superior-medial transcutaneous approach may be utilized.

The superior-medial approach is finding increasing popularity among orbital surgeons, because it obviates the need to disinsert the medial rectus muscle and the orbital surgeon is familiar with the eyelid anatomy. This approach has a variety of uses and may also allow the surgeon to obtain long sections of optic nerve when combined with an enucleation. The superior medial approach is very useful to obtain a biopsy of the superior intraconal space as well as to sample lesions of the optic nerve sheath or decompress a nerve sheath hematoma.

The lateral approach can be applied without bone removal or with bone removal to augment exposure. Despite the benefit of not having to disinsert an extraocular muscle, the lateral approach has a high incidence of postoperative pupillary or accommodative paresis due to injury of the ciliary ganglion. Surgeons at our institution have consequently used the lateral approach less frequently for optic nerve sheath fenestration.

PREOPERATIVE STEPS

1. Order appropriate imaging studies. Consider orbital, sinus, or brain CT and MRI studies (with contrast as necessary), lumbar puncture with CSF pressure analysis, and occasionally angiographic studies.
2. Obtain preoperative informed consent, which in orbital surgery, should routinely include a discussion of the risk of orbital hemorrhage, double vision, periorbital numbness, dry eye, eyelid malposition, pupil or accommodative damage, and ipsilateral blindness. Other potential complications are specific to the surgical approach and listed below.
3. If cessation of antithrombotic agents for systemic disease is necessary, this should be carried out under the guidance of a general medical doctor or an internist. A discussion of the risk and benefit ratio for cessation of anticoagulation is necessary in selected cases.

INSTRUMENTATION AND SUPPLIES

- Headlight, surgical loupes, operating microscope with longer focal length (greater than 220 mm provides clearance between surgical field and scope for orbital instruments)
- Forceps: 0.3-mm and 0.5-mm Castroviejo; Bishop-Harmon; fine-toothed Adson; and long, fine-toothed neurosurgical forceps
- Retractors: Senn double-ended retractors; malleable retractors; orbital Sewell retractors; Desmarres lid retractors; small rakes; single- and double-pronged skin hooks; and self-retaining retractor
- Scissors: assorted (blunt, sharp, straight, curved) Stevens, Westcott, iris, Metzenbaum, and long neurosurgical microscissors
- Clamps: mosquito, Kelly and Serrefine
- Needle holders: Webster, Castroviejo
- Bard-Parker knife handle with Nos. 11, 12, and 15 blades; MVR blade
- Suction catheters: assortment of Frazier tips of varying sizes
- Local anesthetic of choice (1% to 2% lidocaine with epinephrine, bupivacaine 0.25% to 0.75%), topical tetracaine ophthalmic
- Prothrombotic agents: absorbable cellulose mesh (Surgicel) or skin gelatin sponge (Gelfoam), thrombin
- Shielded bipolar cautery, monopolar needle-tip cautery
- Muscle hooks: Jameson, Gass (helpful for slinging muscles)
- Corneal protective shield, surgical cottonoids

SURGICAL PROCEDURES

Superior-Medial Transcutaneous

1. Mark out the medial portion of the upper eyelid crease (Figure 73.1).
2. After induction or sedation, inject the operative site with lidocaine (1% or 2%) or bupivacaine (0.25% to 0.75%) with epinephrine.
3. Perform a single snip superior and medial peritomy by grasping the visible insertion of each corresponding rectus muscle, and snipping the conjunctiva and Tenon's layer down to bare sclera anterior to the grasp. Pass a traction 4-0 silk tie behind the superior and medial recti using a Gass muscle hook. In addition, place an upper eyelid traction suture through the mid-eyelid margin (Figure 73.2).
4. Incise the upper eyelid crease with a No. 15 blade scalpel.
5. Grasp the underlying orbicularis muscle with two 0.5-mm Castroviejo forceps, and buttonhole the muscle. Dissect inferior medial and superior lateral along the direction of the muscle fibers. Repeat the procedure to open the superior medial orbital septum.

Figure 73.1. The medial portion of the upper eyelid crease is incised for approximately 2 cm.

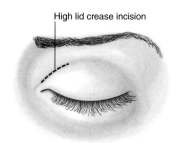

High lid crease incision

Figure 73.2. The conjunctiva just anterior to the insertion of the medial and superior rectus is grasped, lifted, and incised with a Westcott scissors, allowing the passage of a Gass muscle hook to sling the medial and superior recti.

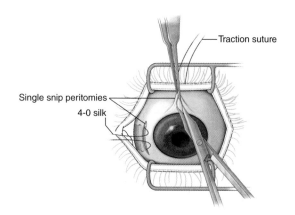

Traction suture

Single snip peritomies

4-0 silk

6. The underlying superior medial orbital fat is now visible. Introduce 2 thin Sewell retractors into the potential space, one nasal to the medial edge of the levator palpebrae superioris, and the other lateral to the superior oblique tendon (Figure 73.3).

7. Dissect bluntly and posteriorly using a combination of cotton-tipped applicators, Sewell retractors, and malleable retractors, toward the optic nerve. The nerve can be directly palpated approximately 1 cm behind the globe by applying traction to the globe via the traction sutures. The eye should be abducted and depressed to bring the nerve into the field of the dissection (Figure 73.4).

8. Take care to avoid vortex veins along the globe and short posterior ciliary nerves at the transition from the optic nerve dura to the posterior apex. In addition, traction sutures and globe retraction are frequently relaxed to prevent vascular occlusion.

9. 3 × 1/4-inch cottonoid sponges may be used to retract fat from the area around the optic nerve. A skilled surgical assistant is indispensable. Bipolar cautery should be used sparingly.

10. Grasp the optic nerve with long, fine forceps, and incise the sheath with an MVR or sickle blade (Figure 73.5). Direct observation is

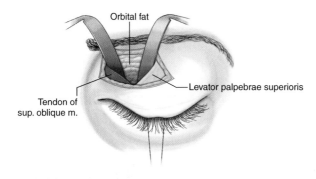

Figure 73.3. The superior medial orbital fat just medial to the medial edge of the levator palpebrae is exposed.

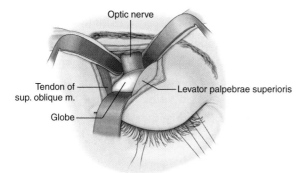

Figure 73.4. A combination of Sewell and malleable retractors is used to bluntly dissect to the optic nerve. Placing the retractor over a moistened 1 x 3-inch cottonoid effectively tamponades the fat from the field.

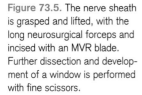
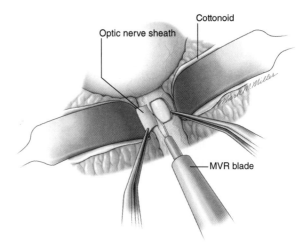

Figure 73.5. The nerve sheath is grasped and lifted, with the long neurosurgical forceps and incised with an MVR blade. Further dissection and development of a window is performed with fine scissors.

facilitated by the use of surgical loupes or the operative microscope at this step. Slits can be extended, or a window within the dural sheath may be developed. The sheath specimen may be sent for histologic analysis if indicated.

11. After adequate hemostasis is obtained, close the lid crease incision with interrupted 6-0 plain gut sutures. The muscle and eyelid traction sutures are removed, and the small peritomies are closed with absorbable 6-0 plain gut sutures.

Medial Transconjunctival Orbitotomy

1. Perform a wide medial peritomy with radial superior medial and inferior medial relaxing conjunctival incisions. Capture the medial rectus with a muscle hook and pre-place a double-armed 5-0 polyglactin (Vicryl) suture prior to disinserting this extraocular muscle (Figure 73.6).

2. Either pass superior and inferior intrascleral traction sutures through the medial rectus stump superior and inferior edge, or capture and sling the superior and inferior recti. These sutures will be used for lateral traction on the globe and should be firmly attached (Figure 73.7).

3. A lateral canthotomy may augment exposure and allow lateral traction of the globe in tight orbits, but it is seldom needed.

4. The underlying medial orbital fat is now visible. Introduce thin Sewell retractors into the potential space, avoiding the vessels between the globe and the posterior surface of the disinserted medial rectus (Figure 73.8).

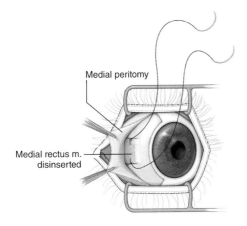

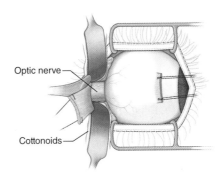

Figure 73.6. A wide peritomy with relaxing wing incisions is made medially from 11 o'clock to 7 o'clock. The medial rectus is slung and disinserted in the standard technique after a 5-0 double-armed polyglactin suture is passed.

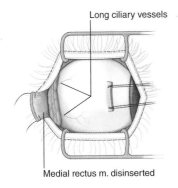

Figure 73.7. After the muscle is disinserted, superior and inferior traction sutures are placed to allow for lateral distraction of the globe.

Figure 73.8. The nerve is exposed using the combination of cotton-tipped applicator blunt dissection plus retractors over cottonoids.

5. Bluntly dissect posteriorly using a combination of cotton-tipped applicators, Sewell retractors, and malleable retractors toward the optic nerve. The nerve can be directly palpated approximately 1 cm behind the globe by applying traction to the globe via the traction sutures. A skilled surgical assistant is indispensable.

6. Take care to avoid vortex veins along the globe and short posterior ciliary nerves at the transition from the optic nerve dura to the posterior apex. In addition, traction sutures and globe retraction are frequently relaxed to prevent vascular occlusion.

7. Cottonoid sponges may be used to retract fat from the area around the optic nerve. Bipolar cautery should be used sparingly.

8. Grasp the optic nerve with long, fine forceps, and incise the sheath with an MVR or sickle blade. Direct observation is facilitated by the

use of surgical loupes or the operative microscope at this step. Slits can be extended, or a window within the dural sheath may be developed.

9. After obtaining adequate hemostasis, remove the muscle traction sutures. The pre-placed, double-armed muscle suture is used to reinsert the medial rectus to its origin.

10. Close the peritomy with absorbable 6-0 gut suture.

POSTOPERATIVE CARE

1. With extensive orbital dissection, overnight observation for vision monitoring, pain, and emesis control may be considered. It is a reasonable practice to ensure the patient has form vision in the few hours following deep orbital dissection. The patient is typically evaluated on postoperative day 1. Serial pupil and intraocular pressure assessment in the immediate postoperative period are occasionally indicated.

2. An icing regimen to the orbit is an important component to postoperative care.

3. Administer systemic postoperative antibiotics or corticosteroids in selected cases.

4. Some surgeons prefer to avoid an occlusive patch because it may mask visual loss in the immediate postoperative period, although it may be necessary to prevent wound leakage when an orbital drain is placed.

5. Instruct the patient to avoid straining (Valsalva) or applying pressure (especially during sleep) to the eye.

COMPLICATIONS

- Infection
- Hemorrhage
- Diplopia or strabismus
- Visual loss or blindness
- Eyelid malposition
- Sensory hypoesthesia
- Dry eye
- Pupillary or accommodative paresis
- Cerebrospinal fluid (CSF) leakage
- Orbital compartment syndrome

To control hemorrhage, use meticulous hemostasis. Methods can include temporary intraoperative packing with surgical gauze, or a variety of pro-thrombotic cellulose materials. Bipolar cautery should be used sparingly. It is appropriate to irrigate out and remove any hemostatic material to prevent mass effect and postoperative compartment syndrome.

Transient diplopia (neurogenic, myopathic) is not uncommon but is usu-ally self-limited and resolves spontaneously. Temporize with prism application or occlusive patching if necessary.

Visual loss or blindness is an unusual complication that most likely occurs from postoperative swelling, bleeding, or vasospasm. Instruct the patient to avoid straining (Valsalva) or applying pressure (eg, sleeping on the operated side) to the eye. Postoperative visual loss may require immediate sight-saving decompression and evacuation of a hematoma. Arterial occlusion causing central retinal or ophthalmic artery occlusion is rare.

Ptosis following upper eyelid surgery is usually temporary.

Mild pupil distortion may be detected intraoperatively, and dissection redirected away from a sensitive area. If damage to the long ciliary nerve is minor, the patient may experience anisocoria, pupillary irregularity, and ipsi-lateral loss of accommodation. If the damage is more complete or affects the lateral ciliary ganglion, the findings will be more permanent and simulate an Adie pupil.

A postoperative CSF-contained cyst may be detected during subsequent scanning or orbital ultrasound studies. It is possible this finding signifies a "functioning" fenestration and usually does not need to be addressed.

Part VII

Trauma

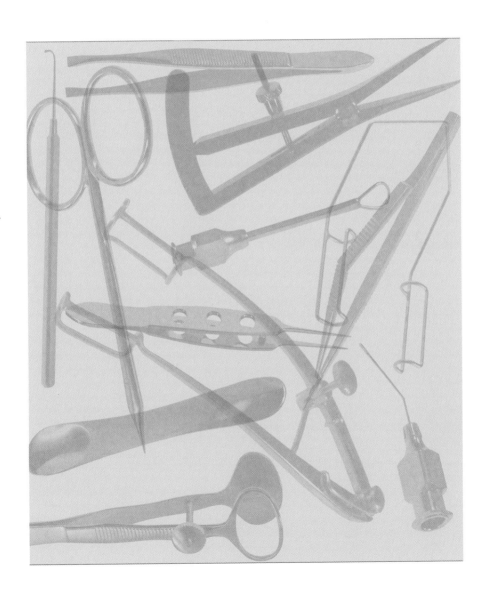

Chapter 74

Repair of Full-Thickness Eyelid Laceration

Paul D. Langer, MD, FACS

The technique for repairing a full-thickness eyelid laceration is employed when an eyelid laceration includes the margin of the eyelid, involving tarsus, orbicularis muscle, and skin. The technique is also used when reapproximating a similar surgical defect in the eyelid, such as one that occurs after a pentagonal wedge excision (Chapter 62). The procedure is usually performed under local anesthesia in an emergency room, but it may be performed under general anesthesia if part of a larger reconstruction. The procedure is best performed under magnification using surgical loupes.

INSTRUMENTATION AND SUPPLIES

- Corneal protector
- Straight, sharp iris scissors
- Locking, medium-jawed Castroviejo needle holder
- Castroviejo 0.5 forceps
- 5-0 polyglactin (Vicryl) suture with spatula needle
- 6-0 nylon suture
- Surgical loupes

SURGICAL PROCEDURE

1. Place topical anesthesia on the eye, and cover the eye with the corneal protector. Infiltrate the wound sterilely using 1% lidocaine with epinephrine 1:100,000. Clean the wound vigorously with soap or an antiseptic, using a scrub brush, if necessary, to ensure all foreign material is removed.

2. Prep and drape the patient in a sterile manner.

3. Using the iris scissors, "freshen" the margins of the wound to create clean, straight parallel edges ready for closure (Figure 74.1).

4. Suture the tarsus with interrupted, parallel, partial thickness bites using 5-0 polyglactin suture on a spatula needle (Figure 74.2).

    • The first suture should be placed close to the eyelid margin (at the inferior edge of the wound in the upper lid, or the superior edge of the wound in the lower lid), and care must be taken to precisely align the margins of the 2 edges with the first suture. The spatula shape will facilitate a partial-thickness passage of the needle through tarsus, avoiding penetration of the palpebral conjunctiva.

    • In the upper eyelid, if the full height of the tarsus is involved, 3 tarsal sutures can be placed. In the lower eyelid with a smaller tarsus, only 2 sutures can be placed if the full height of tarsus is lacerated.

    • All tarsal sutures should be pre-placed and left untied until all of the tarsal sutures are thrown, since the precise placement of further tarsal bites is extremely difficult once a tarsal suture is tied. Once all tarsal sutures are thrown they are then tied, starting with the suture closest to the margin.

5. Close the eyelid margin with 2 interrupted 6-0 nylon sutures. The first suture should reapproximate the eyelash line, as the lashes create a

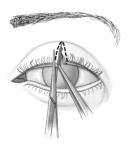

Figure 74.1. The eyelid margin is "freshened" to create straight tissue edges bordering the defect.

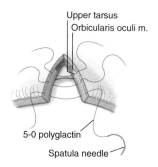

Upper tarsus
Orbicularis oculi m.

5-0 polyglactin

Spatula needle

Figure 74.2. Partial-thickness tarsal bites are placed, but not tied until all tarsal bites are thrown.

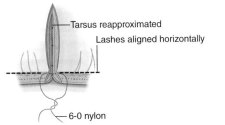

Tarsus reapproximated

Lashes aligned horizontally

6-0 nylon

Figure 74.3. The eyelash line is reapproximated and the suture "tails" left long.

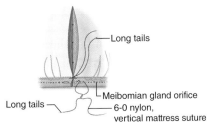

Long tails

Meibomian gland orifice

Long tails

6-0 nylon, vertical mattress suture

Figure 74.4. A vertical mattress suture is placed through Meibomian orifices in the posterior lamella.

natural landmark to realign the lacerated segments of the lid (Figure 74.3). Cut the ends of this suture with long "tails" (about 15 to 20 mm).

6. Place the second marginal nylon suture through the Meibomian gland orifices of the posterior lamella to ensure that the suture incorporates tarsus. A vertical mattress suture ("near-near, far-far") should be employed (Figure 74.4). A vertical mattress suture provides increased strength but, more importantly, will resist the tendency for postoperative contraction that may result in a notch of the eyelid margin. The vertical mattress suture should not be tied overly tight; it should be tightened just until the approximated ends of the lid begin to evert at the margin. Cut the ends of the vertical mattress suture with long "tails" (about 15 to 20 mm).

7. Suture the remainder of the skin incision with 6-0 nylon. The long suture "tails" of the first 2 nylon sutures can be tied down into the knot of the suture placed closest to the lashes (Figure 74.5). After a square knot is placed, the 4 tails (2 from each of the 2 sutures) are laid over the knot and 2 additional throws (a square knot) are placed to secure the suture "tails." Excess suture is then trimmed. This maneuver ensures that the ends of these marginal sutures do not abrade the surface of the cornea.

Figure 74.5. The long suture "tails" of the 2 margin sutures are tied into the knot of the skin suture closest to the eyelid margin.

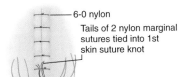

6-0 nylon

Tails of 2 nylon marginal sutures tied into 1st skin suture knot

POSTOPERATIVE CARE

1. Apply antibiotic ointment to the wound.
2. The skin sutures can be removed in 5 to 7 days, but the vertical mattress marginal suture should remain in place for 12 to 14 days.
3. In children or patients in whom suture removal is expected to be difficult, 7-0 polyglactin sutures can be effectively substituted for the 6-0 nylon sutures.

COMPLICATIONS

- Lid notch or uneven apposition
- Wound dehiscence

The most common complication encountered in eyelids that have undergone laceration repair is a depressed notch at the eyelid margin or an uneven juxtaposition of the opposing ends, with an end overriding the other at the margin where the lid was repaired. Notching can usually be prevented with the careful placement of a vertical mattress suture through the posterior portion of the lid margin (ie, through the Meibomian orifices), which will counteract the tendency for postoperative contracture. An uneven lid margin can be prevented by careful apposition of the two tarsal segments. The first tarsal suture, which should be placed very near the lid margin, is especially important in this regard.

If either problem is noticeable, correction would entail reopening the wound and re-closing it, or performing a very thin pentagonal wedge resection around the area of the defect and treating the resulting defect like a fresh wound.

The tarsus heals slowly, and dehiscences can occur at the margin if the margin sutures are removed too early or if trauma is experienced again in the same area of the eyelid. Lid margin dehiscences usually require re-operation if the defect is noticeable. If it is left unrepaired, a notch is likely to result.

Chapter 75

Repair of Corneoscleral Lacerations

Peter S. Hersh, MD
Bradford L. Tannen, MD

Corneoscleral lacerations can be caused by a wide variety of mechanisms and are a major source of ocular morbidity. The primary surgical goals in repairing all corneoscleral lacerations are to achieve a watertight globe and to maintain structural integrity. Secondary goals include repositioning uveal tissues, relieving vitreous incarceration, removing intraocular foreign bodies, and restoring normal anatomic relationships.

PREOPERATIVE STEPS

1. Obtain a careful history and perform a thorough ophthalmic examination. Eliciting the mechanism of injury is helpful in guiding the preoperative workup.
2. Apply only minimal pressure to the globe during examination to avoid iatrogenic disruption of intraocular contents.
3. The presence of a full-thickness corneal laceration can be elicited with Seidel testing using 2% fluorescein.
4. Investigate the possibility of an occult intraocular foreign body using appropriate imaging. CT imaging with thin cuts (1.5 to 3.0 mm) is useful in identifying radiodense foreign bodies. Gentle B-scan ultrasound examination is useful for localizing and identifying both radiodense and radiolucent foreign bodies. MRI, while better than

CT in identifying vegetable matter, glass, wood, and plastic foreign bodies, is contraindicated if a metallic foreign body is suspected.

5. Administer broad-spectrum intravenous antibiotics.

6. As prophylaxis, give a combination of cephalosporin or vancomycin to treat gram-positive bacteria and an aminoglycoside or third-generation cephalosporin to treat gram-negative bacteria. Clindamycin should be added if an intraocular foreign body is present, especially if the wound has been contaminated with vegetable matter.

7. Avoid subconjunctival and topical antibiotic injections preoperatively because they may cause eyelid squeezing.

8. Administer tetanus prophylaxis in accordance with recommendations from the Centers for Disease Control and Prevention.

9. Apply a rigid eye shield to avoid inadvertent pressure on the globe.

10. Administer antiemetics and analgesics as needed to avoid vomiting and agitation.

INSTRUMENTATION AND SUPPLIES

- Castroviejo suture forceps (0.12, 0.3, and 0.5 mm)
- Castroviejo needle holder
- 15° sharp microsurgical knife
- Irrigating canula
- Wescott scissors with blunt tips and Vannas scissors
- Cyclodialysis spatula
- Vitreous sweep
- Viscoelastic
- Small and large muscle hooks
- 10-0 monofilament nylon on a fine spatulated needle for corneal lacerations
- 9-0 nylon suture for limbal lacerations
- 8-0 or 9-0 nylon suture for scleral lacerations
- 4-0 silk used as a rectus bridle suture
- 6-0 silk for limbal fixation
- 8-0 polyglactin (Vicryl) suture for conjunctival repair
- 5-0 Vicryl suture, double-armed on a spatulated needle for rectus muscle disinsertion and reattachment
- Dry cellulose sponges

SURGICAL PROCEDURES

Selected cases of small self-sealing corneal lacerations with good wound apposition may be treated with a bandage soft contact lens in combination with topical antibiotic prophylaxis. The great majority of lacerating anterior segment injuries, however, require the placement of corneal sutures. During repair, cultures should be taken from the wound margins, prolapsed and devitalized tissues, and intraocular foreign bodies.

Isolated Corneal Lacerations

1. General anesthesia is preferred.
2. Prep and drape the patient in a sterile manner. Take care not to put pressure on the globe.
3. If the anterior chamber is formed and the wound is watertight, sutures may be placed directly without entering the anterior chamber with instrumentation. Corneal sutures should be placed in a meticulous fashion: at the point of entry, the curvature of the needle should be perpendicular to the surface of the cornea, and the path of the needle through the tissue should follow the curvature of the needle (Figure 75.1).
4. For less stable wounds, viscoelastic may be irrigated into the anterior chamber either directly through the wound itself or through a separate limbal paracentesis (Figure 75.2).
5. Create a paracentesis, using a 15° sharp microsurgical knife, placing the incision 90° away from the wound.

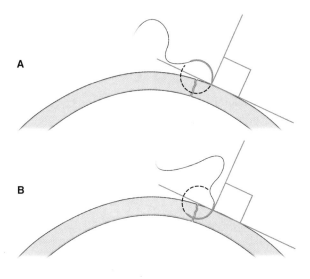

A

B

Figure 75.1. The needle enters the cornea perpendicularly (A), and the pass follows the curvature of the needle (B).

6. A 10-0 monofilament nylon on a fine spatula microsurgical needle is used for corneal sutures. Even finer 11-0 nylon may be used for lacerations near or involving the visual axis.

7. Several methods for suturing corneal lacerations are available.
   - The simplest method is to progressively halve the wound with simple interrupted corneal sutures.
   - Sutures should be placed approximately 90% to 95% depth through the stroma, 1.5 mm in length, of equal depth on each side of the wound, and perpendicular to the wound (Figure 75.3).
   - Placement of sutures through the visual axis should be avoided if possible.
   - Irregular wounds should be divided into straight segments with interrupted sutures. Perpendicular areas of the laceration should be sutured before beveled ones to achieve watertight closure with the fewest number of sutures.
   - Long, deep, relatively tight peripheral wound sutures, in combination with shorter, shallower sutures near the visual axis, may help restore the normal corneal contour (Figure 75.4).

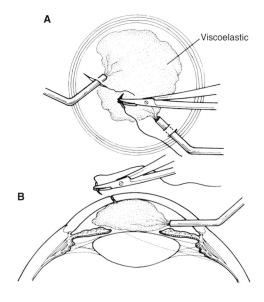

Figure 75.2. Viscoelastic is irrigated into the anterior chamber, either through the wound (A) or through a paracentesis (B). (Reprinted, with permission, from *Duane's Clinical Ophthalmology*, Tasman W and Jaeger EA, eds, Lippincott Williams and Wilkins, Copyright © 1994. www.lww.com.)

A

Viscoelastic

B

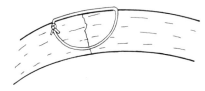

Figure 75.3. Sutures are placed at 90% to 95% of the corneal depth and the knot buried away from the visual axis. (Reprinted, with permission, from *Duane's Clinical Ophthalmology*, Tasman W and Jaeger EA, eds, Lippincott Williams and Wilkins, Copyright © 1994. www.lww.com.)

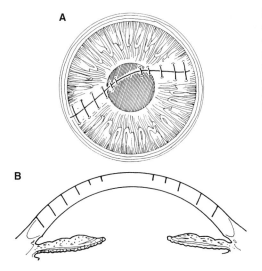

Figure 75.4. Peripheral corneal sutures are placed relatively longer and deeper (A), while sutures nearer the visual axis are shorter and more shallow (B). (Reprinted, with permission, from *Duane's Clinical Ophthalmology,* Tasman W and Jaeger EA, eds, Lippincott Williams and Wilkins, Copyright © 1994. www.lww.com.)

- Using a locked 2-1-1 (2 throws, then one throw, then one throw) knot or a 1-1-1 slipknot facilitates subsequent suture removal.
- The suture knot ends are trimmed short and buried superficially on the side away from the visual axis (Figure 75.3).
- Once the laceration is repaired, deepen the anterior chamber, preferably through the paracentesis port.
- Check the wound for leaks using dry cellulose sponges or 2% fluorescein.
- When stellate corneal lacerations or partial tissue avulsions are present, it may be difficult to obtain a watertight closure. Several techniques may be used, including multiple interrupted sutures, bridging sutures, purse-string sutures, and star-shaped sutures. If closing a stellate laceration is difficult, and leaking persists, tissue adhesive or a corneal patch graft may be used.

8. Iris incarceration and prolapse are commonly seen.
   - Carefully examine the prolapsed iris. Iris tissue that is macerated, feathery, devitalized, depigmented, or that shows signs of surface epithelialization should be excised and sent for histopathologic examination. In general, tissue that has been prolapsed for longer than 24 hours should be excised to avoid infection.
   - Incarcerated iris usually requires mechanical repositioning.
     - Deepen the anterior chamber with viscoelastic agents irrigated through the paracentesis port or the wound adjacent to the involved iris tissue (Figure 75.5).

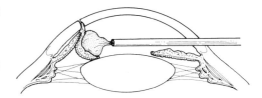

   – A cyclodialysis spatula or irrigating canula can be passed through the paracentesis site and used to directly sweep incarcerated tissue free (Figure 75.6).
   – Once incarcerated or prolapsed tissue is excised or repositioned, suture the corneal laceration as described earlier.

9. Vitreous involvement may be present in isolated corneal lacerations, particularly with lacerations that also involve the lens. The goal in the acute surgical setting is to relieve vitreous incarceration from the wound.
   • Automated microvitrectomy through limbal or pars plana approaches may be performed.
   • Dry cellulose sponges are useful for identifying vitreous strands remaining at the wound. Prolapsed vitreous should be cut flush with the wound.
   • The wound may be then swept with a vitreous sweep through the paracentesis site to dislocate any remaining incarcerated vitreous (Figure 75.7).

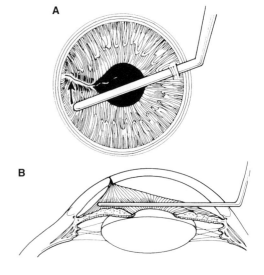

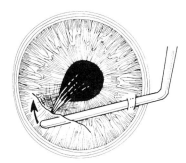

Figure 75.7. A vitreous sweep is used to dislodge incarcerated vitreous from the wound. (Reprinted, with permission, from *Duane's Clinical Ophthalmology,* Tasman W and Jaeger EA, eds, Lippincott Williams and Wilkins, Copyright © 1994. www.lww.com.)

- Pupillary movement and peaking may indicate residual vitreous strands. Acetylcholine may be irrigated into the anterior chamber to constrict the pupil and make peaking more apparent.

Corneoscleral Lacerations

Corneal lacerations extending beyond the limbus require thorough, meticulous evaluation to determine the full extent of the wound. Most ruptures secondary to blunt trauma occur anterior to the equator, often at the limbus. Isolated posterior ruptures may occur. In 10% to 20% of cases, these are often located behind the rectus muscle insertions where the sclera is thinnest.

1. Rectus bridle sutures (4-0 silk) or limbal fixation sutures (6-0 silk) may be helpful for globe manipulation, but they should be placed with caution in an unstable globe.
2. In an unstable globe, repair the limbus before proceeding with further wound exploration, to avoid iatrogenic disruption of intraocular contents.
   - Limbal structures are repaired with 8-0 or 9-0 nylon sutures to restore normal anatomic relationships.
   - Knots should be buried.
3. Corneal lacerations are then repaired as discussed above.
4. The scleral laceration is then explored to ascertain its full extent.
   - In general, a 360° conjunctival peritomy is performed to permit exploration of all 4 quadrants.
   - All quadrants are cleaned of overlying Tenon's capsule with a Westcott scissors.
   - Exploration behind the muscle insertions where the sclera is thin should be particularly meticulous.

5. If necessary, temporary disinsertion of a rectus muscle is performed.
   - Dissect Tenon's capsule and the intermuscular membrane to expose bare sclera posterior to each side of the muscle insertion.
   - Place a large muscle hook under the muscle tendon, posterior to its insertion.
   - Using a double-armed 5-0 polyglactin suture on a spatulated needle, secure the muscle in a locking fashion and disinsert it using Wescott scissors. It is subsequently reattached to the sclera at the site of its original insertion using the same suture.
6. Scleral lacerations are closed with nonabsorbable 8-0 nylon suture.
   - For gaping wounds, advancing the needle completely through one margin and then reloading the needle before making a second pass helps to avoid globe distortion.
7. Prolapsed uveal tissue should be repositioned if possible; excision may cause severe bleeding and risks cutting retinal tissue.
8. For closing sclera over prolapsed uvea, the wound is often most easily closed from the anterior end with closely spaced interrupted sutures that are placed successively in a "zippering" fashion (Figure 75.8).
   - The assistant may use a cyclodialysis spatula to gently depress the uvea into the eye during the suture tightening to avoid tissue incarceration during scleral closure.
   - Alternatively, as with corneal lacerations, sutures may be placed to successively bisect the wound.
9. Prolapsed vitreous, if present, should be secured with dry cellulose sponges and cut flush with the sclera, avoiding traction on the vitreous.
10. It is more difficult to visualize the full extent of posterior wounds and to mechanically remove incarcerated or prolapsed vitreous from them.

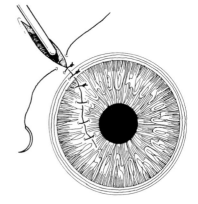

Figure 75.8. The sclera is closed starting anteriorly at the limbus, proceeding posteriorly in a "zippering fashion." (Reprinted, with permission, from *Duane's Clinical Ophthalmology,* Tasman W and Jaeger EA, eds, Lippincott Williams and Wilkins, Copyright © 1994. www.lww.com.)

In these instances, the primary surgical goal is to secure a watertight closure of the globe.

11. For very posterior wounds, complete closure may not be possible; it is better in these cases to leave the most posterior portion of the wound unsutured rather than to cause excessive globe distortion and prolapse of intraocular contents by manipulating the globe to reach the posterior extent of the wound.

12. Where scleral tissue is missing, a patch graft of donor sclera may be used.

13. After scleral repair, the conjunctiva is repositioned and sutured in place with 8-0 polyglactin.

14. Subconjunctival injections of antibiotics (eg, cefazolin) may be used.

Chapter 76

Repair of Internal Orbital Floor Fractures

Paul D. Langer, MD, FACS

An internal orbital floor fracture, also commonly known as a "blow-out fracture," is defined as a fracture of the orbital floor in which the orbital rim remains intact. Such fractures occur when a compressive force is applied to the midface. The force is presumably transmitted posteriorly to the structurally weak inferior wall, resulting in a "buckling" of the bone of the orbital floor without the orbital rim being affected. In some cases, it is theorized that a direct impact to the eye thrusts the globe posteriorly, resulting in a sudden and rapid increase in the intraorbital pressure; this suddenly increased pressure fractures (or "blows-out") the structurally weak orbital floor from hydraulic forces. Both the "buckling" and the "hydraulic" mechanisms may ultimately play a role in the etiology of these fractures.

Not all "blow-out" fractures need to be repaired. The decision whether to repair an individual floor fracture, and during what time period to intervene, has long been a subject of controversy. Herniation of orbital tissue into the bony defect of an orbital floor fracture may result in a permanent motility disturbance, leading to pain on eye movement or frank diplopia, or it may cause cosmetically unacceptable enophthalmos. Both of these problems can often be addressed by surgically repairing the orbital defect. At presentation, however, patients with "blow-out" fractures may have significant orbital edema, which in itself (along with a temporary neuropraxia due to the trauma itself) can result in ocular dysmotility that ultimately resolves without intervention. On the other hand, the same early edema and congestion will mask the final degree of enophthalmos. As a result, as the edema resolves after orbital trauma, ocular motility frequently improves or resolves, while enophthalmos worsens or appears where it previously did not exist. The difficulty facing the surgeon, therefore, is determining which floor fractures, if left unrepaired, will lead to these consequences. To complicate matters, radiologic studies are not predictive in determining which fractures will ultimately lead to significant diplopia.

Traditionally, the timing of repair was said to be optimal around 10 to 14 days after the original injury; this period of time, it was felt, was long enough to allow for edema to resolve, but still early enough so that scarring around the fracture site had not yet occurred, making the repair difficult. However, retrospective series of orbital floor fracture repairs have not validated the premise that, for most patients, undergoing repair within the first two weeks leads to a better outcome than undergoing surgery later. For the great majority of "blow-out" fractures, there is little harm in waiting for most or all of the edema and congestion to resolve and then determining if the patient has disabling diplopia (that is not still improving) or has developed a degree of enophthalmos that the patient finds disturbing.

For patients in whom there is marked clinical entrapment at presentation (such as an eye that has no movement in upgaze), especially when attempted movement is accompanied by significant pain, urgent repair is indicated to prevent the inferior rectus from suffering ischemic damage. Nevertheless, it is prudent to delay repair in most patients until periorbital swelling resolves and any motility disturbance has reached its maximum level of spontaneous improvement. Early repair to "prevent" enophthalmos should probably be discouraged in most cases, since the final degree of enophthalmos is difficult to predict, and judgment concerning the appearance and significance of the final abnormality is best left to the patient.

The goal of repair is to reposition all herniated tissue back into the confines of the orbit and cover the entire bony defect with an implant. The choice of implant depends on the surgeon's preference; a wide variety of materials have been used successfully, including autologous bone grafts, demineralized bone, and alloplastic materials such as silicone or porous polyethylene sheets.

INSTRUMENTATION AND SUPPLIES

- Castroviejo 0.5 forceps
- Corneal protector
- Monopolar cautery
- Desmarres retractor
- Cotton-tipped applicators
- Freer periosteal elevator

- Frazier suction tip
- Sewall orbital retractors
- Mosquito clamps (2)
- Large Mayo scissors
- Hemostat
- Orbital implant material
- 5-0 silk suture, 6-0 plain gut suture

SURGICAL PROCEDURE

1. This procedure is much more easily performed with an assistant.
2. General anesthesia is preferred.
3. Perform a forced duction test: grasp the inferior rectus through the conjunctiva by pressing firmly against the sclera with open 0.5 forceps, about 8 to 10 mm from the limbus inferiorly, and close the tips. Once the inferior rectus is held, gently rotate the globe upwards to gauge the amount of restriction or resistance in the muscle belly; comparison can be made with the normal fellow inferior rectus if necessary (Figure 76.1).
4. Inject the inferior fornix using 1% lidocaine with epinephrine 1:100,000 to assist with hemostasis.
5. Cover the eye with the corneal protector.
6. With the assistant manually retracting the lower eyelid to expose the inferior fornix, make a transconjunctival incision at the base of the tarsus across the entire eyelid with the monopolar cautery, incising through the lower eyelid retractors (Figure 76.2).

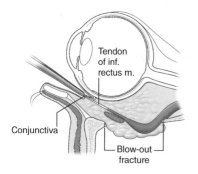
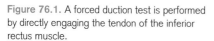
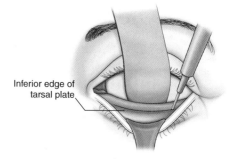

Figure 76.1. A forced duction test is performed by directly engaging the tendon of the inferior rectus muscle.

Figure 76.2. A transconjunctival incision is made with monopolar cautery at the base of the tarsus.

7. Place two 5-0 silk retraction sutures through the inferior edge of the wound. Remove the corneal shield, and pull the conjunctiva over the cornea with the sutures, which are clamped to the head-drape with the mosquito clamps. From this point forward, the assistant should retract the lower lid with a Desmarres retractor (Figure 76.3).

8. Using a cotton-tipped applicator, perform blunt dissection inferiorly in the plane separating the orbicularis muscle and the orbital septum (Figure 76.4A). This plane is virtually bloodless. Continue dissection until the orbital rim is visible (Figure 76.4B).

9. Incise the thickened periosteum at the orbital rim (the arcus marginalis) with the monopolar cautery (Figure 76.5), and dissect the periosteum

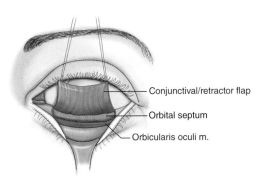

Figure 76.3. The lower eyelid retractor/conjunctiva complex is retracted superiorly to cover the cornea with 2 5-0 silk sutures.

Conjunctival/retractor flap

Orbital septum

Orbicularis oculi m.

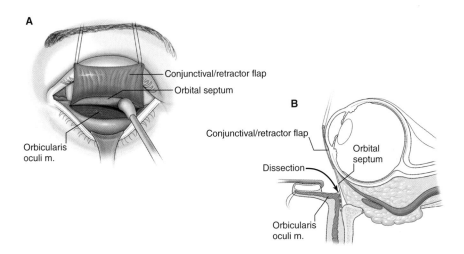

A

Conjunctival/retractor flap

Orbital septum

Orbicularis oculi m.

B

Conjunctival/retractor flap

Orbital septum

Dissection

Orbicularis oculi m.

Figure 76.4. Transconjunctival approach to the orbital rim. (A) Dissection is carried out between the septum and lower eyelid retractors bluntly with a cotton-tipped applicator; the conjunctiva/retractor complex is clamped to the head-drape with traction sutures. (B) Sagittal view of dissection plane through the eyelid toward the orbital rim.

Figure 76.5. The periosteum at the orbital rim is incised with monopolar cautery.

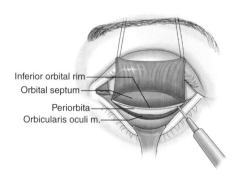

Inferior orbital rim
Orbital septum
Periorbita
Orbicularis oculi m.

off the rim with a Freer elevator. Achieve hemostasis with monopolar cautery, using suction where needed.

10. Lift the incised periosteum off the floor of the orbit posteriorly until the leading edge of the fracture is visible.

11. Free the incarcerated tissue that is herniated into the maxillary sinus, and reposition all tissue into the orbit. The exact technique for accomplishing these maneuvers will vary according to the individual characteristics of each fracture; however, a few technical points can be summarized:

   - The surgeon will usually operate with the suction tip in the non-dominant hand and a dissection instrument (such as a Freer elevator) in the dominant hand.
   - While dissecting, an assistant should retract the orbital tissues superiorly with Sewall orbital (or equivalent) retractors. The edge of the retractors should rest on bone, and as tissues are extracted from the orbital defect, the retractors can be gradually replaced more posteriorly along the edges of the fracture medially or laterally.
   - Both blunt and sharp dissection are frequently necessary.
   - The lateral portion of a "blow-out" fracture almost invariably extends just medial to, or over, the infraorbital neurovascular bundle. The infraorbital nerve is therefore frequently visible; it can be used as a landmark for dissection, as the implant should rest over the nerve and onto the lateral edge of bone with no tissue intervening (recall the nerve usually is covered by a thin bone, so it is not within the orbit normally). Any tissue lying on or adherent to the nerve should be dissected free and ultimately lie above the implant.
   - A small orbital branch or branches of the infraorbital artery penetrate the periosteum of the orbital floor inferiorly entering the orbit.

These vessels must be cauterized and divided to provide a clear subperiosteal space around the defect laterally.

- Sinus mucosa that is adherent to the inferior surface of orbital tissues should be dissected free and repositioned inferiorly into the maxillary sinus.
- Dissection of the incarcerated tissue should proceed posteriorly, with care taken to expose the bony edges for 360° of the fracture site (Figure 76.6).
- The posterior bony edge of the fracture must be visualized, and care taken to ensure no orbital tissue crosses over the posterior edge into the maxillary sinus prior to implant placement. A useful technique when dissection approaches the posterior edge is to palpate the bone directly with the edge of a Freer elevator while the orbital contents are retracted, and then incise onto the rim with the sharp edge of the Freer to directly visualize and expose the bony ledge. This technique ensures no orbital tissue traverses the posterior edge of the fracture, so that after implant placement, there will be no posterior connection between the tissues in the orbit and in the sinus cavity.
- Bleeding during surgery can be controlled with monopolar cautery if it emanates from tissues or bone in the anterior portion of the orbit. Diffuse or posterior bleeding is often controlled by temporary tamponade with 4 × 4-inch gauze, Surgicel, or Gelfoam.

12. Prepare the orbital implant. If an alloplastic material is used, soak it in an antibiotic solution (such as a combination of Bacitracin and Polymyxin), and cut it to size using large Mayo scissors. The implant should be large enough to cover the entire defect and should be wider at its anterior end than the posterior end, with rounded edges throughout, similar to a guitar pick (Figure 76.7).

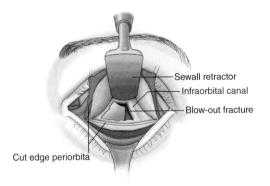

Figures 76.6. The entire orbital floor defect is exposed for 360°.

Sewall retractor
Infraorbital canal
Blow-out fracture

Cut edge periorbita

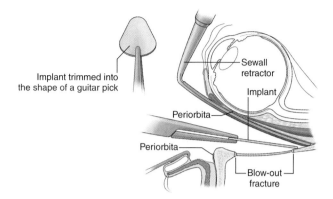

Figures 76.7. The implant is cut in the shape of a guitar pick so that the posterior width is less than the anterior width. The implant is then placed directly on the ledge of bone at the posterior edge of the fracture to insure the entire defect is covered.

13. Clamp the implant in the jaws of the hemostat, and, with the assistant retracting the orbital tissue superiorly with the Sewall retractors, insert the implant along the orbital floor (see Figure 76.7). Place the leading edge of the implant onto the posterior ledge of the fracture under direct visualization. Ensure that the lateral and medial extent of the fracture is also covered by the implant, and that no orbital tissue is trapped beneath the implant.

14. Release the traction sutures and perform a forced duction test (see Figure 76.1). If restriction is present, ensure the implant is not incarcerating tissue. In some cases, inferior rectus muscle edema alone can result in a persistently tight inferior rectus muscle despite the fracture being adequately repaired.

15. Most surgeons prefer to fix the implant to prevent postoperative migration. Fixation can be achieved by a variety of methods including cyanoacrylate adhesive, screws, or sutures, depending on the implant material and the surgeon's preference. If fixation is desired, re-clamp the traction sutures, expose the implant, and fix the implant at this stage.

16. Remove the traction sutures and close the conjunctiva with 2 interrupted 6-0 plain gut sutures. Some surgeons prefer to simply reapproximate the conjunctival incision with cotton-tipped applicators but do not suture the incision.

17. Apply Bacitracin ophthalmic (or equivalent) ointment into the inferior fornix.

POSTOPERATIVE CARE

1. Check vision in the recovery room to ensure the patient can at least count fingers at 4 to 5 feet.
2. Advise the patient to apply ice packs to the periorbital area several times per day, for 20 minutes at each setting, for the first 5 days after surgery; prescribe pain medication.
3. Most surgeons administer intraoperative intravenous corticosteroids and postoperative oral corticosteroids for 3 to 5 days to reduce orbital edema.

COMPLICATIONS

- Lower eyelid malposition (retraction or entropion)
- Postoperative diplopia or enophthalmos
- Persistent enophthalmos
- Visual loss

Lower eyelid malposition most commonly results from scarring within the eyelid when the surgical dissection has disrupted multiple planes of the lid or traumatized the orbicularis muscle; it occurs not uncommonly when a transcutaneous approach is used. Blunt dissection in the plane between the orbicularis and the septum following a conjunctival incision greatly decreases the frequency of this complication. Treatment of symptomatic cases often requires eyelid reconstruction with a posterior lamellar graft.

Diplopia commonly occurs in the immediate postoperative period due to transient weakness (or restriction) of the inferior rectus muscle coupled with orbital edema. Frequently, the diplopia resolves over the course of several weeks to months after surgery. In some cases, however, even when an orbital fracture is repaired correctly and in a timely fashion, permanent diplopia may result from irreparable muscle injury, nerve damage, or fibrosis of the inferior rectus muscle that limits its distensibility. When diplopia does not resolve, a postoperative CT scan should be obtained (with coronal and sagittal views) to ensure that all of the herniated orbital tissue has been replaced into the orbit, and that the implant is correctly placed, resting on the edge of intact bone at the posterior edge of the fracture. If the implant does not cover the posterior portion of the fracture site, it may be advisable to remove the implant and replace it with one that is correctly positioned.

Persistent enophthalmos can also occur when a portion of the fracture site is not covered, leading to persistent herniation of tissue into the maxillary sinus. Again, a postoperative CT is critical in assessing the placement of the implant; an incorrectly positioned implant may need to be replaced. It should be noted that some degree of enophthalmos may persist even when a floor fracture is correctly repaired due to fat atrophy or the traumatic loss of the supportive septa of the orbit. Since both diplopia and enophthalmos, alone or in combination, may persist following an appropriately repaired "blow-out" fracture, patients should be counseled of such a possibility prior to surgery.

Though rare, acute loss of vision is the most ominous complication of orbital fracture repair. It is most commonly due to compressive ischemic damage of the optic nerve from postoperative hemorrhage or edema involving the posterior portion of the orbit. Meticulous attention to hemostasis and judicious use of intraoperative and postoperative corticosteroids are important to prevent this complication. If compressive visual loss is suspected in the postoperative period, immediate imaging (to check for hemorrhage and to ascertain the precise location of the implant), removal of the implant, and corticosteroid treatment may be necessary. A calcium channel blocker such as nimodipine should be administered to counteract vasospasm in the optic nerve. If orbital hemorrhage is suspected, immediate canthotomy and cantholysis (Chapter 70) can sometimes dramatically restore vision if performed soon after vision is lost.

Index

Page numbers followed by *f* denote figures.